Dental Materials Science

Dental Materials Science

Rama Krishna Alla
Assistant Professor
Department of Dental Materials
Vishnu Dental College
Bhimavaram, Andhra Pradesh, India

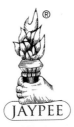

JAYPEE BROTHERS MEDICAL PUBLISHERS (P) LTD

New Delhi • London • Philadelphia • Panama

Jaypee Brothers Medical Publishers (P) Ltd.

Headquarters

Jaypee Brothers Medical Publishers (P) Ltd.
4838/24, Ansari Road, Daryaganj
New Delhi 110 002, India
Phone: +91-11-43574357
Fax: +91-11-43574314
Email: jaypee@jaypeebrothers.com

Overseas Offices

J.P. Medical Ltd.
83, Victoria Street, London
SW1H 0HW (UK)
Phone: +44-2031708910
Fax: +02-03-0086180
Email: info@jpmedpub.com

Jaypee Brothers Medical
Publishers (P) Ltd.
17/1-B, Babar Road, Block-B
Shaymali, Mohammadpur
Dhaka-1207, Bangladesh
Mobile: +08801912003485
Email: jaypeedhaka@gmail.com

Jaypee-Highlights Medical
Publishers Inc.
City of Knowledge, Bld. 237, Clayton
Panama City, Panama
Phone: +507-301-0496
Fax: +507-301-0499
Email: cservice@jphmedical.com

Jaypee Brothers Medical
Publishers (P) Ltd.
Shorakhute
Kathmandu, Nepal
Phone: +00977-9841528578
Email: jaypee.nepal@gmail.com

Jaypee Medical Inc.
The Bourse
111, South Independence Mall East
Suite 835, Philadelphia
PA 19106, USA
Phone: + 267-519-9789
Email: joe.rusko@jaypeebrothers.com

Website: www.jaypeebrothers.com
Website: www.jaypeedigital.com

Dental Materials Science

First Edition: **2013**

ISBN 978-93-5090-671-2

Printed at: S. Narayan & Sons

Dedicated to

*my Parents, Teachers and
to the Almighty*

Preface

The dental materials science is a combination of science of biology, chemistry and physics. Dental materials science is advancing day by day with the research and development of new materials and technology. Though many materials have been in use, new materials are being developed giving more importance to long-lasting service and esthetics. In addition, attention towards the biological compatibility of the materials locally or systematically is being extensively investigated. The performance of dental materials in the oral environment is one of the factors influencing the quality of dental treatment. Therefore, knowledge of chemical makeup, properties and handling of the materials is a must for the dental practitioner in order to obtain optimum results.

This book is divided into basic dental materials science, laboratory and clinical dental materials and detailed information about each material has been provided along with the figures wherever necessary. This book also gives the information about the modifications, developments and recent advances in dental materials.

Section I: Basic Dental Materials Science: This section describes the relationship between the structure and the properties of materials. Also, explains why different materials exhibit different properties in relation to their clinical usage.

Section II: Clinical Dental Materials: The materials used in dental operatory are discussed in this section. The composition, chemistry, handling characteristics, and properties appropriate to clinical use are discussed. Modifications and recent advances are also discussed.

Section III: Laboratory Dental Materials: The materials used by the dental technicians to construct prosthesis are discussed in this section.

This book is drafted with a simple language aiming at the undergraduate dental students to understand the subject easily and at the same time the intricate details on the recent advances will be useful for the postgraduate students.

Rama Krishna Alla

Acknowledgments

Kishore Ginjupalli MSc PhD
Senior Lecturer
Department of Dental Materials
Manipal College of Dental Sciences
Manipal University, Manipal, Karnataka, India

Nagaraj Upadhya MSc PhD
Senior Lecturer
Department of Dental Materials
Manipal College of Dental Sciences
Manipal University, Manipal, Karnataka, India

Rama Krishna Ravi MDS
Professor
Department of Conservative Dentistry and
Endodontics, SB Patil Dental College
Bidar, Karnataka, India

Ravichandra Shekhar Kotha MDS
Professor and Head
Department of Pedodontics
Dr Sudha Nageswararao Sidhartha Institute of
Dental Sciences, Gannavaram
Andhra Pradesh, India

Srinivas P MDS
Professor and Head
Department of Community and Preventive
Dentistry, Sibar Institute of Dental Sciences
Guntur, Andhra Pradesh, India

Srinivas P MDS
Professor
Department of Prosthodontics
Narayana Dental College
Nellore, Andhra Pradesh, India

Koteswara Rao Patchava MSc (Dent Mate.)
Senior Lecturer
Department of Dental Materials
Kamineni Institute of Dental Sciences
Narketpalli, Andhra Pradesh, India

Savita Bhat MSc (Dent. Mate.)
VS Dental College and Hospital
Bengaluru, Karnataka, India

Anusha Alla MSc (Chemistry)

Vijaya Lakshmi G MSc (Dent. Mate.)

Ajay Dev MDS
Professor and Head
Dr Sudha Nageswararao Sidhartha Institute of
Dental Sciences
Gannavaram, Andhra Pradesh, India

M Sujesh MDS
Professor
Department of Prosthodontics
Mamata Dental College
Khammam, Andhra Pradesh, India

T Rambabu MDS
Professor
Department of Conservative and Endodontics
Vishnu Dental College
Bhimavaram, Andhra Pradesh, India

Subash M Reddy MDS
Professor
Department of Prosthodontics
Rajah Muthaiah Dental College and Hospital
Annamalai University
Chidambaram, Tamil Nadu, India

Madan R MDS
Reader
Department of Prosthodontics
Rajah Muthaiah Dental College and Hospital
Annamalai University
Chidambaram, Tamil Nadu, India

Sathyanarayana Reddy MDS
Senior Lecturer
Department of Orthodontics
Rajah Muthaiah Dental College and Hospital
Annamalai University
Chidambaram, Tamil Nadu, India

Shammas Mohammed MDS
Professor
Department of Prosthodontics
Sri Rajiv Gandhi College of Dental Sciences
and Hospital
Bengaluru, Karnataka, India

x | Dental Materials Science

Raghavendra Swamy MDS
Professor
Department of Prosthodontics
JSS Dental College and Hospital, JSS University
Mysore, Karnataka, India

Fatima Abussam BDS MS PhD
Assistant Professor
Department of Dental Materials
University of Tripoli, Tripoli, Libya

Suresh Sajjan MC MDS
Professor and Head
Department of Prosthodontics
Vishnu Dental College
Bhimavaram, Andhra Pradesh, India

AV Rama Raju MDS
Professor
Department of Prosthodontics
Vishnu Dental College
Bhimavaram, Andhra Pradesh, India

Srinivas Raju MDS
Professor
Department of Prosthodontics
Vishnu Dental College
Bhimavaram, Andhra Pradesh, India

Jithendra Babu MDS
Professor
Department of Prosthodontics
Vishnu Dental College
Bhimavaram, Andhra Pradesh, India

Subbarayudu MDS
Reader
Department of Prosthodontics
Vishnu Dental College
Bhimavaram, Andhra Pradesh, India

Bheemalingeswara Rao MDS
Reader
Department of Prosthodontics
Vishnu Dental College
Bhimavaram, Andhra Pradesh, India

Naveen Reddy MDS
Reader
Department of Prosthodontics
Vishnu Dental College
Bhimavaram, Andhra Pradesh, India

Sathyanarayana Raju Mantena MDS
Senior Lecturer
Department of Prosthodontics
Vishnu Dental College
Bhimavaram, Andhra Pradesh, India

Indumathi Siva Kumar MDS
Senior Lecturer
Department of Prosthodontics, Vishnu Dental
College, Bhimavaram, Andhra Pradesh, India

Sowjanya G MDS
Senior Lecturer
Department of Prosthodontics, Vishnu Dental
College, Bhimavaram, Andhra Pradesh, India

Sidharth Gosavi MDS
Reader
Department of Prosthodontics
Krishna School of Dental Sciences
Malkapur, Karad, Maharashtra, India

Sulekha Gosavi MDS
Reader
Department of Prosthodontics
Krishna School of Dental Sciences
Malkapur, Karad, Maharashtra, India

Umesh Palekar MDS
Associate Professor
Department of Prosthodontics
Faculty of Dentistry
Al-Fateh University, Tripoli, Libya

Prudhvi BDS

Ahalya BDS
Lecturer
Department of Dental Materials
Vishnu Dental College
Bhimavaram, Andhra Pradesh, India

Altaf Hussain BDS
Lecturer
Department of Dental Materials
Vishnu Dental College
Bhimavaram, Andhra Pradesh, India

RV Raju BDS
Assistant Professor
Department of Prosthodontics
Vishnu Dental College
Bhimavaram, Andhra Pradesh, India

Srinivasara Rao Yellaneni B Tech

Lingeswar Rao Punati M Pharm

Contents

SECTION | 1

Basic Dental Materials Science

- Properties of Tooth Structure
- Standards for Dental Materials
- General Properties of Dental Materials
- Chemistry of Synthetic Resins
- Physical Metallurgy

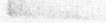

Properties of Tooth Structure

A brief outline of the structure and the properties of the tooth are required as any conservative treatment is to replace the missing part of tooth or missing teeth with artificial materials that ideally should have similar properties.

CROWN AND ROOT

Crown is the visible part of the tooth above gingiva, which is about 1/3rd of the total length. The remaining 2/3rd is the root, which is stably positioned in the alveolar bone sockets.

ENAMEL

Enamel is a highly calcified substance covers that part of the tooth, which is visible. It is the hardest tissue in the body. The mineral phase has hydroxyapatite structure and it is in the form of rod-shaped units termed enamel prisms. Small quantities of organic matter consist of soluble proteins, peptides, insoluble proteins and citric acid.

The organic material is mostly present on the enamel surface. The prismatic rods have different refractive indices, dispersed at different densities; the structure is optically anisotropic medium, which shows different color parameters in different directions for different wavelengths. Hence it is impossible to do perfect matching of color parameters with artificial materials.

DENTIN

The bulk of the tooth substance is dentin, which resembles base in many respects. As with enamel the mineral content is hydroxyapatite and organic matter about 20% by weight is mostly collagen and small quantities of citric acid, insoluble protein, mucopolysaccharide and lipid.

PULP

The pulp of the tooth is soft tissue containing nerves and blood vessels. The pulp is very sensitive to chemical, thermal and electrical stimulation.

CEMENTUM

Cementum is the mineralized dental tissue covering the anatomic roots of human teeth. It begins at the cervical portion of the tooth at the cementoenamel junction and continues to the apex.

Composition

Cementum contains 45–50% inorganic substances and 50–55% organic material and water. Inorganic portion consists of calcium and phosphate in the form of hydroxyapatite. Cementum has the highest fluoride content of all the mineralized tissues. Organic portion consists of type-I collagen and protein polysaccharides.

Physical Properties

- The hardness of fully mineralized cementum is less than that of dentin.
- It is light yellow in color.
- Lighter in color than dentin.

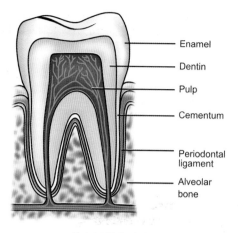

Fig. 1.1 Cross-section of tooth structure

Table 1.1 Properties of tooth

Property	Enamel	Dentin
Density (cm³)	2.97	2.14
Proportional limit (MPa)	224	148
MOE (MPa)	88,900	18,600
Ultimate compressive strength (MPa)	380	300
UTS (MPa)	10	57
Shear strength (MPa)	90	135
Modulus of resilience (MJ/m³)	0.55	0.94
Surface hardness (KHN) (Kg/mm²)	343	68
Specific heat (cal/gm/°C)	0.18	0.28
Thermal conductivity (cal/sec/cm²)	0.0022	0.0015
Thermal diffusivity (mm²/sec)	0.469	0.783
COTE (X10⁻⁶ or ppm)	11.4	8.3

PERIODONTAL LIGAMENT

The periodontal ligament is a fibrous connective tissue that is noticeably cellular and contains numerous blood vessels. The periodontal ligament occupies the periodontal space, which is located between the cementum and the periodontal surface of the alveolar bone. The majority of the fibers of the periodontal ligament are collagen, and the matrix is composed of variety of macromolecules.

Functions

- Attachment and support
- Nutrition
- Synthesis and resorption
- Proprioception.

PROPERTIES

The properties of enamel may vary somewhat with its position on the tooth, i.e. cuspal enamel being stronger than enamel on the sides of the tooth. The proportional limit, ultimate compressive strength, modulus of elasticity of enamel are greater than corresponding values for dentin. However, dentin is capable of sustaining significant plastic deformation under compressive loading before fracture. Thus, enamel is stiffer and more brittle material than dentin. Dentin is more flexible and tougher. The high modulus of elasticity results in less resilience of enamel in comparison with dentin (Table 1.1).

Dentin is considerably stronger in tension than enamel. The low thermal conductivity of enamel and dentin aids in preventing thermal shock and pulpal pain when hot or cold foods or drinks taken into the mouth. Enamel is translucent and exhibits a property called fluorescence.

SUGGESTED READING

1. Bertassoni LE, Habelitz S, Kinney JH, Marshall SJ, Marshall GW Jr. Biomechanical perspective on the remineralization of dentin, Caries Res. 2009;43:70-7.
2. Chai Y, Slavkin HC. Prospects for tooth regeneration in the 21st century: a perspective. Microsc Res Tech. 2003;60(5):469-79.
3. Dhoble A, Padole P, Dhoble M. Bone mechanical properties: a brief review, trends biomater. Artif Organs. 2012;26(1):25-30.
4. Du C, Moradian-Oldak J. Tooth regeneration: challenges and opportunities for biomedical material research. Biomed Mater. 2006;1(1): R10-7.

5. Harold C Slavkin. The future of dentistry. Dent Today. 2006; 25(10):90-2.
6. Hassan R, Caputo AA, Bunshah RF. Fracture toughness of human enamel. J Dent Res. 1981; 60(4):820-7.
7. Ho SP, Balooch M, Goodis HE, Marshall GW, Marshall SJ. Ultrastructure and nanomechanical properties of cementum dentin junction. J Biomed Mater Res A. 2004;68(2):343-51.
8. Ho SP, Goodis HE, Balooch M, Nonomura G, Marshall SJ, Marshall GW. The effect of sample preparation technique on determination of structure and nanomechanical properties of human cementum hard tissue. Biomaterials. 2004;25(19): 4847-57.
9. Ho SP, Marshall SJ, Ryder MI, Marshall GW. The tooth attachment mechanism defined by structure, chemical composition and mechanical properties of collagen fibers in the periodontium. Biomaterials. 2007;28(35):5238-45.
10. Solheim T. A new method for dental age estimation in adults. Forensic Science International. 1993;59:137-47.
11. Thesleff I, Tummers M. Stem cells and tissue engineering: prospects for regenerating tissues in dental practice. Med Princ Pract. 2003;12(Suppl 1):43-50.
12. Vasudeva G, Pawah S. Dentistry in the 21st century: a look into the future. J Oral Health Comm Dent. 2009;3(1):9-14.
13. Vystrèilová M, Novotný V. Estimation of age at death using teeth. Variability and Evolution. 2000;8:39-49.

Standards for Dental Materials

2

The science of dental materials involves a study of the composition and properties of materials and the way in which they interact with the oral environment. The success or failure of a treatment depends on the selection of materials with adequate properties and their manipulation.

The materials used in dentistry are rigid polymers, elastomers, metals, alloys, ceramics, inorganic salts and composite materials. Many dental materials are fixed either permanently in the patient's mouth or removed intermittently for cleaning; such materials have to withstand the effects of a most hazardous environment.

SELECTION OF DENTAL MATERIALS

The process of dental materials selection involves analysis of the problem, consideration of requirements, comparison of available materials and their properties, and choice of material.

EVALUATION OF MATERIALS

The most manufacturers of dental materials operate an extensive quality assurance program. The materials are thoroughly tested before being released to the general practitioners.

Specification and standardization of both national and international standard organization have been developed to aid producers, users and consumers in the evaluation of the safety and effectiveness of dental products. Such specifications—

- Maintain quality levels for dental materials.
- Give details for the testing of certain products, methods of calculating results and minimum permissible results, which is acceptable.

e.g.: American Dental Association (ADA)
International Standard Organization (ISO)
Fédération Dentaire Internationale (FDI).

A series of similar specifications are also available for products in Australia, Japan, and other several countries throughout the world. Recently a program for international specification was established that induces the combined efforts of Fédération Dentaire Internationale (FDI) and the International Organization for Standardization (ISD). Through the specification the quality of each product is maintained and improved.

AMERICAN DENTAL ASSOCIATION (ADA)

The work at American Dental Association research division is divided into a number of categories, including the determination of those physical and chemical properties of dental materials based on their clinical significance, and the development of new materials, instruments and test methods.

The first ADA specification was for amalgam alloy, formulated and reported in 1930. The details of first 25 specifications were included in a book, "American Dental Association Guide to Dental Materials and Devices" (1974). More recent specifications and revisions are published in the "Journal of American Dental Association" (JADA).

A close examination of each of the specifications reveals a general pattern of standardization common to each material.

- These features include an item on scope and classification of the material. This defines the application and general nature of each material.
- Each specification includes information on other applicable specification.
- The requirements of each material take note of such factor as uniformity color or general working characteristics of material and general limitation of test values.
- The method of sampling, inspection, and testing procedure including details of sample preparation and physical test to be performed.
- Each specification includes information on preparation for delivery with instructions concerning packaging, instructions for use and marking with a lot of numbers and date of manufactures.
- Each specification is included notes that provide additional information on intended uses and references to the special items.

Certification and Acceptance Program

ADA through the Council on Dental Material instruments and Equipment maintains a program for certification of dental material and devices. Under this program the manufacturers certify that the product comprises with ADA specification and the manufacturer is in compliance with the ADA advertising and exhibition standard.

Research division collects the samples randomly and tests the qualities of the material such as physical and other properties. If it has sufficient values equal to ADA specification values, they will give the standardization mark. Then the manufacturer can distribute the material.

ADA specification numbers of selected dental materials were mentioned in Table 2.1.

INTERNATIONAL STANDARDS

For many years, these standards have been great interest in the establishment of specifications

Table 2.1 ADA Specification numbers of dental materials

ADA specification number	Materials
1	Dental amalgam
2	Gypsum bonded investment
3	Impression compound
4	Inlay casting wax
5	Dental casting alloys
6	Dental mercury
7	Dental wrought gold alloy
8	Zinc phosphate cement
9	Silicate cement
10	Dental rubber (obsolete)
11	Agar impression material
12	Denture base resins
13	Cold-curing repair resin
14	Base metal casting alloys
15	Synthetic resin teeth
16	Zinc oxide eugenol impression paste
17	Denture base temporary relining resin
18	Alginate impression material
19	Elastomeric impression material
20	Duplicating material
21	Zinc silicophosphate cement
23	Excavating burs
24	Base plate wax
25	Gypsum products
27	Direct filling resins
28	Endodontic files and reamers
30	Zinc oxide eugenol and noneugenol cements
32	Orthodontic wires not containing precious metals
37	Dental abrasive powders
38	Metal ceramic system
39	Pit and fissure sealants
42	Phosphate bonded investment
46	Dental chairs
55	Dispensers of alloy and mercury for amalgam
57	Endodontic filling materials
58	Root canal files (H-files)
61	Zinc polycarboxylate cement
66	Glass ionomer cement
69	Dental ceramics
72	Endodontic spreaders
87	Impression trays
106	Dental amalgam capsules

for dental materials on an international level. It includes the combined efforts of "Fédération Dentaire International" (FDI) and "International Standards Organization" (ISO).

Federation Dentaire International

Initiated and supported a program for the formulation of international specifications for dental materials. As a result, several specifications for dental materials and devices have been adopted.

International Standards Organization (ISO)

ISO is an international, nongovernmental organization. Primary objective is the development of international standard. ISO standard led to the formation of an ISO committee. The responsibility of this committee is to standardize terminology, test methods and specifications for dental materials, instruments, appliances and equipment.

OTHER STANDARDS AND ORGANIZATIONS

The work at the National Institute and Technology (NIST) has stimulated comparable programs in other countries, Australia, Japan, and other countries throughout the world.

Specifications and standards have been developed to aid producers, users and consumers in the evaluation of the safety and effectiveness of dental materials.

General Properties of Dental Materials

3

INTRODUCTION

Dental materials are available in the form of powder, liquid, pastes and gels. Many of the dental materials in use today are manipulated by the dentist in a plastic or semi-liquid state. Either in the plastic or semi-liquid condition they are formed to the required shape, then by a physical change or chemical reaction, they become a solid. The suitability of a dental material depends upon its properties in the finished or solid condition.

The internal structure of solids and liquids affects the way in which they react to the environment in which they are placed. Before going to study dental materials science, one should have the basic knowledge of the forces, which hold the atoms or molecules of materials in a certain relation and which resist changes of shape of that material.

LIQUIDS

An essential feature of liquid state is irregularity and undefinition of structure, so liquids have little or no ordered arrangement of atoms. The atoms are attracted to each other within the liquid, whilst those at its free boundaries are attracted more by the same atoms within the liquid than to the air, produces a boundary between the atmosphere and the surface of the liquid.

Within a liquid, the thermal energy is sufficient to keep the atoms in constant relative motion. Change in atomic relations, results in flow or deformation.

SOLIDS

Based on the internal structure, solids are classified into amorphous and crystalline solids. Amorphous solids have haphazard atomic arrangement, e.g. glasses, whereas crystalline solids have a highly regular and well-defined atomic structure, e.g. metals.

CHANGE OF STATE

Atoms and molecules are held together by atomic interactions. When water boils, energy is needed to transform to vapor. This energy is known as heat of vaporization. The same amount of energy is required for condensation of water vapor, i.e. matter is made of atoms and for these atoms to be held together there must be a force.

Matter exists in three forms such as solids, liquids and gases. The difference in these forms is mainly due to differences in energy.

For example, when 1 gm of water is to be changed into gaseous state at 100°C, 540 cal of heat is needed. Thus gaseous state has more energy than liquid state. Although molecules in gaseous state exert a certain amount of mutual attraction they can readily move because of high kinetic energy. This also explains why gaseous molecules need to be confined to avoid dispersion.

Although atoms may also diffuse in liquid state, their mutual attraction is greater, and energy is required for this separation. If kinetic energy (KE) of liquid decreases sufficiently when its temperature is decreased, liquid changes into solid during which KE is released in the form of heat. This energy released is known as latent heat of fusion. The temperature at which solid changes into liquid is known as melting temperature.

INTERATOMIC BONDS

The forces of attraction between atoms or molecules may be divided into:
- Primary bonds
- Secondary bonds.

Primary Bonds

They may be of three types:
- Ionic
- Covalent
- Metallic.

Ionic Bond

It occurs as a result of mutual attraction of positive and negative charges.
For example, NaCl.

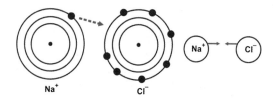

Covalent Bond

In many chemical compounds, adjacent atoms share two valence electrons.
For example: H_2 molecule, in this single outer most electron in each hydrogen atom is shared with that of other.

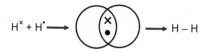

Metallic Bond

The valence electrons from each metallic atom form an electron cloud. The positive ions formed by the loss of electrons and the electron cloud

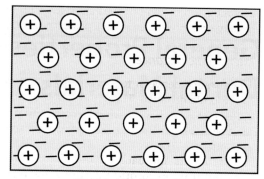

Fig. 3.1 Metallic bonding

itself produce strong forces of attraction bonding the metal together (Fig. 3.1).

In general, metal atoms which have only a few loosely held valence electrons are more metallic in their bonding.

For example: Na, K, Cu, Ag, Au have high electrical and thermal conductivity since their valence electrons are very mobile.

As the number of valence electrons increases, the bonding becomes less metallic and more covalent.

For example: Fe, Ni, W, and Ti.

Tin exists in two forms of bonding, one mostly metallic and the other mostly covalent.

Interatomic Secondary Bonds

In contrast with primary bonds, secondary bonds do not share electrons but charge variations among molecules or atomic groups induce polar forces that attract the molecules.

Hydrogen Bonding

For example in H_2O molecule two hydrogen atoms are attached by oxygen atom. These bonds are covalent as they share electrons. The hydrogen bond, which has associated positive charge of hydrogen caused by polarization.

van der Waals Forces

These forces form the basis of dipole attraction in a symmetric atom example inert gas a fluxuated dipole is formed, which will attract other similar dipoles that is within an atom there is accumulation of atoms in one half which leads to negative polarity and other half, positive polarity.

Interatomic Distance

The distance between two atoms is known as interatomic distance. These forces are of two types, attractive and repulsive forces. The net force between two atoms is sum of both repulsive and attractive forces.

The atoms approach too closely they are repelled from each other by their electron charges. On the other hand, forces of attraction tend to draw the atoms together. The passion at which these forces of repulsion and attraction become equivalent magnitude (opposite in direction) is the equilibrium passion of the atoms. At this passion, atoms are with minimum energy and maximum stability. The interatomic distance can be increased or decreased by application of mechanical forces.

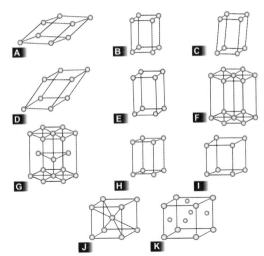

Figs 3.2A to K Different crystal arrangements (A) Rhombohedral (B) Orthorhombic (C) Monoclinic (D) Triclinic (E) Tetragonal (F) Simple hexagonal (G) Close packed hexagonal (H) Rhombic (I) Simple cubic (J) Body centered cubic (K) Face centered cubic

CRYSTALLINE STRUCTURE

Space lattice or crystal lattice can be defined as an arrangement of atoms in space such that in every atom it is in similar relation to every other atom. Space lattice may be the result of primary or secondary bonds. There are 14 possible types of lattice forms, but three relatively cubic crystal structure of lattice are found for most of the metals.

E.g.:
1. Simple cubic
2. Face centered cubic
3. Body centered cubic.

The solid circles in the Figures 3.2A to K represent the passion of atoms. There passions are located at the points of intersection of three sets of parallel planes, each set being perpendicular to other plane. These planes are referred as crystal planes.

NONCRYSTALLINE STRUCTURE

Noncrystalline solids lack a systematic and regular arrangement of atoms over relatively large atomic distances. Sometimes such materials are also called amorphous that means materials without any form.

In crystalline structure, the arrangement of atoms in the lattice is in order and follows a particular pattern. In non-crystalline structures or amorphous structures, e.g. waxes, used in dentistry, the molecules are distributed randomly.

However, there is tendency for arrangement of atoms or molecules to be regular. For example glass is considered to be non-crystalline solid, yet its atoms bind to form short-range order rather long-range order lattice. Since such an arrangement is also typical of liquids such solids are referred to as super-cooled liquids. Polymer may be completely crystalline, or noncrystalline or mixture of two.

The success or failure of many forms of treatment depends on the correct selection of materials possessing adequate properties combined with careful manipulation.

The various types of materials used in dentistry are rigid polymers, elastomers, metals, alloys, ceramics, inorganic salts and composite materials. Many dental materials are fixed permanently into the patient's mouth or are removed intermittently for cleaning; such materials have to withstand the effects of a most hazardous environment.

Temperature variations, wide variations in acidity or alkalinity and high stresses all have an effect on the durability of materials. Normal temperature variations in the oral cavity lie between 32°C–37°C depending upon whether the mouth is open or closed. The ingestion of hot or cold food or drink extends this temperature range from 0°C–70°C. Alkalinity or acidity of fluids in the oral cavity as measured by pH varies from around pH 4–pH 8.5. Whilst the intake of acid fruit juices or alkaline medicaments can extend this from pH 2–pH 11.

SURFACE PROPERTIES

ADSORPTION

This is a reaction involving attraction of a substance onto the surface of a material.
- It is common for both liquids and solids to adsorb gases or other liquids on their surface.
- This is because of certain forces (intermolecular or van der Waals forces), the surface of the material has the tendency to attract and retain molecules of other species, with which it is brought into contact.
- The molecules remain only at the surface and do not go deeper into the bulk.

Adsorbent: The material, which takes up or adsorbs the molecules onto its surface is called as "adsorbent".

Adsorbate: The molecules, which get adsorbed onto the surface of material are called as "adsorbate".

Adsorption process is of two types. They are:
- 1. Physical adsorption or physisorption
  2. Chemisorption.
- In physisorption, the process consists of just a physical phenomenon where just the van der Waals force is in action.
- In chemisorption, it involves a chemical process where exists a chemical interaction between the surface atoms of adsorbent and the atoms of adsorbate.
- Differences between physisorption and chemisorption are given in Table 3.1.

Applications in dentistry: Applications can be categorized as constructive and destructive applications.

Constructive applications: The process of adsorption to the surface of the substance is important in the wetting process in which the substance is coated or wetted with a foreign substance, such as liquid for example, the degree to which the saliva will wet or adhere to the surface of a resin denture depends on the tendency for surface adsorption.

Destructive applications:
1. *Gold foils:* Gold like most metals attracts gases to its surface. This causes temporary noncohesiveness, i.e.; any adsorbed gas film prevents the intimate atomic contact between the sheets.
2. *In oral cavity:* Many problems arise due to the deposits on the surface of teeth/resto-

Table 3.1 Differences between physisorption and chemisorption

Physisorption		Chemisorption	
1.	It occurs only at low temperatures.	1.	Occurs at all temperatures.
2.	Magnitude of physisorption decreases with rise in temperatures.	2.	Magnitude of chemisorption increases with rise in temperature.
3.	Heat evolved in this is very high (40-400 kJ/mol).	3.	Heat evolved is quite low (4-40 kJ/mol).
4.	Process is reversible, i.e.; the adsorbate can be separated from the adsorbent.	4.	Process is irreversible, i.e. the adsorbate cannot be recovered from the adsorbent.

rations. Deposits are nothing but the strong adsorption of various materials onto the surface of the tooth.

- Deposits are of two types:
  a. Hard deposit
     e.g. calculus
  b. Soft deposits
     e.g.: Plaque: food particles containing micro-organisms.
- These deposits might be the initial stage finally leading to caries.

ABSORPTION

In this process, the substance adsorbed is sucked into or penetrates in a type of diffusion process.
- Basically the process of absorption is a combination of adsorption and penetration or diffusion.
- When the dry grapes are being kept immersed in water, it imbibes water and hence swells.

Application in dentistry:
1. When the hydrocolloid impression is being stored in the presence of moisture (water), they absorb water and swell. Thus it is the factor, which reduces dimensional stability. Immersion of impression materials in the disinfectant solution for long time also causes absorption of the disinfectants by the materials.
2. Calcium sulfate hemihydrate is hygroscopic material and easily absorbs moisture from the humid atmosphere to form calcium sulfate dihydrate. Formation of dihydrate on the hemihydrate powder results in lengthening of the setting time.

SORPTION

This is a process in which both adsorption and absorption are known to exist and it is not clear which process is predominating.

Application in dentistry: The sorption of water alters the dimensions of acrylic dentures. This change in dimension is reversible and plastic may go through numerous expansions and contractions when alternately soaked in water and dried. However, the patient should avoid

repeated wetting and drying of finished dentures because irreversible warpage of the denture bases may result.

DIFFUSION

Diffusion is the movement of solvent molecules from a region of higher concentration to a region of lower concentration.

Application in dentistry:
- Salts and dyes diffuse through dentin.
- Stains and discoloring agents will diffuse through plastic restorative materials.

SURFACE TENSION

Surface tension may be defined as the force acting tangentially to the liquid surface and perpendicular to the unit length of an imaginary line drawn on the surface.

$$\text{Surface tension } (\gamma) = \frac{\text{Force}}{\text{Length}}$$

Units: Newton/meter or Dynes/cm
- The increase in energy per unit area of a surface is referred to as the surface energy.
- Greater the surface energy, greater the capacity for adhesion.
- The surface tension and adhesive qualities of given solid can be reduced by any surface impurities.
- The surface tension values of different liquids at 20°C are as follows:
  Water   = 72.8 dynes/cm
  Benzene = 29 dynes/cm
  Alcohol = 22 dynes/cm
  Ether   = 17 dynes/cm
  Mercury = 465 dynes/cm

Factors affecting surface tension:
1. *Temperature*: As temperature rises, surface tension decreases.
   Temperature $\propto$ 1/Surface tension
   For example, surface tension of water at

0°C	–	76 dynes/cm
25°C	–	72 dynes/cm
50°C	–	68 dynes/cm
100°C	–	59 dynes/cm

2. *Purity:* Surface tension of liquids is also reduced by the presence of impurities.

    For example, detergents such as sodium lauryl sulfate or the ingredients of soaps including sodium stearate or sodium oleate, which have long hydrocarbon chains attached to hydrophobic groups, are partially effective in reducing surface tension.

3. *The functional chemical group* or *the type of crystal plane* of a space lattice present at the surface may affect the surface energy.

Applications in dentistry: **In dentifrices**, detergents such as sodium lauryl sulfate or sodium-N-lauroylsarcosinate are added as surface-active agents. In the paste form its composition is about 1–2% and in powder form the composition of detergents is about 1–6%. These detergents improve the ability of the dentifrice to wet the tooth surface and thus it aids in removing debris from tooth surface.

WETTING

To produce adhesion, the liquid must flow easily over the entire surface and adhere to the solid; this character is referred to as "wetting".

Factors affecting wetting:
1. The surface of the adherent should be clean.
2. The surface energy of the adherent should be high so that the liquids wet their surface.
3. There should not be any irregularities.

ANGLE OF CONTACT

The contact angle is the angle formed by the adhesive with the adherent at their interface.
- The extent to which an adhesive wets the surface of an adherent may be determined by measuring the contact angle between adhesive and the adherent.

If the adherent is having more surface energy and less surface tension the contact angle would be zero, which results in complete wetting of adherent surface and will take place by the adhesive (Fig. 3.3A). If the energy of the surface of the adherent is reduced slightly by contamination or by the increase in surface tension of solid results a slight increase in the contact angle (Fig. 3.3B). A very high contact angle may be formed in the case of solids with low surface energy, such as "polytetra fluoro-ethylene" (Teflon) (Fig. 3.3C).

The tendency for the liquid to spread increases as the contact angle decreases and thus contact angle is a useful indicator of spreadability or wettability.

Factors affecting contact angle:
1. The surface of the adherent should be clean.
2. The surface energy of the adherent should be high so that the liquids wet their surface.
3. There should not be any irregularities.

Applications in dentistry: In rubber impression materials, wettability may be assessed by measuring the advancing contact angle of water on the surface of the set impression material. The hydrophilic addition silicones and polyethers are wetted best and the condensation silicones and hydrophobic addition silicones the least.

Material	Advancing contact angle of water (degree)
Polysulfide	82
Condensation silicones	98
Addition silicone	
Hydrophobic	98
Hydrophilic	53
Polyether	49

Wetting is more important in the retention of a denture under static conditions. The

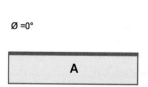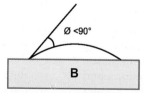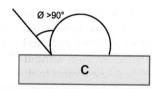

Ø =0°   Ø <90°   Ø >90°

A   B   C

Figs 3.3A to C Contact angles of different solids with different surface energies

wetting of the plastic surface depends on the energy relationship between solid and liquid. If complete wetting occurs, the liquid will spread on the solid. If partial wetting occurs, the liquid forms droplets on the surface. The plastics used in dentistry are only partially wetted by saliva, but the wetting may improve after contact with oral fluids because of the adsorption of certain components of the saliva by the plastic denture.

ADHESION

Adhesion occurs when two unlike molecules join together on being brought into contact due to force of attraction between them.

An "adhesive" is a material used to produce adhesion and the substance to which adhesive is applied is called "adherent". The attachment of plaque or calculus to tooth structure can be partially explained by an adhesion mechanism.

Bonding may be achieved by one of the two mechanisms:
1. Mechanical bonding
2. Chemical bonding.

In mechanical attachment the adhesive simply engages in undercuts in the adherent surface. When the surface irregularities responsible for bonding have dimensions of only a few micrometers, the process known as "micromechanical attachment". This is different from macromechanical attachment, which forms the basis of retention for many filling materials, using undercut cavities.

In the case of chemical attachment, the adhesive has a chemical affinity for the adherent surface.

If the attraction caused by van der Waals forces or hydrogen bonds, the resultant bond may be relatively weak. On the other hand, the formation of ionic or covalent links may result in stronger bond.

Applications in Dentistry

Polyacrylate cement: An interesting feature of polyacrylic cement is its bonding to enamel and dentin, which is attributed to the ability of the carboxylate groups in the polymer molecule to chelate calcium. The bond strength of enamel is several times to dentin. Optimum bonding requires cleaned tooth surfaces.

Zinc polycarboxylate cement: This cement also adheres chemically to the tooth structure. The polycarboxylic acid is believed to react via carboxyl groups with calcium hydroxyapatite. The inorganic content and homogeneity of enamel are greater than those of dentin. Thus, the bond strength to enamel is greater than that of dentin.

Zinc phosphate cement: The zinc phosphate cement does not involve any chemical reaction with surrounding hard tissue or other restorative materials. Therefore, primary bonding occurs by mechanical interlocking at interfaces and not by chemical interactions.

COHESION

Cohesion occurs when two like molecules or substances join together on being brought into contact due to the force of attraction between them.

Application in dentistry: Pure gold either in foil or in other forms is cohesive and can be welded to itself at mouth or room temperature simply by the application of force. The surface should be completely clean if welding is to be done. Pure uncontaminated foil, when properly annealed is always cohesive. Since gold foil can be produced in a sufficiently clean and pure condition, it can be cold-welded.

MECHANICAL PROPERTIES

Mechanical properties are defined by the laws of mechanics, i.e. the physical science that deals with energy and forces and their effects on bodies.

Force

"Force is that which alters the state of rest or motion possessed by a body."

A force is defined by three characteristics:
1. The point of application
2. The magnitude
3. The direction of application.

Unit: Pound or Newton.

Work

Whenever force acting on a body causes it to move; the force is said to do work and work is measured by the product of force and a distance moved by the body along the line of action of that force.

Power

It is the rate at which work is done.

Energy

It is the capacity of a body to perform work and it is measured by the work. It is capable of doing by virtue of its velocity or position.

Mechanical energy is of two types:
1. Kinetic energy
2. Potential energy.

STRESS

Whenever force acts on a body tending to produce deformation, a resistance that is developed to the external force application. The internal reaction is equal in intensity and opposite in direction to the applied external force and is called as stress. Both the applied force and internal resistance are distributed over a given area of the body and so the stress in structure is designated as force/unit area.

"Stress is the force per unit area acting on millions of atoms or molecules in a given plane of material".

Units: PSI (pounds per square inch), Pa, MPa.
1 Pa	=	$1\ N/m^2$
MPa	=	MN/m^2
1Mpa	=	10^6 or 150 PSI

$$\text{Stress } (\sigma) = \frac{\text{Force}}{\text{Unit area}}$$

Types of Stress

1. *Compressive stress:* Compression results when the body is subjected to sets of forces in the same straight line that are directed towards

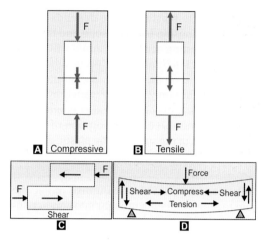

Figs 3.4A to D (A) Compressive stress (B) Tensile stress (C) Shear stress (D) Flexural stress, where F is force

each other. When compression is applied they resist being forced more closely together (Fig. 3.4A).

2. *Tensile stress:* Tension results in a body, when it is subjected to two sets of forces directed away from each other in the same straight line.

When tension is applied, the molecules must resist being pulled apart (Fig. 3.4B).

3. *Shear stress*
   • A shear stress tends to resist the sliding of portion of a body over another.
   • Shear stress is a result of two sets of forces being directed towards each other but not in the same straight line (Fig. 3.4C).

4. *Flexural (bending) stress:* Bending a beam at 3-point loading produces flexural stress. This situation is commonly encountered in the construction of a fixed bridge in prosthetics (Fig. 3.4D).

STRAIN

When external force or load is applied to a material the phenomena of strain occurs; i.e. the change in the dimensions of the material described as change in length (deformation) per original unit length of the body when it is subjected to a force or stress.

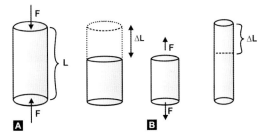

Figs 3.5A and B (A) Compression results in shortening of body (B) Tension results in elongation of the body, where F is force, L is length of the sample, and ΔL is change in the length (deformation)

Strain is denoted as 'ε'

$$\text{Strain} = \frac{\text{Change in length } (\Delta L)}{\text{Original length } (Lo)}$$

$$= \frac{L - Lo}{Lo} = \frac{\Delta L}{Lo}$$

- Has no unit of measurement.
- Strain under tensile stress is an elongation in the direction of loading (Fig. 3.5A).
- Strain under compression is shortening of the body in the direction of loading (Fig. 3.5B).

Types of Strain

1. May be elastic or recoverable, i.e. the material is returned to its original length after removal of the applied force.
2. The material may remain deformed in which case the strain is not recoverable is called "plastic".
3. A third possibility is that strain may be partially recoverable. The extent to which the strain is recovered as a function of the elastic properties of materials.

Importance of Stress and Strain

Most applications of materials in dentistry have a minimum mechanical property requirement. For example, certain materials should be sufficiently strong to withstand biting forces without fracture. Others should be rigid enough to maintain shape under force. Such properties are generally characterized by the stress-strain relationship.

Since the stress in a structure varies directly with the force and inversely the area, so it is necessary to recognize that the area over which the force acts is a most important factor of consideration. Thus for a given force the smaller the area over which it is applied (small restoration), the larger the value of the stress.

The importance of strain in dentistry for example, orthodontic wire or a clasp in a metal partial denture should withstand a large amount of strain before failure as it can be bent and adjusted with less chance of fracture.

THE STRESS-STRAIN RELATIONSHIP OR S-S CURVE

A convenient means of comparing the mechanical properties of materials is to apply various forces to material to determine the corresponding values of stress and strain. A plot of the corresponding values of stress and strain is referred to as "s-s curve" (Fig. 3.6). This diagram provides quantities used to describe the material properties, such as:

1. Proportional limit
2. Elastic limit
3. Yield strength
4. Ultimate strength

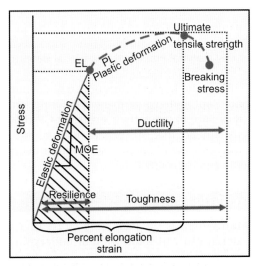

Fig. 3.6 S-S curve (*Abbreviations:* EL: Elastic limit; PL: Proportional limit; MOE: Modulus of elasticity)

5. Breaking stress or fracture stress
6. MOE
7. Modulus of resilience
8. Ductility and malleability.

PROPORTIONAL LIMIT

Proportional limit may by defined as the greatest stress that a material will sustain without a deviation from the proportionality of stress to strain.

It is found by plotting the s-s diagram and determine the point at which first deviation from linearity is noticeable (Fig. 3.6). The region of the s-s curve before the proportional limit is called the "elastic region". So within this range of stress application the material is elastic in nature and no permanent deformation occurs in the structure.

The region of the curve beyond this proportional limit is called as "plastic region" and any application of a stress greater than the proportional limit results in permanent strain or deformation in the sample.

Application

When a restoration is stressed, the stress should not be greater than the proportional limit. If the proportional limit is exceeded, the deformation is permanent and the restoration no longer fits. Therefore a high proportional limit is indicated for any material employed in a partial denture or crown and bridge application.

For example, connectors of partial denture should not undergo permanent deformation, if they have to retain their shape. Cr-Co alloy is usually popular for this application since it can withstand high stresses without being permanently distorted.

ELASTIC LIMIT

"Elastic limit is the maximum stress that a material can withstand without undergoing permanent deformation."

Elastic limit corresponds to the stress beyond which strains are not fully recovered

(describes elastic behavior of materials). A high value of elastic limit is necessary requirement for materials used for making appliances or restorations, since the structure is expected to return after it has been stressed (Fig. 3.6).

Elastic limit deals only with the elasticity of the material, but proportional limit deals with proportionality stress and strain. Theoretically, the values will be same.

YIELD STRENGTH (PROOF STRESS)

"Yield strength is defined as the stress at which a material exhibits a specified limiting deviation from proportionality of stress to strain" or "It is defined as the stress at which the material begins to function in a plastic manner."

Selecting a desired offset, and drawing a line parallel to the linear region of the s-s curve as shown in Figure 3.7, determine the yield stress. The point at which the parallel line intersects the s-s curve is the "yield stress" (a value of 0.1 or 0.2 of the plastic strain is often selected and is referred to as "percent offset" or "proof stress").

Applications

1. *Constructive application:* In the process of shaping an orthodontic appliance or adjusting a clasp on a cast removable partial denture it is necessary to induce a stress into the structure in excess of the yield strength, if the material is permanently bent or shaped.

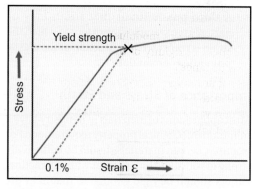

Fig. 3.7 Yield strength of a material measured at 0.1% offset

2. *Destructive application:* Any dental structure or restoration for example crown and bridge, which is permanently deformed during services through the forces of mastication and use is usually a functional or chemical failure to some degree. The restoration or appliance may no longer fit as original design (proper occlusion relationship is lost). Any alloys used for making the crowns and bridges should have highyield strength.

POISSON'S RATIO

When a test sample is stressed by a uniaxial force, it is strained in the direction of force and also in a direction of perpendicular to the direction of the force.

The strain in the direction of force is known as "longitudinal strain", and that perpendicular to it is known as "lateral strain". The ratio between the lateral strain and longitudinal strain is called as "Poisson's ratio".

$$\text{Poisson's ratio} = \frac{\text{Lateral strain}}{\text{Longitudinal strain}}$$

Under compressive loading there is an increase in the cross-section of the material. Under tensile loading the material elongates in the direction of load, there is a reduction in cross-section.

MODULUS OF ELASTICITY (MOE) OR ELASTIC MODULUS

"The term elastic modulus represents the relative stiffness or rigidity of the material within the elastic range".

If any stress value equal to or less than the proportional limit is divided by its corresponding strain value, a constant of proportionality will result (Fig. 3.6).

$$\text{MOE} = \frac{\text{Stress}}{\text{Strain}}$$

Elastic quality of a material represents a fundamental property of a material. The interatomic or intermolecular forces of the material are responsible for the property of elasticity. The stronger the basic attraction forces, the greater the values of the elastic modulus and the more rigid is the material.

$$\text{Young's modulus (E)} \atop \text{(Tension)} = \frac{\text{Longitudinal stress}}{\text{Elongation strain}}$$

$$\text{Bulk modulus (K)} \atop \text{(Compression)} = \frac{\text{Compressive force}}{\text{Volume strain}}$$

$$\text{Rigidity modulus (G)} \atop \text{(Shear)} = \frac{\text{Shearing stress}}{\text{Shearing strain}}$$

Applications

Orthodontic wires: A wire (active components) should have a value of stiffness as indicated by low MOE (flexible), which enables it to apply a suitable force for tooth movement to an orthodontic movement. A flexible component will be able to apply lower and a more constant force over a great distance.

Reactive components: These anchor the appliance to teeth, which are not to be moved, should not deform wires used for this purpose should have higher MOE.

Restorative materials: Stiffness is important in the selection of restorative materials. Since large deflections under stress are not desired. For example a restoration or filling must not alter the shape within the tooth when the patient bites on it otherwise the tooth will break and the filling will become loose. Therefore a material, which is placed in the mouth, should have higher MOE coupled with a high proportional limit.

Rigidity or stiffness: Stiffness is the resistance of the material to elastic deformation, i.e. a material, which suffers a slight deformation under a given load, has a high degree of stiffness.

For example, stiffness is important in the selection of restorative materials since large deflections under stress are not desirable.

FLEXIBILITY

Maximum flexibility is defined as the strain, which occurs when the material is stressed to its proportional limit.

The relationship between the maximum flexibility, proportional limit and MOE may be expressed mathematically as follows:

$$\text{MOE (E)} = \frac{\text{Proportional limit}}{\text{Maximum flexibility}}$$

Applications

Elastic impression materials should be flexible for easily removable over undercuts.

RESILIENCE (CUSHION LIKE)

"It can be defined as the amount of energy absorbed by a structure when it is stressed to its proportional limit" or "it is the energy needed to deform the material to its proportional limit".

Modulus of Resilience

The resilience of a material is usually measured in terms of its modulus of resilience. This is the amount of energy stored in a body when 1 unit volume of a material is stressed to its proportional limit, or it is measured by the area under the elastic portion of the stress-strain curve (Fig. 3.8).

Units: MJ/m^3.

Applications

1. *Resilient liner:* These are the soft cushions like liners given to the denture base to

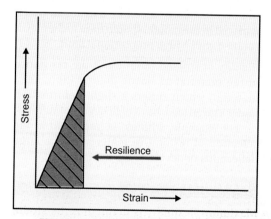

Fig. 3.8 Area of resilience in the s-s graph

absorb considerable amounts of energy without being permanently distorted. The energy is stored and released when the material springs back to its original shape after removal of the applied stress. Hence such liner serves as a "shock absorber" between occlusal surfaces of denture and the underlining oral tissues, and will protect the affected soft tissues from impact energies of mastication.

2. *Orthodontic wire:* Resilience has particular importance in the evolution of orthodontic wires. Since the amount of work expected from a particular spring in moving a tooth movement when the wire is located to the maximum elastic force or stress value.

3. The modulus of resilience of dentin is greater than that of enamel, thus is able to absorb impact energy. Enamel is a brittle substance with a comparably high MOE, PL and a low modulus of resilience however supported by the dentin with its ability to deform elastically (high modulus of resilience) teeth seldom fracture under normal occlusion.

DUCTILITY AND MALLEABILITY

Ductility

Ductility represents the ability of a material to sustain a large permanent deformation under a tensile load without rupture or it is the ability of a material to draw into a wire under a force of tension.
- A material with a high value of plastic deformation is generally ductile.

Malleability

Malleability represents the ability of a material to sustain a large permanent deformation under a compressive load without rupture or it is the ability of a material to hammer into sheets under compression.

Applications

1. *Orthodontic wires:* Alloys used for wires, show a high degree of ductility since they

are extended considerably during production process. In addition, clasps of denture constructed from ductile alloys can be altered by bending.

2. *Direct filling gold:* Due to its high ductility and malleability it is capable of adapting to cavity walls.

3. The malleability of stainless steel is utilized when forming a denture base by swaging technique. So, this involves the adaptation of a sheet of stainless steel over a preformed cast.

ELONGATION

"The deformation that results from the application of a tensile force is elongation".

- The total percentage elongation includes both the elastic elongation and plastic elongation (Fig. 3.9).

$$\% \text{ Elongation} = \frac{\text{Increase in length}}{\text{Original length}} \times 100$$

Application

An alloy that has a high value for total elongation can be bent permanently without danger of fracture, i.e.; clasps can be adjusted, orthodontic appliance can be prepared, if they are prepared from alloy have high values of elongation.

TOUGHNESS

"Toughness is the ability of the material to absorb energy during plastic deformation up to fracture"

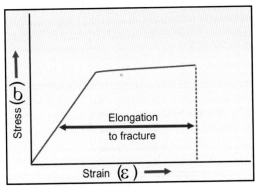

Fig. 3.9 Percentage of elongation

or "It is the amount of energy required to stress the material to the point of fracture".

Measurement

Toughness is measured by the amount of energy that a unit volume of the material has absorbed after being stressed up to point of fracture.

Unit: Mega Joule/m^3 (MJ/m^3).

BRITTLENESS

"It is defined as a tendency to fracture without appreciable deformation is therefore opposite of ductility".

- Brittle material is liable to fracture at or near to its proportional limit.
- Brittle materials are good under compression but not under tension.
  For example: Gypsum products, dental cements, dental amalgam, dental ceramics, etc.

ULTIMATE STRESS

"Ultimate stress is the maximum stress that a material can withstand before failure".

Ultimate Tensile Stress

"A maximum stress that a material can withstand before failure in tension".

Ultimate Compressive Stress

"A maximum stress that a material can withstand before failure in compression".

$$\text{Ultimate stress} = \frac{\text{Maximum load}}{\text{Original C/S area}}$$

Application

The ultimate stress of an alloy has been used in dentistry to give an indication or the size or cross-section required for a given restoration. An alloy that has been stressed to near the ultimate stress will be permanently deformed.

BREAKING STRESS

"The stress at which the material fractures is called as fracture stress or breaking stress".

A material does not necessarily fracture at the point at which the maximum stress occurs. After a maximum stress is applied the test bar shows a reduction in c/s area called "necking". As a result the load carrying capability of the test bar is reduced until the fracture occurs. Accordingly, the stress at the end of the curve is less than that some intermediate point on the curve.

True Stress

"It is defined as a ratio of load to the actual or instantaneous area of cross-section".

True Strain

"It is defined as a ratio of increase in length to the instantaneous length of the specimen".

True Breaking Stress (TBS)

After the ultimate stress the sample develops a neck, i.e. a local decrease in cross-sectional area at which further deformation is concentrated. The load now acts on a diminishing area and produces a stress sufficient to fracture the material. "The stress is obtained by dividing the breaking load by actual cross-sectional area known as the true breaking stress". Theoretically, it would be higher than the ultimate stress.

STRENGTH

"Strength is the capability of the material to withstand stress without undergoing fracture".

Unit: MPa or PSI.

Applications

Dental materials should have good strength to withstand stresses due to forces of mastication. For example, among all the cements the silicate cement (180 MPa) is having high strength and zinc oxide eugenol cement is the weakest (20 MPa).

TYPES OF STRENGTH

1. Tensile strength
2. Compressive strength
3. Shear strength
4. Flexural strength (modulus of rupture)
5. Impact strength
6. Fatigue strength
7. Tear strength.

TENSILE STRENGTH

"Tensile strength is defined as the maximum stress that a material can withstand before fracture in tension".

- Tensile strength is measured when maximum load in tension is delivered on the original cross-sectional area of the sample.
- Tension strength is generally determined by subjecting a rod, wire, or dumb-bell-shaped specimen to tensile loading.
- Such a test is difficult to perform for brittle materials. Another test is used for determining tensile strength is called "Diametral compression test".

Diametral Compression Test

Also called as "Indirect tensile test" for brittle materials.

In this method a disk of the brittle material is compressed diametrically in a testing machine until fractures. The compressive stress applied to the specimen that introduces a tensile stress in the material perpendicular to the plane of the force application of the test machine (Fig. 3.10).

FATIGUE STRENGTH

A subject that has been subjected to a stress below the proportional limit and subsequently relieved of this stress should return to its original form without any change in its properties or

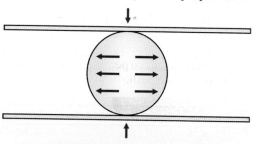

Fig. 3.10 Diametral test for brittle materials

internal structure. When the stress is repeated a great number of times, the strength of materials may be drastically reduced and causes ultimate failure. This is called "Fatigue failure".

Applications

In denture base resin, denture breaks due to fatigue from repeating loads during service.

SHEAR STRENGTH

"The maximum stress that a material can withstand before fracture in a shear mode of loading".
- A common method of testing the shear strength of the dental material is the "punch method". Stress distributed caused by this method is not pure shear.

$$\text{Shear strength} = \frac{F}{\pi dh}$$

where F = Compressive force
d = Diameter of punch
h = Thickness of specimen

IMPACT STRENGTH

"Impact strength is the capability of the material to withstand fracture under an impact force" or "energy required to fracture a material under an impact force". Impact strength can be tested by—
1. Charpy type impact tester
2. Izod impact tester.

TEAR STRENGTH

"Tear strength is the capability of a material to withstand fracture under tearing forces".

Applications

Impression material should be sufficiently elastic to be drawn over undercuts. Tearing occurs when severe undercuts are present. So removal should be at a sharp to reduce permanent deformation and maximize strength.

HARDNESS

Hardness is defined as resistance to permanent scratching or indentation or penetration. Among the properties that are related to hardness of a material are strength, proportional limit, ductility, etc.

Hardness tests are included in numerous ADA specifications for dental materials. Any test method will involve complex stresses in the material. Each of these differs slightly from the others and each presents certain advantages, and disadvantages. They have a common quality; each depends on the penetration of some small symmetrically shaped indenters onto the surface of object being tested. The indenter may be steel cone, steel ball, diamond pyramid or similar form.

A standardized force or weight, which varies with each test method, is applied to the penetrating point through an appropriate mechanism. Such a force application to the indenter produces a symmetrically shaped indentation, which can be measured for depth, area or width of the indentation, produced. With a fixed load applied to a standardized intender, the dimension of the indentation will vary inversely with the resistance to penetration of material being tested.

Methods

1. Moh's scratch test method
2. Indentation method
3. Penetration method.

Moh's Scratch Method

It is very crude method. This method is done by scratching one with other. The hardness is indicated in Moh's scale, value ranges from 0.2 to 10.

Recently, Bier Baum developed a scratching method to compare surface hardness.

Indentation Method

Indentation test is further divided into two types based on the size of the indenter used:
a. *Macrohardness test*
   - Brinell's hardness test
   - Rockwell hardness test.
b. *Microhardness test*
   - Vicker's hardness test
   - Knoop's hardness test.

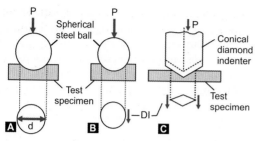

Figs 3.11A to C (A) Brinell's hardness test: spherical steel ball indenter; (B) Rockwell's hardness test: spherical steel ball indenter; (C) Rockwell test: conical diamond indenter. Where P is applied load, d is diameter of indentation and DI is depth of indentation

Brinell's hardness test: It is the oldest method used to test alloys and metals. As shown in Figure 3.11A, the test involves a spherical hardened steel ball of suitable diameter (10 mm) "D" is pressed on the surface of a test material by applying a load "P" for certain time and removed. The diameter of indentation "d" is measured. The force acting per unit area expressed as kg/mm^2 is calculated and is known as Brinell's hardness number "BHN". 'd' is measured with a calibrated marking on eyepiece of microscope. BHN is computed by a formula

$$BHN = \frac{2P}{\pi D [D-(D^2-d^2)^{1/2}]}$$

Smaller the area of indentation, harder is the material, larger is BHN.

To measure the hardness of small samples of materials used in dentistry, a smaller version of instrument known as "Baby Brinell's" has a small spherical ball of 1.6 mm diameter and load of 123N. BHN of selected dental material were mentioned in the Table 3.2.

Disadvantages:
- Cannot be used for very hard metals, as 'd' cannot be measured properly.
- Cannot be used for brittle materials.
- Cannot be used for elastically recovering material.
- It does not give a more reliable or correct value due to large depth of indentation, however the instrument and method is simple.

Table 3.2 Hardness numbers of selected dental materials

Material	Hardness
Tooth enamel	270-380 KHN
Dentin	60-70 BHN
Porcelain (fused)	415 VHN
Yellow cast gold alloys (hardened)	260 BHN
White gold (as cast)	150 BHN
Hard inlay gold	92-140 BHN
Amalgam	90 BHN
Stainless steel (soft)	180 KHN
Stainless steel (cold worked)	350 BHN
Co-Cr alloys	270-370 BHN
Yellow wrought gold alloys (work hardened)	250-350 BHN
Silicate cement	58 BHN
Hardened carbon steel	700-850 BHN
Zinc phosphate cement	36 BHN
Pure gold	18-30 BHN
Composite filling	25-35 BHN
Acrylic polymer (heat-cure)	18-22 BHN
Acrylic polymer (self-cure)	16-18 BHN
Vinyl denture base	14-20 BHN
Gold foil restoration	20-60 BHN
Soft inlay gold	40-75 BHN

Rockwell's hardness test: It was developed as a rapid method for hardness determination. It is mainly used for brittle and not very hard materials. The indenter is hardened steel ball (Fig. 3.11B) or conical diamond indenter (Fig. 3.11C). Depth of indentation is measured and Rockwell Hardness Number (RHN) is calculated.

First, minor load of 3 kg is applied; the "0" on scale is adjusted. Load is increased to major load of any suitable value like 10, 20, 40 kg and large diameter ball (12.7 mm) and RHN is found on proper corresponding scale. This test method has direct value reading, i.e. no formula is needed (Fig. 3.11B).

Another advantage is it can be used for measuring percentage elastic recovery of materials by

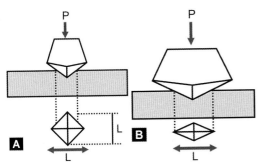

Figs 3.12A and B (A) Vicker's hardness test (B) Knoop's hardness test. Where P is applied load, L is length of diagonals

keeping the indenter with certain load on sample for 10 min. This is useful for plastic, elastomers, and viscoelastic materials.

Disadvantages
- Cannot be used for very hard.
- It does not give real surface hardness.

Vicker's hardness test: It is also called as 136° diamond pyramid, as diamond pyramid indenter is forced into the material with a load varying from 1 to 120 kg. As shown in Figure 3.12A, the indenter produces a square indentation; the length of diagonals are measured.

The hardness number calculated is called as "Vicker's hardness number" (VHN).

To get real value for surface hardness, the depth of indentation must be minimum. This produces an indentation to a depth of 10-15 μ on a well-polished metal surface.

This method is convenient to use for very hard materials like chrome cobalt, stainless steel, and alumina.

Disadvantages
- Cannot be used for elastically recovering materials as "length of diagonals (L)" becomes smaller when the indenter is removed.
- As high polished surface of material is required, the surface hardness may be greater than the actual value since the polishing causes increase in hardness due to work hardening.

Knoop's hardness test: It was developed to fulfill the needs of microindentation test method. Load is applied with a carefully prepared diamond-indenting tool (indenter has its opposite face inclined at a 130° to 172.5°). It produces indentation of orthorhombic shape and length of indentation is measured as shown in Figure 3.12B.

The elastic contraction takes place along minor diagonals and not along major diagonals. Hence major diagonals are measured. Higher the value of KHN, harder is the material.

This is the most popular method and is used for almost all dental materials even if they are available in small quantities. Only disadvantage is its high cost and requiring a highly polished surface.

Penetration Method or Shore A— Durometer Test

This method is particularly useful to compare the hardness of rubber in industry and elastomeric impression materials in dentistry.

The instrument consists of a blunt pointed indenter 0.8 mm in diameter that tapers to a cylinder 1.6 mm. With the help of a spring it can be loaded to any suitable value. It is connected to a pointer with lever arrangement. The pointer moves over a semicircular scale giving enlarged reading of depth of penetration. Initially the reading of the pointer is adjusted to a zero when tip of indenter touches the bottom and a maximum 100 reading is given when tip is on the surface.

The elastomeric mix is loaded in a small conical vessel and penetrometer is lowered at every ½ minute interval. Because rubber is viscoelastic, it is difficult to obtain an accurate reading, since the indenter continues to penetrate the rubber as a function of time. The usual method is to press down firmly and quickly on the indenter and record the maximum reading as shore A – hardness.

Abrasion Resistance

Like hardness, abrasion is influenced by a number of factors. Hardness has often been used to indicate the ability of a material to resist abrasion.

THERMAL PROPERTIES

MELTING AND FREEZING TEMPERATURE

The temperature at which a material melts or freezes is an important quality. Materials should have a melting or softening point at a temperature only slightly above the body temperature, but in no case should it be less than the temperature of the mouth.

Many times this temperature of softening or melting is the main factor in determining the choice of or selection of a material for use in the mouth or laboratory. The melting temperature likewise is important in the fabrication of materials outside the mouth.

- The melting temperature of metals and alloys used for restoration is important in that it limits the qualities of mold materials into which the metals may be cast.
- Knowledge of melting temperature of solders in relation to that of the structure being soldered is necessary if proper assembly is to be obtained.

Most materials used in dentistry have melting ranges rather than melting points because they are not single elements or components.

HEAT OF FUSION

The heat of fusion, L, is the heat in calories or joules, J required to convert 1 gm of a material from the solid to the liquid state at the melting temperature.

Equation for the calculation of heat of fusion is

$$L = Q/m$$

where Q = Total heat absorbed.

m = Mass of substance melted.

The heat of fusion is closely related to the melting or freezing point of the substance because when the change in state occurs, it is always necessary to apply the additional heat

to the mass to cause liquefaction and as long as the mass remains molten, the heat of fusion is retained by the liquid state is liberated. The difference in energy content is necessary to maintain the kinetic molecular motion, which is characteristic of the liquid state. Heat of fusion and melting point of various metals are mentioned in the Tables 3.3 and 3.4.

Table 3.3 Heat of fusion

Materials	Heat of fusion (Cal/gm)
Gold	16
Silver	26
Copper	49
Chromium	75
Aluminum	94

Table 3.4 Melting point and densities of various metals

Materials	Melting point (°C)	Density (g/cm³)
Gold	1063	19.30
Mercury	−39	13.55
Nickel	1455	8.90
Platinum	1774	21.45
Tin	232	7.28
Zinc	419	7.14
Aluminum	660	2.70
Cadmium	321	8.64
Cobalt	1495	8.90
Chromium	1890	7.20
Copper	1083	8.92
Gallium	30	5.90
Indium	156	7.30
Lead	327	11.34
Iron	1535	7.86
Molybdenum	2620	10.20
Palladium	1549	11.97
Silver	961	10.50
Iridium	2454	22.40
Titanium	1668	4.43

THERMAL CONDUCTIVITY

The thermal conductivity (K) of a substance is the quantity of heat in calories or joules per second passing through a body of 1 cm thick with a cross-section of 1 cm^2 when the temperature difference is 1°C.

Units: Cal/sec/cm^2 or °C/cm.

The conductivity of a material changes slightly as the surrounding temperature is altered but generally the difference resulting from temperature changes is much less than the difference that exists between different types of materials.

Applications

Restorative materials: When a large gold or amalgam restoration is used in the deep cavity and an inadequate thickness of dentin is present, a layer of cement called as base is placed under the permanent restoration to protect the pulp from thermal shock because these restorative materials are good conductors of heat.

Denture base materials: The difference in thermal conductivity of denture base materials likewise may cause differences in soft tissue response. A good thermal conductor is preferred for denture bases to maintain good health in the supporting tissues by having the heat readily conducted to and from the tissue by the denture base.

SPECIFIC HEAT

The specific heat (Cp) of a substance is the quantity of heat required to raise the temperature of a unit mass of substance by 1°C.

The heat required to raise the temperature of 1 gm of water from 15° to 16°C is 1 cal, which is used as the basis for the definition of heat unit.

Unit: Cal/g/°C

When the mass of a body is disregarded, the heat capacity of a substance is the quantity of heat required to raise the temperature of a body 1°C and is controlled by the mass of the substance. Thus the total heat required depends on the total mass and the specific heat of the substance.

In general, the specific heat of liquids is higher than the specific heat of solids.

Applications

During the melting and casting process the specific heat of the metal or alloy is important because of the total amount of heat that must be applied to the mass to raise the temperature to the melting point.

Specific heat of gold and the materials used in gold alloys is low, so prolonged heating is necessary.

THERMAL DIFFUSIVITY

The value of thermal diffusivity of a material controls the time rate at temperature change as heat passes through a material.

It is a measure of the rate at which a body with a non-uniform temperature reaches a state of thermal equilibrium.

$$h = K/Cp.$$

Where h = thermal diffusivity
         K = thermal conductivity
         Cp = temperature dependent specific
               heat capacity.
             = temperature dependent density

Units: m^2/sec or cm^2/sec or mm^2/sec.

Applications

Restorative materials: Many restorative materials are metallic, because of free electrons present in metal; these materials are good thermal conductors that the tooth pulp may be adversely affected by thermal changes. In many instances, it is necessary to insert a thermal insulator between the restoration and the tooth structure. In this respect, a restorative material that exhibits a low thermal conductivity is more desirable.

Denture base materials: Artificial teeth are held in a denture base that is ordinarily constructed of a synthetic resin, a poor thermal conductor. In upper denture, the base usually covers most of the roof of the mouth (hard palate). Its low thermal conductivity tends to prevent heat exchange between the supporting soft tissues and the oral cavity itself. Thus patient partially loses the sensation of hot and cold while eating and drinking. The use of metal denture base may be more comfortable and pleasant from this standpoint as it has high thermal diffusivity when compared to acrylic denture bases.

COEFFICIENT OF THERMAL EXPANSION (COTE)

The increase in the size of material on heating is called thermal expansion. This property is seen in solids, liquids, and gases.

Coefficient of Linear Expansion

The change in length per unit length of a material for a 1°C change (rise) in temperature is called as coefficient of linear expansion. It is denoted by 'α'.

Units: /°C.

This type of expansion is seen in solids.

$$\alpha = \frac{\text{(L final- L original)}}{\text{L original - (°C final}^- \text{ °C original)}}$$

Coefficient of Superficial Expansion

The change in area per unit area of a material for a 1°C change (rise) in temperature is called as coefficient of superficial expansion. It is denoted by 'β'.

Units: /°C.

$$\beta = \frac{\text{A final- A original}}{\text{A original x (°C final}^- \text{ °C original)}}$$

This type of expansion is seen in solids. It is observed that β is twice its α.

$$\beta = 2\alpha$$

Coefficient of Cubical Expansion

The change in volume per unit volume of a material for a 1°C change (rise) in temperature is called as coefficient of cubical expansion. It is denoted by 'γ'.

Units: /°C.

$$\Upsilon = \frac{\text{V final- V original}}{\text{V original x (°C final}^- \text{ °C original)}}$$

This type of expansion is seen in solids, liquids and gases. It is observed that 'γ' is thrice its α.

Finally, it can be written as $\alpha: \beta: \gamma = 1: 2: 3$.

Applications

Impression materials: COTE should be minimum to minimize contraction or dimensional change when cooled from mouth temperature to room temperature. On being withdrawn from the patient's mouth which is at a temperature of 32-37°C to a room temperature of around 23°C, the impression undergoes approximately 10°C cooling. This results in thermal contraction, the magnitude of which depends on the value of COTE of that particular impression material used and the impression tray to which it is attached.

Dental waxes (pattern waxes): The COTE of wax is higher than that of any other dental material. In the direct technique, softened wax is forced into the tooth cavity and held under pressure till it hardens. So the technique is carried out at around 37°C. Before investment, the wax pattern pulls down from 37°C–23°C (room temperature), which causes a linear shrinkage of 0.6%.

In the indirect technique, softened wax is forced into cavity on the gypsum die. Since this procedure is carried out at room temperature rather than mouth temperature, inlay wax for indirect pattern may soften at a lower temperature than direct pattern waxes. Thus the value of α is much lower, in the range of 0.2-0.4%.

Denture base resins: Denture base and the artificial teeth should have same values of COTE. Acrylic resin teeth are more compatible with acrylic denture base than porcelain teeth. There is a severe mismatch in COTE and modulus of elasticity between porcelain and acrylic resin. This may lead to crazing of denture base in the region around the base of porcelain teeth.

Restorative materials: The COTE should be minimum or zero to minimize percolation. When a patient takes hot drinks or cold drinks,

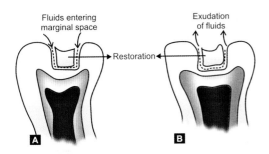

Figs 3.13A and B (A) Imbibition of fluids
(B) Exudation of fluids

restorative materials will be subjected to temperature changes in mouth that results in dimensional changes. Due to this expansion or contraction of the restorative material, the restoration may leak or it may debond from the tooth.

During contraction, depending on the value of α of restoration comparative to tooth a gap will develop at the junction. This will lead to imbibition of fluids containing bacteria, and then exuding them as the temperature rises. This pumping action of alternately imbibing and exuding fluids has been termed as percolation (Figs 3.13A and B).

If the values of α of tooth and restorative material match then the magnitude of gap formed will be less.

Among all the restorative materials, acrylic has the highest COTE; it will shrink or expand almost 7 times that of tooth structure for every degree change in temperature.

To minimize the marginal leakage, the walls of the cavity are lined with or coated with cavity varnish.

Electrical Properties

ELECTRICAL CONDUCTIVITY OR RESISTIVITY

The ability of a material to conduct an electric current can be stated either specific conductance or conductivity or conversely as the specific resistance or resistivity.

It can be determined experimentally that the resistance of a homogeneous conductor of uniform cross-section at a constant temperature varies directly with the length and inversely with the cross-sectional area of the sample, according to the equation as follows:

$$R = \rho \frac{l}{A}$$

Where
R = Resistance in ohms
ρ = Resistivity in ohm-centimeters
l = Length of the sample in centimeters
A = Section area in cm^2

The change in electrical resistance has been used to study the alteration in internal structure of various alloys as a result of heat treatment.

For example: In gold-copper alloy system, change in internal structure caused by an accompanying change in conductivity.

Resistivity is important in the investigation of the pain perception threshold resulting from applied electrical stimuli and of displacement of fluid in teeth caused by ionic movements.

When electrical resistance of normal and carious teeth is observed, less resistance observed by the carious teeth. Enamel is relatively poor conductor of electricity whereas dentin is somewhat better.

DIELECTRIC CONSTANT

Material that provides electrical insulation is known as a dielectric.

The dielectric constant or relative permittivity 'ε_r' compares the permittivity 'ε' of the dielectric to the permittivity 'ε_0' of empty space.

$$\varepsilon_r = \varepsilon/\varepsilon_0$$

where 'ε_0' of vacuum is 8.854×10^{-12} Farad/m.

Dielectric constant varies with temperature, bonding, crystal structure and structural defects of the dielectric.

The dielectric constant of dental cements generally decreases as the material hardens.

ELECTROMOTIVE FORCE

The electromotive force series is a listing of electrode potentials of metals according to the order of their decreasing tendency to oxidize in solution.

Metals and alloys used for dental restorations or instruments that are susceptible to corrosion. Some understanding of the relative position of the metal in the electromotive series is desirable.

- This serves as the basis of composition of the tendency of metals to oxidize in air.
- Those metals with large negative electrode potentials are more resistant to tarnish than those with a high positive electrode potential.

GALVANISM

The presence of dissimilar metals in the oral cavity may cause a phenomenon called as "galvanic action" or "galvanism". This results from a difference in potential between dissimilar fillings in opposing or adjacent teeth.

These fillings in conjunction with saliva or bone fluid as electrolytes make up an electric cell. Here the two metal restorations act as electrodes.

For example, many patients occasionally experience a mild electrostatic discharge when a metallic restoration is contacted by metallic spoon.

Galvanic shock can be experienced as a pain sensation caused by electric current generated by a contact between two dissimilar metals, forming the battery in the oral environment. The flow of current takes place through the pulp, the patient experiences pain and corrosion.

Galvanism When Two Fillings are Brought in Contact

When the two fillings are brought into contact the potential is suddenly short circuited through the two alloys. The result may be sharp pain.

For example, when amalgam restoration is placed on the occlusal surface of an upper tooth directly opposing a gold inlay in a lower tooth. Since both restorations are wet with saliva an electrical couple exists, with a difference in potential between the dissimilar restorations, it can be shown in the Figure 3.14A.

It is known that gold and amalgam restorations in the same mouth will develop a greater

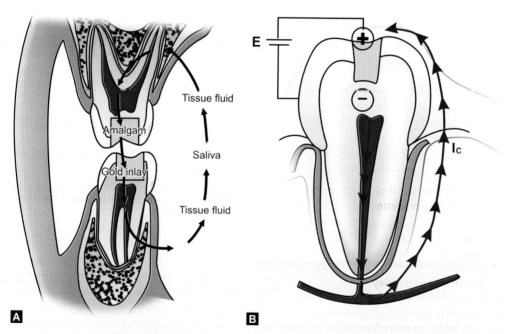

Figs 3.14A and B (A) Possible path of Galvanic current in the mouth (B) Possible pathway of Galvanic current in the single restoration

electrical potential than amalgam-amalgam or gold-gold combinations.

Galvanism When Two Fillings are not in Contact

When teeth are not in contact the difference in electrical potential between the two fillings still exists, a circuit exists. Saliva forms the electrolyte and the hard and soft tissues can constitute the external circuit.

For example, when an amalgam restoration is placed in the occlusal surface of the upper tooth which opposites a gold crown in a lower tooth. The electric current measured under these conditions between a gold crown and an amalgam restoration in the same mouth but not in contact; appear to be approximately 0.5 to 1 μA.

Galvanism in Single Isolated Metallic Restorations

The current is even present although it is of less intense. In this condition, the cell is generated by the potential difference created by two electrolytes such as saliva and tissue fluids as shown in Figure 3.14B. The interior surface of restoration exposed to the dental fluid have more active potential.

Clinical Significance of Galvanic Currents

Small galvanic currents associated with electro-galvanism are continuously present in oral cavity.

- Cements are good electrical insulators. But once they are wetted with dentinal fluids or oral fluids by marginal leakage they will become poor insulator.
- Postoperative pain occurs immediately after insertion of a new restoration and generally it subsides in few days.
- Coating with varnish can prevent electrical conductivity.
- Galvanic current could account for dyscrasias (lichenoid reaction, ulcer, cancer, etc.) but no evidence has been found.

ZETA POTENTIAL

A charged particle suspended in an electrolytic solution attracts ions of opposite charge to those at its surface. The layer formed by these ions is called the "stern layer". To maintain the electrical balance of the suspending fluid, ions of opposite charge are attracted to the stern layer. The potential at the surface of that part of the diffuse double layer of ions is called as "the electrokinetic" or "zeta potential".

Zeta potential may affect the near surface mechanical properties such as wear of the material.

RHEOLOGICAL PROPERTIES

'Rheology' is the study of the flow and deformation of materials. This term can be applied to both solids and liquids. This is of importance in dental materials in the following instances.

- Many dental materials are mixed as fluid pastes, which subsequently solidify.
- The mixed pastes are adapted to the required shape.
- The setting of such materials initially involves a change in viscosity with time and then the development of elastic modulus as solidification proceeds. From the physical analysis of these properties a working time and setting time can be defined.
- Flow and deformation of solids is also important. In practice, some solids are viscoelastic, such materials combine with viscous flow and elasticity and their properties are time dependent.

FLOW

Flow is the ability of a material to undergo plastic deformation by the external force or by its own weight.

Flow is a property usually attributed to the amorphous state as in this type of stress; the forces of attraction between atoms are not as great as in crystalline state.

Factors Affecting Flow

- Temperature.

- Load applied.
- Time for which force is applied.

Applications

Flow is an essential property for all impression materials. When the impression material is first inserted into the mouth they should have high flow property to record accurate and fine impression of the oral cavity and should have minimum flow after hardening to minimize the possibility of distortion of the impression during removal from the mouth.

Similarly dental inlay waxes should have high or maximum flow before hardening to get all the fine details of the cavity and should have minimum flow after hardening to minimize the possibility of distortion of the pattern during removal from the tooth cavity or die.

CREEP

Creep is a rheological behavior of a solid material under certain combination of stress and temperature. All materials that are subjected to a constant stress exhibit an increase of strain with time. This phenomenon of time dependent plastic deformation in crystalline materials is called as 'creep'.

If a metal is held at a temperature near its melting point and is subjected to a constant applied force, the resulting deformation or strain will be found to increase as a function of time.

Types of Creep

Static Creep

Static creep is the time dependent plastic deformation produced in a completely set solid subjected to a constant stress.

Dynamic Creep

Dynamic creep is the time dependent plastic deformation produced in a completely set solid when subjected to a fluctuating stress, such as fatigue type or cyclic stresses.

Applications

Dental amalgam has components with melting points only slightly above the room temperature. Because of its low melting range, dental amalgam can slowly creep from a restored tooth site under periodic sustained stress. The creep produces continuing plastic deformation so the process can be destructive to dental restoration.

VISCOSITY

Viscosity (η) is the resistance of a liquid to flow and equal to shear stress divided by shear strain rate.

$$\text{Viscosity } (\eta) = \frac{\text{Shear Stress } (\sigma)}{\text{Shear strain rate } (E)}$$

For example, the two parallel layers of the liquid are moving with different velocities, the experience tangential forces which tend to retard the faster layer and accelerate the slower layer, these forces are called as forces of viscosity.

The forces of viscosity on a layer is found to be proportional to the area (A) of the layer and velocity gradient, i.e. dv/dn of the layer in the normal direction.

Units: Poise

100 centipoises (cp) = 1 poise.

1 poise = 1 degree $\times$ sec/cm^2

Newtonian Viscosity

It is an ideal fluid demonstrates of shear stress that is proportional to shear rate and then the plot is a straight line as shown in Figure 3.15. Such behavior is called Newtonian.

Pseudoplastic

Viscosity decreases with increase in shear rate as shown in Figure 3.15, e.g. addition polysilicones.

Dilatant (Shear Thickening)

Viscosity increases with increase in shear rate. These types of liquids become more rigid as the rate of deformation increases (Fig. 3.15), e.g. Fluid denture base resins.

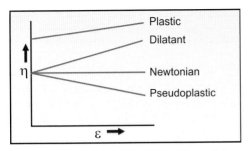

Fig. 3.15 Relationship between viscosity and shear strain rate

Plastic

Plastic materials behave like a rigid body until some minimum value of shear stress is applied. They began to flow until a certain minimum amount of stress applied (Fig. 3.15).

Applications

Viscosity is an essential property for all impression materials. When the impression material is being removed from the mouth they should have high viscosity to minimize the possibility of distortion of the impression.

Impression compound is the most viscous of the impression materials. The very high viscosity of impression compound is significant in two ways:

- Firstly, it limits the degree of fine details, which can be recorded in an impression.
- Secondly, it characterizes the compound as a mucocompressive impression material.

VISCOELASTICITY

In practice, many materials show a combination of both elastic and viscous properties. This phenomenon is termed as viscoelasticity.

Applications

Reversible hydrocolloid: In the sol form Agar is sufficiently fluid to allow detailed reproduction of hard and soft oral tissues. Its low viscosity classifies it as a mucostatic material, as it does not compress or displace soft tissues. In the gel form, Agar is sufficiently flexible to be withdrawn from undercuts. The materials are viscoelastic and the elastic recovery can be optimized by using correct technique. These materials are viscoelastic and are likely to undergo permanent deformation if subjected to stresses for more than a few seconds.

OPTICAL PROPERTIES

Each restorative material has some properties that are necessary to permit a material to restore the function of damaged or missing natural tissues. Another important goal of dentistry is to restore the color and appearance of natural dentition. Esthetic considerations in restorative and prosthetic dentistry have assumed a high priority within the past several decades.

Light is an electromagnetic radiation that can be detected by the human eye. Visible light (Table 3.5) is a very small part of the electromagnetic spectrum (Table 3.6), being that region of the spectrum of the wavelength approximately 380-780 nm. White light is made up of mixtures of color.

For an object to be visible, it must reflect or transmit light incidents on it from an external source. The latter is the case for objects that are of dental interest. The incident light is usually polychromatic, i.e. some mixture of the various wavelengths.

The phenomenon of vision and certain terminology can be illustrated by considering the

Table 3.5 Wavelength of different regions of visible spectrum

Color	Approximate wavelength
Violet	380-430 nm
Blue	430-460 nm
Blue-Green	460-500 nm
Green	500-570 nm
Yellow	570-590 nm
Orange	590-610 nm
Red	610-710 nm

Table 3.6 The electromagnetic spectrum

Nomenclature	Frequency (Hz)	Approximate wavelength (m)
γ-rays	3×10^{19}–3×10^{22}	10^{-14}–10^{-11}
X-rays	3×10^{16}–3×10^{19}	10^{-11}–10^{-8}
Ultraviolet rays	6×10^{14}–3×10^{16}	10^{-8}–5×10^{-7}
Visible light	3×10^{14}–6×10^{14}	4×10^{-7}–8×10^{-7}
Infrared	3×10^{12}–3×10^{14}	10^{-6}–10^{-4}
Microwaves	3×10^{8}–3×10^{12}	10^{-3}–1
Radiowaves	$< 3 \times 10^{8}$	>1

response of the human eye to light coming from an object. Light from an object that is incident on an eye is focused on the retina and is converted into nerve impulses that are transmitted to the brain. Cone-shaped cells in the retina are responsible for color vision. These cells have threshold intensity required for color vision and also exhibit a response curve related to the wavelength of the incident light, because a neural response is involved in color vision, constant stimulation by a single color may result in color fatigue and a decrease in the eye's response.

The signals from the retina are processed by the brain to produce the psychophysiologic perception of color. Defects in certain portions of the color-sensing receptors result in the different types of color blindness and thus, people vary greatly in their ability to distinguish colors.

COLOR

The perception of the color of an object is the result of a physiological response to a physical stimulus. The sensation is a subjective experience, whereas the beam of light, which is the physical stimulus that produces the sensation is entirely objective. The perceived color response results from either a reflected or a transmitted beam of white light or a portion of that beam.

According to Grassmann's laws, the eye can distinguish differences in only three parameters of colors. The parameters are as follows:
- Hue
- Value
- Chroma.

Hue

Hue is commonly referred to as color. It is the dominant wavelength of a color and is the wavelength of a monochromatic light that when mixed in suitable proportions with an achromatic color will match the color perceived.

Light having short wavelengths (350 nm) is violet in color, and light having long wavelengths (700 nm) is red, between these two wavelengths are those corresponding to blue, green, yellow, and orange colors. This attribute of color perception is also known as hue.

Value

Value is the luminous reflectance. It is the lightness or darkness of a color. Value is the most important color factor in tooth color matching. The value of a color permits an object to be classified as equivalent to a member of a series achromatic objects ranging from black to white for light diffusing objects and from black to perfect clear and colorless for transmitting objects.

A black standard is assigned a luminous reflectance of zero; whereas a white standard is assigned 100. This attribute of color perception is described as value in one visual system of color measurement.

Chroma

Chroma is excitation purity and is a measurement of color intensity, i.e. the amount of a saturation of hue in a color (degree of saturation of a particular hue). The higher the chroma more intense

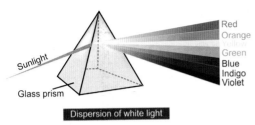

Fig. 3.16 Light transmission through a prism

is the color (dark). So chroma, it can not exist itself but it is always associated with hue and value. The excitation purity of a color describes the degree of its difference from achromatic color perception more resembling it. Numbers representing excitation purity 'range 0-1, this attribute for color perception is also known as chroma.

COLORS AND COLOR MIXING

White Light

White light contains a mixture of colors. It is dispersed into components by passing it through a prism (Fig. 3.16).

Primary, Secondary and Complementary Colors

Primary Colors

Blue, green and red are primary colors, combining of suitable proportions of these colors results in white color (Fig. 3.17).

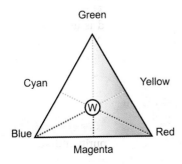

Fig. 3.17 Equilateral triangle representing color mixing where 'w' is white color

Secondary Colors

A secondary color is obtained by the addition of two primary colors (Fig. 3.17).

E.g.:   Blue + Green = Cyan (peacock blue).
Green + Red = Yellow.
Red + Blue = Magenta.

Complementary Colors

Two colors are said to be complementary if they are combined to produce white color (Fig. 3.17).

E.g.:   Blue + Yellow
Green + Magenta
Red + Cyan

Transmitted Color

It is the resultant color of light transmitted by the object and the color, which is not transmitted is an absorbed color (Fig. 3.18), e.g. a yellow color filter absorbs blue and transmits yellow, similarly green filter transmits green color and absorbs magenta.

Reflected Color

Materials gain their reflected colors by reflecting them and absorbing other colors. For example, blue object reflects only blue color and absorbs all other colors (Fig. 3.18).

- A white object reflects all incident colors and a black object absorbs all incident light and does not reflect any color.
- An object appears black when no light is reflected.

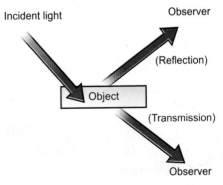

Fig. 3.18 Light transmission and reflection

COLOR MIXING

Addition or Additive Mixing

This process applies only to colored lights reflecting from white surface, the resultant is an additive combination of colors.

It can be represented by an equilateral triangle (Fig. 3.17). In which primary colors are at the corners and secondary colors at the midpoint of sides. Two colors said to be complement if they combine to produce white.

Subtractive Mixing

This process applies to pigments and paints. Each component reflects its own color and absorbs other color, resultant is the color, which is nonabsorbed.

PIGMENTATION

Pleasing esthetic effects are sometimes produced in a restoration by the incorporation of colored pigments in non-metallic materials such as composite resins, dental acrylics, dental porcelain and silicone maxillofacial materials.

Usually inorganic pigments rather than organic dyes are used. Since the pigments are more permanent and durable in their color qualities. When the colors are combined with proper translucency, the restorative materials may be made to match closely the surrounding tooth structure or soft tissue.

To match tooth tissue; various shades of yellow and gray are blended into the white base material. To match the pink soft tissues of the mouth various blends of red and white are necessary, with occasional need for blue, brown and black in small quantities. The color and translucency of human tissue shows a wide variation from patient to patient and from one tooth or area of the mouth to another.

MEASUREMENT OF COLOR

The color of dental restorative materials is most commonly measured in reflected light by two techniques.

- **Instrumental technique**, done with the help of spectrophotometers and colorimeters (Figs 3.19A and B).
- **Visual technique**, a popular system for visual determination of color is the Munsell color system (Fig. 3.19C).

LIGHT AND INTERFACES

When a beam of light strikes on an object the following things can happen:
1. Reflection
2. Refraction
3. Transmission
4. Absorption
5. Scattering of light.

Reflection

When a light, traveling in a homogeneous medium, falls on the surface of another medium, a part of incident light is sent back to the first medium (Fig. 3.20A).

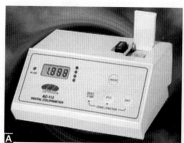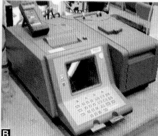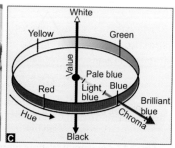

Figs 3.19A to C (A) Colorimeter, (B) Spectrophotometer, and (C) Munsell color system

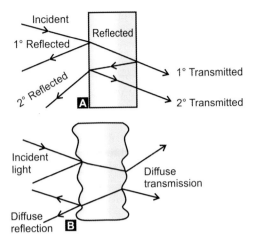

Figs 3.20A and B Light transmission and reflection through the objects with smooth and rough surfaces respectively

Refraction

When a ray of light traveling in a homogeneous medium, enter into another medium there will be change in direction or in path of ray (Fig. 3.20A).

Reflection results from the difference in the refractive indices of two mediums.

Transmission

Substances, which are transparent, can transmit light (Figs 3.20A and B). Rough surfaces give rise to diffuse light, i.e. transmitted light emerges in all directions; diffusion transmission gives a translucent appearance.

Absorption

Lambert's law of absorption states that each specific light of substance absorbs an equal fraction of light passing through it.

$$I_X/I_0 = e^{-Kx}$$

Where I_X = Intensity of light after passing through the distance of materials.

I_0 = Initial intensity

K = Absorption coefficient of material.

Scattering of Light

Presence of scattering centers such as opacifiers (e.g.: TiO_2), air bubbles in the medium causes light to emerge in all directions.

The effect of scattering is dependent on size, shape, and refractive index of the material and the amount of scattering centers present. Opacity increases with increase in scattering.

Opacity

Opacity is the property of materials that prevents the passage of light. When all the colors of spectrum from a white light source such as sunlight are reflected from an object with same intensity as received, the object appears white.

An opaque material may absorb some of light and reflect the remainder. For example, red, orange, yellow, blue and violet are absorbed, the material appears green in reflected white light.

Translucency

The translucency of an object is the amount of incident light transmitted by the object that scatters part of the light.

- A high translucency gives a lighter color appearance.
- Translucency decreases with increase in scattering in the material.
- Some translucent materials used in dentistry are porcelain, composite resins, plastics, etc.

Transparency

Transparent materials allow the passage of light in such a manner that little distortion takes place and objects may be clearly seen through them, e.g. glass.

Refractive Index or Index of Refraction

The index of refraction for any substance is the ratio of the velocity of light in a vacuum or air to its velocity in the medium.

When a ray of light travels from one medium to another, the ratio between 'sin' of angle of incidence and 'sin' of angle of reflection is called

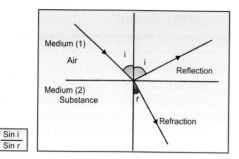

Fig. 3.21 Representation of light traveling from one medium to another

refractive index of second medium with respect to first medium (Fig. 3.21).

The refractive index is a characteristic property of the substance and is used extensively for identification.

METAMERISM

The change in color matching of two objects under different light sources is called metamerism. Two objects that are matched under one light source but are not matched under other light sources are called a metameric pair (Fig. 3.22).

An example of metamerism is when a shade guide tooth matches the tooth under incandescent light.

Metamerism results from possible differences in illumination between the dental clinic and the dental laboratory, causing poor matching in a fabricated restoration such as a porcelain crown.

The ideal situation is to have objects possess the same color reflectance. The objects are

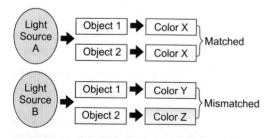

Fig. 3.22 Metamerism—a pair of objects color is matched under light source A and does not match under light source B

then called as an isomeric pair; they are color matched under all light sources.

FLUORESCENCE

Fluorescence is the emission of light by an object at different wavelengths from those of the incident light.

When the molecules of a substance absorb radiation they are raised to a high energy state and the excess energy is emitted out with greater wavelength within short time (approximately 10^{-8} seconds), this phenomenon is called as fluorescence.

The wavelength of the emitted light usually is longer than that of the exciting radiation.

Natural teeth fluoresce in the blue region when illuminated by ultraviolet light. Some anterior restorative materials and dental porcelains are formulated with fluorescing agents to produce the natural appearance of teeth structure.

BIOCOMPATIBILITY

The term biocompatibility is used to describe the state of affairs in a biomaterial exists within a physiological environment, without either the material adversely and significantly affecting the body, i.e. biomaterials being harmonious with life and not having toxic or injurious effects on biologic junctions. Outwardly there are two broad aspects of biocompatibility, such as

- The effects on the material.
- The effects on the tissues.

These are, however, very much interrelated for it is often an adverse effect on a material by the physiological fluid, leading to the release of particulate or soluble matter from the material that can cause adverse response from the tissues. Biocompatibility is largely about the chemical interaction that takes place between the material and the body fluids and the physiological responses to these reactions. Thus for example the biocompatibility of metallic materials is the electrochemical interaction due to release of metal ions or some cases the release of insoluble particles into the tissues.

BIOMATERIALS

The biomaterial may be defined as material that is used in the treatment of patients and which at some stage interferes with the tissues for a significant length of time so that the interaction between the tissue and the material is an important factor in the treatment.

In broad sense, a biomaterial can be any substance other than a drug that can be used for any period of time, as a part of system that treats, augments or replaces any tissues, organs or function of body. For example dental materials are used in humans for a short or long period of time they function in close contact with human tissues.

CONCEPT OF BIOCOMPATIBILITY

The application of biomaterials in medical disciplines is varied ranging from its usage in orthopedics to urology and dentistry to gynecology. Likewise the materials vary from hard Co-Cr alloy to soft hydrophilic polymers and from inert alumina ceramics to degradable collagenous products. However, same type of materials can be used differently in different situations. For example use of acrylic PMMA in dentistry, neurosurgery, and orthopedic surgery and also in ophthalmology all have different functions and are used in different anatomical locations.

The concept here, therefore, is that problems of biocompatibility are subtle and complex, but not necessarily totally different from one application to another or from one material to another.

Thus, in general, biocompatibility is measured on the basis of the localized cytotoxicity, systemic responses, allergenicity, hypersensitivity, estrogenicity and carcinogenicity.

FACTORS INFLUENCING THE BIOCOMPATIBILITY ASPECTS/RESPONSES

- Oral health conditions
  For example chronic medical problems, requiring long-term treatments like radiation, chemotherapies, etc.
- Age of the person.
- Products of corrosion of alloys or degradation of materials.
- Context of placement of restorations.
  For example a crown and bridge alloy shows different biological responses when used as an implant.
- Surface characteristics: Rough surface causes accumulation of food debris – act as a seat for µ-organisms to grow and produce biohazardous materials and causing inflammations, etc.

REQUIREMENTS OF BIOCOMPATIBILITY

Should not
1. Produce allergic reactions.
2. Harmful to the tooth or soft tissues.
3. Be containing toxic substances.
4. Be carcinogenic.
5. Undergo biodegradations.
6. Show estrogenicity.
7. Create immunotoxicity.

TESTS FOR EVALUATION OF BIOCOMPATIBILITY

The purpose of biocompatibility tests is to eliminate any potential product or component of products that can cause harm or damage to oral or maxillofacial tissues.

Before conducting biocompatibility tests, the following aspects must be carefully considered:
1. Location of the material.
2. Nature of the tissues (soft/hard).
3. Exposure of the material to the oral situations, saliva, blood, tissue fluids, etc.
4. Types of contact (direct/indirect).
5. Duration of contact (few minutes – impression materials and several years – restorations).
6. Chemical nature: Compositions, degradations and corrosion products of restoratives.
7. Physical conditions: Stresses, fatigue resistance, wearing, etc.
8. Surface modifications (coated, electroplated) and surface characteristics.

Biocompatibility tests are classified on three levels or at three stages of testing:

1. Group I: Primary-screening tests
2. Group II: Secondary–animal tests
3. Group III: Preclinical–usage tests.

Primary Screening Tests

Cytotoxicity Tests

Dental materials in a fresh or cured state are placed directly on tissue culture cells or on membranes overlying tissues. Manufacturer can modify them if they are cytotoxic.

Genotoxicity Tests

Mammalian or nonmammalian cells, bacteria, yeast or fungi are used to determine the gene mutations, changes in chromosomal structure or other de-oxyribonucleic acid or genetic changes caused by the dental material, devices or extracts from materials. Cytotoxic tests employed are:
- Cell plating and growth tests.
- Cell membrane permeability tests.
- Agar overlay method.
- Chemotaxis assay.
- Assay for immune reaction.
- Mutagenesis assay.

Mutagenesis Assay

Mutagenic assays detect changes in the morphology or metabolic function of a particular cell type that is caused by genotoxicity. Most widely used short-term mutagenesis tests are as follows:
- The Anne's test, and
- Style's transformation tests.

The Anne's test is more specific, technically easier to conduct, often conducted in screening program. These studies suggest that not all carcinogens are genotoxic (mutagenic) and not all mutagens are carcinogenic.

Advantages of Cytotoxicity Tests

- Screening large number of samples quickly and inexpensively.
- Quantifying results.
- Greater sensitivity to toxic material than usage tests.
- Testing for specific function of cell metabolism.

Disadvantages of Cytotoxicity Tests

- Limitation of testing to only one cell type at a time
- Dissimilarity of test cells and host cells.
- Lack of inflammatory and other tissue protective mechanism in tissue culture.

Secondary Tests

At this level, a series of long-term tests are conducted to identify agents that cause inflammatory response or immune reactions. They are performed mainly on rodents, rabbits, or guinea pigs, i.e. at this level the products are evaluated for its potential to create systemic toxicity, inhalation toxicity, skin irritation, sensitization and implantation tests.

Mucous Membrane Irritation Tests

This test is important because many chemical substances from the dental products can come in contact with the mucous membrane. This test is conducted by placing the test material in contact with mucous membrane in positive and negative control animals either on cheek pouch tissue or with oral tissues for several weeks.

Skin Sensitization Test

The agents are intradermally or the test material is held in contact with the skin for a longer period of time from one exposure to repeated exposures. The degree of reaction and the percentage of animals showing the reactions are basis for scoring the allergenicity of the material.

Implantation Tests

In these tests, the test material is implanted into the subcutaneous tissue or into the bone. The location of implant site is determined for inflammation of other reactions.

Advantage

- In vivo tests are quite reliable as the biological responses are investigated directly.

Disadvantages

- Expensive and difficult to control the experiment in long duration.
- Reliability of the fact whether the animal represents fully the human species.
- Ethical concern of animal sacrifice.

Preclinical Usage Tests

Once the test material successfully possesses the screening and secondary tests, these pre-clinical usage tests can be conducted on subhuman primates (dogs, pigs, etc). Usage tests are performed to identify the effects of various types of dental materials on tissue environment in which they will be used. The tissues generally used are the dentin, pulp, gingival, mucosal tissues and periodontal tissues. Most usage test involves presumably intact and noncarious teeth without inflamed pulp.

Dentin – Pulp Usage Tests

Materials to be tested are placed in class V cavities prepared on intact, noncarious teeth of nonrodent mammals and the test compounds were then evaluated with the control at 3 days, 5 weeks and 8-week interval. These teeth were then removed and subjected for microscopic examination for inflammatory response, prevalence of reparative dentin formation in the pulp and the microleakage.

Mucosal and Gingival Usage Tests

Because various dental materials are placed into cavity preparation with subgingival extensions, the gingival responses to these materials were also measured. The test cavities are prepared class V cavities; the material is mixed as per the manufacturers recommendations and placed in the cavities with subgingival extension. The material effect on gingival tissues was then observed at an interval of few days to few weeks. The tissue was then proposed and subjected for microscopical examination.

Pulp Capping and Pulpotomy Usage Tests

In this, the pulp is merely exposed for pulp capping evaluation and the test material is placed. Observe the formation of dentinal bridge adjacent to the test material (capping material) The quality or structure of the covering dentinal bridge is determined.

Endodontic Usage Test

In this test the pulp is completely removed from the pulp chamber and root canals are replaced by the obturating test material and control material. The teeth were removed together with surrounding apical periodontal soft and hard tissues and subjected for microscopical examination.

For a biocompatible material one should observe minimal or no response and the shortest resolution time of response is detected.

ALLERGIC RESPONSE TO DENTAL MATERIALS

Allergic Contact Dermatitis

This is commonly seen first by primary physicians. This forms one of the most occupational diseases. The interval between exposures of causative agent is the reoccurrence of clinical manifestations usually varies between 12-48 hours.

Dermatitis usually occurs where the body surface makes direct contact with allergen.

Personnel and patients involved in orthodontics and pediatric dentistry have the high incidence of side effects. An allergic contact dermatitis associated with numerous monomers of bonding agents frequently involves the distal parts of the fingers and palmar aspects of the fingertips.

Allergic Contact Stomatitis

This is the most common adverse reaction to dental materials. The reaction may be observed as local or contact type of lesions, but reactions distant from material site (such as itching on the palms of the hand, etc.). The long-term reaction is dependent on the composition of the materials, the toxic components, the degradation products, the concentration of absorbed and accumulated components and other factors associated with substances leached from the materials.

Dental materials contain many components known to be common allergens such as chromium, cobalt, mercury, eugenol, resin-based materials and formaldehyde. Various studies demonstrated that free residual monomer from autopolymerized acrylic dentures or appliances can cause allergic reactions.

Chemicals that may produce allergic contact stomatitis and short-term basis can also be found with mouthwashes, dentifrices and topical medications. They can cause burning sensation, swelling and ulceration of oral tissues.

Composite Fillings

These materials consist of tiny glass particles suspended in a *resin* (plastic) matrix.

However, they are more natural looking, require less tooth reduction to place, and are bonded in place for a better seal. Composites are not totally compatible either. Most are made of the petrochemical bisphenol, which some research indicates leaches out estrogen-like substances. Some composites are less biocompatible than others because of the amount of iron oxide, aluminum oxide, barium, and other materials in them.

Gold Alloys

Most "gold" crowns placed today contain from 1–40% gold and have nickel in them, which is inappropriate for those with a compromised immune system.

Amalgam

Amalgam is the most commonly used material for posterior teeth. It contains approximately 50% mercury and varying amounts of silver (30%), tin, zinc, and copper. The controversy is that it contains mercury, a known neurotoxin (poison to the nervous system).

Galloy

Galloy is a brand new material containing silver, tin, copper, indium, and gallium. It is meant to be mercury-free alternative to amalgam. Studies of gallium alloys have reported problems with corrosion, durability, tooth fracture, and tooth sensitivity.

Base Metal Alloys

It is especially important for patients with metal sensitivities to avoid the base alloys since these usually contain toxic metals such as nickel and chromium. But even the high noble materials can be incompatible for patients and even toxic; palladium, for example, is toxic.

Nonprecious Alloy

Nonprecious alloys are used when maximum strength is desired, appearance is not a factor, but cost is most important. There are two basic formulations, one that contains nickel and one that is nickel-free. The controversial issue is that nickel, beryllium, cobalt, chromium, and palladium may cause immune problems and/or toxicity.

Electrogalvanism

Dissimilar metals in the mouth, including different formulations of the "same" metal, create micro amps of current which could cause oral pain, corrosion of the metal (black mercury amalgam fillings), dry mouth, metallic taste, erythema (red and swollen gums), and possible dysfunction of other organ systems, endocrine glands, etc. on that meridian.

Denture Materials

Dentures are usually made from acrylic, stainless steel, chromium-cobalt, nylon, a gold alloy, or titanium. Most pink-colored acrylics and vinyl's contain cadmium, which is considered toxic and/or immune reactive. The alternative is to use cadmium-free pink or clear materials. Metals are used to increase rigidity and increase retention of the prosthesis in the mouth during function. If metals are not used, the opposite is true, which is not desirable from a functional perspective. For more information, refer Denture Base Resins Chapter of this book.

Breakthroughs in the development of dental materials and techniques are occurring on a regular basis. We have yet to find one single material that is compatible for everyone. Debate continues about how to best restore a patient's mouth to optimal health and no perfect solution has yet presented itself. The best we can do is to keep an open mind and keep searching for answers. Only by thorough testing can it be determined which is most compatible for any one person.

TARNISH AND CORROSION

Metals undergo chemical or electrochemical reaction with the environment resulting in dissolution or formation of chemical compounds; corrosion products.

These chemical compounds may accelerate, retard or have no influence on the subsequent deterioration of the metal surface. Corrosion is undesirable and sometimes it is helpful like in the case of dental amalgam, where there is limited amount of corrosion around amalgam as corrosion products seal marginal gap and inhibit ingestion of oral fluids and bacteria.

TARNISH

Tarnish is surface discoloration on a metal or even as a slight loss or alteration of the surface finish or luster.

It is a process by which metal surface is dulled in brightness or discolored through the formation of chemical film such as sulfide and an oxide.

Causes for Tarnish

- Occurs from the formation of hard and soft deposits on a surface of the restoration.
  - Calculus—light yellow to brown hard deposit.
  - Plaque—soft deposit and films composed of microorganisms and mucin.
- May also arise on metal from the formation of thin films such as oxides, sulfides and chlorides.

- Stain or discoloration arises from pigment producing bacteria, drugs containing chemicals such as iron and mercury and adsorbed food debris.

CORROSION

Corrosion is a process in which deterioration of a metal is caused by reaction with its environment.

Causes of Corrosion

- The corrosion of metal may take place due to the action of moisture, atmosphere, various acidic (phosphoric acid, lactic acid and acetic acid) at proper concentrations and pH, alkaline solutions and certain chemicals (hydrogen sulfide, ammonium sulfide, etc).
- Tarnish always leads to corrosion.
- Saliva contains water and ions like chlorine and oxygen also may contribute to corrosion.

Rusting of iron is one of the examples for corrosion, in this iron combines oxygen and water to form hydrated oxide.

$$Fe + O_2 (H_2O) \rightarrow Fe (OH)_2 + FeO \text{ 'or' } Fe_2O_3.H_2O.$$

Factors Affecting Corrosion

Rate of corrosion increases over time, especially with surfaces subjected to stress; with intergranular impurities in the metal ion with corrosion products that do not completely convey the metal surface.

Effects of Corrosion

- Corrosion causes severe and catastrophic disintegration of the metal body.
- In addition, corrosion is extremely localized and may cause rapid mechanical failure of a structure, even though the actual volume loss of material is quite small.

CLASSIFICATION OF CORROSION

Corrosion can be classified into chemical and electrochemical corrosion. The detailed classification is given in Flow chart 3.1.

Flow chart 3.1 Classification of corrosion

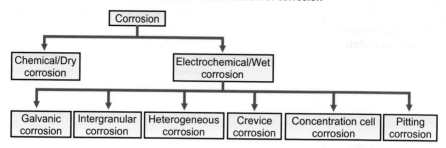

Chemical or Dry Corrosion

In chemical corrosion, there is a direct combination of metallic and nonmetallic elements to yield a chemical compound through processes such as oxidation, halogenation or sulfurization reactions. A good example is discoloration of silver by sulfide; forms by chemical process of corrosion can also be a corrosion product of dental gold alloys.

$$2Ag + S \rightarrow Ag_2S$$

This mode of corrosion is also called as "dry corrosion" as it occurs in the absence of water or another fluid electrolyte.

Oxidation of alloy particles in dental amalgam is another example.

Oxidation of eutectic alloy in dental amalgam may reduce the reactivity of the silver and copper alloys with mercury. Hence it may affect the amalgamation. Therefore, alloy should not be placed in a cool, dry location to ensure an adequate shelf life.

Electrochemical Corrosion or Wet Corrosion

The metal with lower electrode potential value undergoes oxidation and acts as anode and that with higher electrode potential has a reduction reaction and acts as cathode.

Apparatus: Anode, cathode, electrolyte and voltmeter.

From Figure 3.23 Anode: Dental amalgam restoration. Cathode: Gold alloy restoration. Electrolyte: saliva.

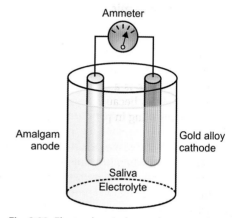

Fig. 3.23 Electrochemical corrosion in amalgam

Procedure

- Anode is the surface where positive ions are formed. This is the metal surface that corrodes, as at this electrode electrons are lost.
- The reaction is sometimes referred to as corrosion caused by oxidation.

$$M° \rightarrow M^+ + e^-$$

- At the cathode a reaction must occur that will accept the free electrons produced at the anode.
- The following reduction reactions take place at the cathode.

$$M^+ + e^- \rightarrow M°$$
$$2H^+ + 2\ e^- \rightarrow H_2$$
$$2H_2O + O_2 + 4\ e^- \rightarrow 4\ (OH)^-$$

- The cathode consumes the electrons, which are lost by the anode, in presence of electrolyte. This completes circuit.
- Anode gets corroded due to the loss of electrons.

Electrode Potential

The potential, which is exhibited by a metal electrode when it is placed in a solution of its own ions, is known as electrode potential.

Types of Electrochemical Corrosion

Galvanic Corrosion

It is also called as electrogalvanism. It occurs when electro-chemically two dissimilar metals are in contact. There is a sudden, sharp pain called galvanic shock because of *short* circuit to the two alloys resulting in patient experiencing shock.

Galvanism when two metals are brought into contact, Galvanism when two metals are not in contact and Galvanism in single isolated metallic restorations were discussed in the electrical properties chapter of this book.

Clinical significance of galvanic currents was discussed in the electrical properties chapter of this book.

Intergranular Corrosion

It is due to difference in grain structure. Even homogenized solid solution is susceptible to corrosion at the grain boundaries, which are anodic to cathodic interiors, became atomic arrangement at grain boundaries are less regular and have high energies. Impurities in alloy enhance corrosion, which is segregated at the grain boundaries.

Stress Corrosion

Occurs in fatigue, cyclic loading in oral environ-ment. This increases internal energy of alloys, which results in the displacement of atoms.
- A metal, which has been stressed by cold working, becomes more reactive at the site of maximum stress.

- If stressed and unstressed metals are in contact in an electrolyte, the stressed metal will become the anode of a galvanic cell and will corrode.
- If an orthodontic wire has been cold worked, stress corrosion may occur and cause the wire to break.

Heterogeneous Type of Corrosion

This type of corrosion is due to the heterogeneous composition of the metal surface. Commercial dental alloys contain more than three alloys, which are more heterogeneous.

For example, solder joints may corrode due to the inhomogeneous composition of the alloy.

Impurities in any alloy enhance corrosion.

Concentration Cell Corrosion

This is due to variations in the electrolytes or in the composition of an electrolyte in a system. This is of two types:
1. Electrolyte concentration cell: In a metallic restoration, which is partly covered by debris, the composition of electrolyte under the debris will differ from that of saliva and this can contribute to the corrosion of the restoration. Here food–debris at the interproximal areas produce electrolytes that are anodic and saliva on occlusal surface.
2. Oxygen concentration cell. A difference in oxygen tension in between parts of same restoration causes corrosion of restoration. Greater corrosion occurs in the part of the restorations having lower concentration of oxygen.

Crevice Corrosion

Corrosion occurs in narrow spaces or crevices such as in dental prosthesis. This occurs due to changes in electrolyte and oxygen concentration by the presence of deposits as in case of the concentration cell corrosion.

Pitting Corrosion

It can be seen in chromium passivated metals. Patients should be warned not to use household bleaching materials to cleanse partial denture frameworks.

- Interior of pit becomes anode or pits on restorations are anodic. It is due to less oxygen and surface is cathodic.
- Corrosion is very rapid in pit areas since the area availability is less.

Prevention of Corrosion

- Can be prevented by electroplating ex.: With nickel and chromium for corrosion protection and esthetic reasons.
- Passivation, e.g. stainless steel contains sufficient amount of chromium added to iron.
- Use of nobel metals – since they resist tarnish and corrosion due to their high positive electropotential values.
- Coating with varnish.
- Polishing of metal restorations.
- Homogenization treatment for the alloy.
- Restoration should adapt properly to cavity walls otherwise cement becomes electric conductor.
- Avoid using dissimilar metallic restorations.
- Unnecessary burnishing of margins is avoided which might induce localized stress.
- Maintaining oral hygiene.
- Use of metallic and nonmetallic coatings.

SUGGESTED READING

1. Al-Hiyasat AS, Tayyar M, Darmani H. Cytotoxicity evaluation of various resin based root canal sealers. Int Endodont J. 2010; 43:148-53.
2. Anantha Ramakrishna S. Physics of negative refractive index materials. Rep Prog Phys. 2005;68:449-521.
3. Ancowitz S, Torres T, Rostami H. Texturing and polishing: the final attempt at value control. Dent Clin Am. 1998;42(4):607-13.
4. Antonucci JM, Toth EE. Extent of polymerization of dental resin by differential scanning colorimetry. J Dent Res. 1983;62:121.
5. Atai Z, Atai M. Side Effects and complications of dental materials on oral cavity. Am J Applied Sci. 2007;4(11):946-9.
6. Cao Z, Sun X, Yeh CK, Sun Y. Rechargeable infection responsive antifungal denture materials. J Dent Res. 2010;89(12):1517-21.
7. Cattaneo PM, Dalstra M, Melsen B. The finite element method: a tool to study orthodontic tooth movement. J Dent Res. 2005; 84(5):428-33.
8. Clark GCF, Williams DF. The effects of proteins on metallic corrosion. J Biomed Mater Res. 1982;16:125.
9. Cornell D, Winter R. Manipulating light with the refractive index of an all-ceramic material. Prac Proced Aesthet Dent. 1999;11(8): 913-7.
10. Dhoble A, Padole P, Dhoble M. Bone mechanical properties: a brief review. Trends Biomater Artif Organs. 2012;26(1):25-30.
11. Gardiner TH, Waechter JM Jr, Wiedow MA, Solomon WT. Glycidyloxy compounds used in epoxy resin systems: A toxicology review. Regul Toxicol Pharmacol. 1992;15(Part 2):S1-S77.
12. German RM, Wright DC, Gallant RF. In vitro tarnish measurements on fixed prosthodontics alloys. J Prosthet Dent. 1982;47: 399.
13. Gladys S, Van Meerbeek B, Lambrechts P, Vanherle G. Evaluation of esthetic parameters of resin modified glass-ionomer materials and a poly-acid modified resin composite in Class V cervical lesions. Quint Inter. 1999;30(9):607-14.
14. Gupta A, Sinha N, Logani A, Shah N. An ex vivo study to evaluate the remineralizing and antimicrobial efficacy of silver diamine fluoride and glass ionomer cement type VII for their proposed use as indirect pulp capping materials – Part I. J Con Dent. 2011; 14(2):113-6.
15. Hanks CT, Wataha, JC, Sun Z. In vitro models of biocompatibility; a review. Dent Mater. 1996;12:186-92.
16. Ho SP, Goodis HE, Balooch M, Nonomura G, Marshall SJ, Marshall GW. The effect of sample preparation technique on determination of structure and nanomechanical properties of human cementum hard tissue. Biomaterials. 2004;25(19):4847-57.
17. Holland RI. Galvanic currents between gold and amalgam. Scand J Dent Res. 1980;88:269.
18. Hu X, Johnston WM, Seghi RR. Measuring the color of maxillofacial prosthetic material. J Dent Res. 2010;89(12):1522-7.
19. Jolanki R, Kanerva L, Estlander T, Tarvainen K, Keskinen H, Eckerman M. Occupational dermatoses from epoxy resin compounds. Contact Dermatitis. 1990;23:172-83.
20. Kanerva L, Jolanki R, Estlander T. Allergic and irritant patch test reactions to plastic and glue allergens. Contact Dermatitis. 1997; 37(6):301-2.
21. Lackovic KP, Wood RE. Tooth root color as a measure of chronological age. J Forensic Odonto-Stomatology. 2000; 18(2): 37-43.

22. Lefever D, Mayoral JR, Mercade M, Basilio J, Roig M. Optical integration and fluorescence: A comparison among restorative materials with spectrophotometric analysis. Quintessence Int. 2010;41:837-44.
23. Lloyd CH. The determination of specific heats of dental materials by differential thermal analysis. Biomaterials. 1981;2:179.
24. Magni E, Ferrari M, Hickel R, Ilie N. Evaluation of the mechanical properties of dental adhesives and glass-ionomer cements. Clin Oral Invest. 2010;14:79-87.
25. Marcucci B. A shade selection technique. J Prosthet Dent. 2003; 89:518-21.
26. Mohsen NM, Craig RG, Filisko FE. The effects of different additives on the dielectric relaxation and the dynamic mechanical properties of urethane dimethacrylate. J Oral Rehabil. 2000;27:250.
27. Murray PE, Godoy CG, Godoy FG. How is the biocompatibilty of dental biomaterials evaluated? Med Oral Patol Oral Cir Bucal. 2007;12:E258-66.
28. O'Brien W. Double layer effect and other optical phenomena related to aesthetics. Dent Clin Nort Am. 1985;29(4):667-73.
29. Oliver WC, Pharr GM. An improved technique for determining hardness and elastic modulus using load and displacement sensing indentation experiments. J Mater Res. 1992;7(6):1564-83.
30. Park S, Quinn JB, Romberg E, Arola D. On the brittleness of enamel and selected dental materials. Dent Mater. 2008;24(11): 1477-85.
31. Pharr GM, Oliver WC, Brotzen FR. On the generality relationship among contact stiffness, contact area, and elastic modulus during indentation. J Mater Res. 1992;7:613-7.
32. Provenzano JC, Oliveira JCM, Alves FRF, Rôças IN, Siqueira JF Jr, de Uzeda M. Antibacterial activity of root-end filling materials. Acta Stomatol Croat. 2011;45(1):3-7.
33. Quinn JB, Quinn GD. Indentation brittleness of ceramics: a fresh approach. J Mat Sci. 1997;32(16):4331-46.
34. Quinn GD, Bradt RC. On the Vickers indentation fracture toughness test. J Am Ceram Soc. 2007; 90(3):673-80.
35. Ray NJ. Some aspects of colour and colour matching in dentistry. J Irish Dent Assoc. 1994; 40(1):16-9.
36. Sakar-Deliormanli A, Guden M. Microhardness and fracture toughness of dental materials by indentation method. J Biomed Mater Res: Appl Biomat. 2006;76(2):257-64.
37. Shammas M, Rama Krishna Alla, Color and shade matching in dentistry. Trends Biomater. Artif Organs. 2011;25(4):172-5.
38. Wang L, Perlatti D'ALPINO PH, Lopes LG, Pereira JC. Mechanical properties of dental restorative materials: relative contribution of laboratory tests. J Appl Oral Sci. 2003;11(3):162-7.
39. Wennberg A, Mjor IA, Hensten-Pettersen A. Biological evaluation of dental restorative materials- a comparison of different test methods. J Biomed Mat Res. 1983;17:23-36.
40. Willems G, Celis JP, Lambrechts P, Braem M, Vanherle G. Hardness and Young's modulus determined by nanoindentation technique of filler particles of dental restorative materials compared with human enamel. J Biomed Mater Res. 1993;27(6): 747-55.
41. Witte J, Jacobi H, Juhl-Strauss U. Suitability of different cytotoxicity assays for screening combination effects of environmental chemicals in human fibroblasts. Tox Letters. 1996;87:39-45.

Chemistry of Synthetic Resins

4

POLYMER

A polymer is a large molecule built by repetition of small, simple chemical units.

Or

Polymer is a large molecule made up of many parts.

The term polymer derives from Greek meaning "many parts" (Poly = many, mer = Unit).

MONOMER

The individual small molecules from which the polymer is formed are known as monomers, meaning "single unit" (mono = single, mer = unit).

POLYMERIZATION

The process by which the monomer molecules are linked to form a polymer molecule is called polymerization.

CLASSIFICATION OF POLYMERS

Polymers can have different chemical structures, physical characteristics, mechanical behavior, thermal characteristics, and thermal characteristics. Polymers can be classified in different ways. They are as follows:

According to Origin

1. *Natural polymers:* Polymers, which are isolated from natural materials.
   A. Polysaccharides
      For example: Starch, cellulose, etc.
   B. Polyamides
      For example, Molecules containing $\overset{\overset{\displaystyle O}{\displaystyle \|}}{C}$ – NH groups.
   C. Polyisoprenes
      For example, Vulcanite, rubber, gutta-percha
   D. Polynucleic acids
      For example, DNA, RNA
2. Synthetic polymers: Polymers synthesized from low molecular weight compounds.
   For example, Polyethylene, PVC, nylon, etc.

According to their Backbone Structure

1. *Organic polymers:* A polymer whose backbone chain is essentially made of carbon atoms is termed as organic polymers. However, the atoms attached to the side valancies of the backbone carbon atoms are usually hydrogen, oxygen, nitrogen, etc.
2. *Inorganic polymers:* The molecules of inorganic polymers generally contain no carbon atoms in their backbone.
   For example, silicone rubber.

According to their Thermal Response

1. *Thermoplastic polymers:* Some polymers soften on heating and can be converted into different shapes and retain their shapes on cooling. The process of heating, reshaping and retaining the same on cooling can be repeated several times. Such polymers that undergo a physical change when heated or cooled are termed as thermoplastic.
   For example, Polyethylene, nylon, etc.

2. *Thermoset polymers:* They undergo chemical change on heating to convert themselves into an infusible mass.

Or

Thermoset polymers are those that change irreversibly under the influence of heat from a fusible and soluble material into one that is infusible and insoluble through the formation of covalently cross-linked, thermally stable network. Such polymers that become an infusible and insoluble mass on heating are called thermosetting polymers. For example, Polymethyl methacrylate.

According to Method of Polymerization

1. *Addition polymers:* Addition polymers are formed from monomer containing double bonds (unsaturated molecules) without change in composition is called addition polymers. The process of formation of addition polymers is called as addition or chain polymerization. No byproduct is formed during the reaction.

    The structure of monomer is repeated many times in a polymer. The molecular weight of the polymer is roughly equal to that of the molecules, which combine to form polymer.

    For example, Polymethyl methacrylate, addition polysilicones, etc.

2. *Condensation polymers*
   - Condensation polymers are formed due to reaction between the functional groups of the monomers are called condensation polymers and the process of formation of such a polymer is called as condensation polymerization or step growth polymerization.
   - While forming the polymer, small molecules get eliminated as byproducts.
   - Condensation or step growth polymerization is brought about by monomers containing two or more reactive functional groups such as hydroxyl, carboxyl or amino groups.
   - In condensation polymers, the molecular weight of the polymer is lesser by the weight of simple molecules eliminated during the condensation process.

    For example, Polysulfides, condensation polysilicones, nylon, etc.

According to their Ultimate Form and Use

1. *Plastics:* When a polymer is shaped into hard tough utility articles by the application of heat and pressure, it is used as a plastic.

    For example, Polystyrene, PVC, polymethyl methacrylate, etc.

2. *Elastomers:* When vulcanized into rubbery products exhibiting good strength and elongation, polymers are used as elastomers.

    For example, Natural rubber, silicone rubber, etc.

3. *Fibers:* If the polymers drawn into long filament like materials whose length is at least 100 times its diameter such polymers are said to have been converted into fibers.

    For example, Nylon, Terylene, etc.

4. *Liquid resins:* Polymers in a liquid form are described as fluid resins. They are used as adhesives and sealants.

    For example, Epoxy adhesives and polysulfide sealants.

Applications of Polymers in Dentistry

1. *Dental cements:* Glass ionomer cement and Zn polycarboxylate cement contains polyacrylic acid, which is responsible for chemical bonding with tooth structure.

2. *Restorative or composite resins:* For example, Bis phenol a Glycidyl dimethacrylate, polyurethanes.

3. *Bonding agents:* Used to attach composite resin to tooth enamel and dentin.

    For example, Bis GMA, NPGGMA, NTGGMA, etc.

4. *Cavity varnish:* It is used to minimize marginal leakage around amalgam restorations. These contain natural resins such as copal resin and resin dissolved in a suitable volatile solvent.

5. *Impression materials:* For example, Elastomers and hydrocolloids.

6. *Denture base resins:* For example, Poly-methyl methacrylate, nylon, bakelite, vulcanite, epoxy resins, cellulose, vinyl polymers, etc.
7. *Resilient lining materials:* For example, heat cure, self-cure, hydrophilic acrylics, heat and self-cured silicones.
8. *Artificial teeth:* For example, cross-linked polymethyl methacrylate.
9. *Maxillofacial materials:* For example, Vinyl plastics, polyurethanes, PMMA, etc.
10. *Special tray materials:* For example, Self-cure acrylic resins.
11. *Denture repair resins:* For example, Heat or self-cure acrylic resins.
12. *Orthodontic appliances:* For example, Heat or self-cure acrylic resins.
13. *Die materials:* For example, Epoxy resins, polyethers, self-cure acrylics, epimines, etc.
14. *Pattern material:* For example, Dental waxes.
15. *Polymeric crown and bridge materials:* For example, Acrylic resins.
16. *Implant materials:* For example, Composites, etc.
17. *Miscellaneous materials:* For example, Toothbrushes, disposable syringes, etc.

Degree of Polymerization

Degree of polymerization is defined as the total number of monomers in a polymer molecule.

Degree of polymerization (DP) = number of monomers.

Molecular weight of polymer = molecular weight of monomer × DP

Therefore,

$$DP = \frac{\text{Molecular weight of polymer}}{\text{Molecular weight of monomer}}$$

The growth of the polymer chain is a random process. Some chains grow faster than others. Therefore not all chains have same length, i.e. they have a distribution of molecular weights.

In general, the molecular weight of a polymer is reported as the average molecular weight. Since the number of repeating units may vary greatly from one molecule to another.

Polymers of low degree of polymerization are called "resole" (low molecular weight). At this stage it is thermoplastic and alcohol soluble. Similarly, polymers with high degree of polymerization are called "resite" (high molecular weight), which is its final form. At this stage, it is both insoluble and infusible. They have higher strength, hardness, and softening temperatures.

TYPES OF POLYMERIZATION

There are two types of polymerizations they are condensation and addition polymerization (Flow chart 4.1).

Condensation Polymerization

- Condensation polymerization is brought by monomers containing two or more reactive functional groups (poly functional) such as hydroxyl, carboxyl or amino groups.
- In this type of polymerization, the polymers build up proceeds through a reaction between functional groups of monomers accompanied by the elimination of small molecules. The reaction takes place in a stepwise manner and the polymer build up is therefore slow.
- Condensation reaction between molecules tends to stop before the molecules have reached a truly giant size because as the chain grows, they become less mobile and numerous.

Flow chart 4.1 Classification of polymerization

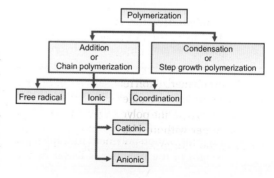

- Since reaction is slow, longer reaction times are required to get a high molecular weight polymer.
- The polymer formed still contains both the reactive functional groups at its chain ends

(as end groups) and hence is active and not dead.

- The molecular weight of the polymer formed is lesser by the weight of the simple molecules eliminated during the condensation process, for example, water and alcohols.

For example:

i. *Polysulfides*

ii. *Condensation polysilicones*

Addition Polymerization

Addition polymerization is characterized by a self-addition of the monomer molecules to each other very rapidly through a chain reaction without simultaneous production of byproducts.

Chain polymerization reactions usually occur with unsaturated molecules containing double bonds. In this type, the polymers are formed from the monomer without change in composition because the monomer and the polymer have the same empirical formulas. In other words, the structure of the monomer is repeated many times in the polymer.

Since majority of these monomers fall under the vinyl category, chain polymerization is also termed as vinyl polymerization.

Chain polymerization consists of three major steps namely initiation, propagation and termination and the process can be brought about by a free radical, ionic or coordination mechanism.

Requisites for Addition Polymerization

Presence of Unsaturated Groups

Molecules containing unsaturated groups can undergo addition polymerization.

For example, Molecules containing double bonds ($H_2C = CXY$), such as polyethylene, polyvinyl chloride, polystyrene, polyacrylic acid, polymethacrylic acid, polymethyl methacrylate, etc.

Presence of Initiators

They can be free radicals, anions or cations.

Initiators
- Initiators are unstable compounds containing a very weak bond, which can be broken by supplying energy to produce products called as free radicals.
- A free radical is an atom or a group of atoms possessing odd electrons.
- When energy is supplied initiator decomposes to form two reactive species, each carrying an unpaired electron called free radicals. This type of decomposition is called hemolytic decomposition.

   For example, if R-R is an initiator its decomposition can be represented as:

$$R : R \rightarrow \overset{.}{R} + \overset{.}{R} \quad or \quad 2\,\overset{.}{R}$$

- The free radicals formed have electron withdrawal ability because it possesses an unpaired electron. When this free radical attacks the monomer molecule, it forms a sigma bond by combining with one of its "π" electrons and the other "π" electron is transferred to the other end of the molecule.
- Thus, the original free radical bonds to the monomer molecule one side, the remaining "π" electron at the other end, then acts as a new free radical site which can further attack other monomer molecules to propagate the reaction.
- Decomposition of initiators into free radicals is called as "activation".

   For example, the most commonly used initiator in dentistry is Benzoyl peroxide, this decomposes to produce free radicals.

Table 4.1 Different types of initiators and activators used in dentistry

Material	Initiator	Activator
Heat cured PMMA	Benzoyl peroxide	Heat
Self-cure/cold cure/auto cure PMMA	Benzoyl peroxide	N,N – Dimethyl p-toluidine/ 3° amine
UV light activated composites	Benzoin methyl ether	UV Light λ = 365 nm
Visible light activated	Camphoro-quinone	Visible light λ = 450 nm

Various initiators systems are given in Table 4.1 for different resins.

Benzoyl peroxide free radical

Activators

- Activators decompose the initiators to form free radicals. Activation of initiators can be brought about by the heat energy, light energy or by using catalysts (Table 4.1)

Free Radical Polymerization

In free radical polymerization, the initiation of polymer chain growth is brought about by free radicals produced by the decomposition of initiators.

Polymerization process occurs in four stages. They are:

1. Initiation
2. Propagation
3. Termination
4. Chain transfer.

Initiation

- Polymerization reaction is initiated when the free radicals formed on activation reacts with a monomer molecule.

- The reaction can be illustrated for benzoyl peroxide radical and the methyl methacrylate monomer as follows:

Initiation

- The time during which the molecules of the initiator become energized or activated and start to transfer their energy to the monomer molecule is called induction or initiation period.

- The initiation energy required to activate each monomer is 16,000-29,000 cal/mole in the liquid phase.
- The induction period is greatly influenced by the purity of the monomer. Any impurity in the monomer that can react with free radicals will inhibit the polymerization reaction.
- The impurity can react either with the activated growing chain to prevent further growth. For example:
  i. Addition of a small amount of hydroquinone to the methyl methacrylate monomer will inhibit polymerization.
  ii. Presence of oxygen often causes retardation of the polymerization,
  Since oxygen can react with the free radicals.
- It is common practice to add a small amount (approximately 0.0006% or less) of hydroquinone or methyl ether of hydroquinone to the monomer to avoid accidental polymerization during production and storage and to prolong shelf-life of the monomer.
- After the consumption of an inhibitor, the polymerization follows the normal course.

Propagation

Following initiation, the new free radical is capable of reacting with a fresh monomer unit resulting in the linking up of the second monomer unit to the first and transfer the radical site from the first monomer unit to the second by unpaired electron transfer process which is capable of reacting with further monomer molecules.

The process involving a continuing attack on fresh monomer molecules that in turn keep successively adding to the growing chain one after another is termed as propagation.

Propagation

The process lasts till the chain growth is stopped by the free radicals being killed by some impurities or by a termination or there is no monomer available for the reaction.

When once activation starts, smaller activation energy of 4,000–5,000 cal/mole is sufficient for propagation. Propagation is exothermic and heat liberated during reaction is 12,900 cal/mole.

Termination

Any further addition of the monomer units to the growing chain is stopped and growth of the polymer chain is arrested.

It is of two types:
a. Termination by direct coupling
b. Termination by disproportionation.

Propagation

Termination by disproportionation

Termination by Direct Coupling

In this, the two growing chains unite by the coupling of the lone pair electron present in each chain to form an electron pair and thus nullify their reactiveness. Since this process involves the coupling of the two lone electrons, this kind of termination is known as termination by coupling.

$$RM_n^• + RM_m^• \longrightarrow RM_{(n+m)}$$

Termination by direct coupling

Termination by Disproportionation

In this type, one hydrogen atom from one growing chain is abstracted by the other growing chain and utilized by the lone pair electron for getting stabilized, while the chain which had donated the hydrogen gets stabilized by the formation of double bond. This termination results in the formation of two polymers of shorter length.

In this termination process, the product molecules do not contain any free radical site and hence cannot grow any further. The polymer formed can be referred to as dead polymer chain.

Chain Transfer

This is yet another method of chain termination which takes place by the transfer reaction. In this, the growth of one polymer chain is stopped forming a dead polymer with simultaneous generation of new free radical capable of initiating a fresh polymer chain growth.

Types of Chain Transfer

a. Activation energy is transferred from the activated molecule to an inactive monomer molecule.
b. Activation energy is transferred from the activated molecule to an already terminated molecule.

Chain transfer

HOMOPOLYMERS AND COPOLYMERS

- Polymers, which contain only one kind of monomer as repeating unit, are called as homopolymers. They can be linear or branched.
- The polymer, which is composed of more than one type of repeat units, is called as copolymers and its process of formation is known as copolymerization. The monomers from which the copolymer is made are called comonomers.

$$nA + nB \rightarrow - A - B - A - B - A - B -$$

Homopolymers can exist in three different types:

1. Linear

   $$- A - A - A - A - A - A - A - A - A - A -$$

2. Branched

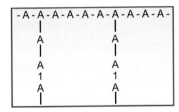

3. Cross-linked.

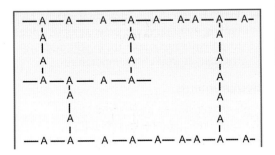

Types of Copolymers

1. Alternating Copolymers

The two different types of monomers in a polymer are distributed alternatively throughout the chain.

$$nA + nB \rightarrow A - B - A - B - A - B -$$

2. Random Copolymers

When two different monomer units in a polymer are distributed in random throughout the chain the polymer is called random copolymer.

$$nA + nB \rightarrow A - B - A - A - A - B -$$
$$A - A - A - B - B - B -$$

3. Block Copolymer

When a block of one repeat unit is followed by a block of another repeat unit, which in turn is followed by the first repeat unit and the polymer is called block polymer.

$$nA + nB \rightarrow A - A - A - B - B - B -$$
$$A - A - A - B - B - B -$$

4. Graft Copolymer

Graft copolymers are branched molecules where the main chain is made entirely of one repeat unit, while the branched chains are made of yet another repeating end.

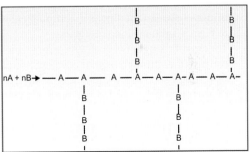

Advantages: Copolymerization may alter the physical properties of resulting polymer such as impact strength, hardness, flexibility, water sorption and wettability.

1. Copolymerization of polymethyl methacrylate with butadiene – styrene rubber results in a copolymer is more resistant to fracture by impact forces – high impact strength acrylic.

2. Copolymerization of methyl methacrylate with octyl methacrylate results in a polymer, i.e. soft and flexible at mouth temperature and has been used as soft liner.

3. Copolymerization of methyl methacrylate with hydroxy ethyl methacrylate results in a copolymer that increases the water sorption. This material is called hydrophilic acrylic and is used as a soft liner for dentures.
4. Vinyl and acrylic monomers are also copolymerized by manufacturer resulting in a powder, which is later mixed with methyl methacrylate monomer to fabricate dentures.
5. In glass ionomer cements, the liquid contains 50% aqueous solution of acrylic acid in the form of a copolymer with itaconic and maleic acids. These acids tend to increase the reactivity of the liquid, decrease viscosity and reduce tendency for gelation.

CROSS-LINKING

- Formation of chemical bonds between linear polymer molecules commonly referred to as cross-linking, can lead to infinite network of molecules.
- Cross-linking provides a sufficient number of bridges between the linear macromolecules to form a 3-dimensional network.
- The cross-linking between polymer molecules can be either through regular covalent bonds or through secondary valence type such as hydrogen bonds. The former type is called chemical cross-linking or irreversible cross-linking and latter type is called physical or reversible cross-linking.
- Cross-linking agent should have double bonds at both ends of the molecule, e.g. Ethylene glycol dimethacrylate is used as a cross-linking agent in acrylic denture base

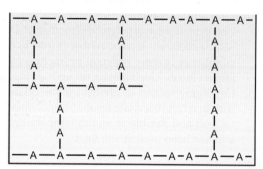

materials. Cross-linking agent may be in small amounts of about 2–40% can be used.

Advantages

- The effect of cross-linking on physical properties varies with the composition, concentration of cross-linking agent and the polymer system.

Increases	Decreases
• Strength	• Water sorption
• Hardness	• Permanent deformation
• Resistance to solvents	• Solubility
• Resistance to crazing	

PLASTICIZERS

- Plasticizers have low molecular weight, high boiling point, and are water soluble, added to polymers to make them soft and more resistant at workable temperatures.

Requirements

A plasticizer should have/should be
1. High boiling point, less volatility.
2. Compatible with the polymer to which it is added.
3. Chemically inert, resistant to moisture, nontoxic and non-fuming.
4. Impart flexibility and show permanent retention.
5. Water insoluble.

Action of Plasticizer

- Plasticizers partially neutralize secondary bonds or intermolecular forces that normally prevent the resin molecule from slipping past one another when the material is stressed.

- Plasticizers penetrate between the polymer chains and increase the intermolecular spacing.
- It reduces strength and hardness.
- It reduces glass transition temperature of a polymer.
- It increases polymer flexibility and flow characteristics.

Types of Plasticizers

External Plasticizers

These plasticizers are physically blended with the polymer and do not enter the polymerization reaction but are distributed throughout the polymerized mass. In this way they interfere with the interaction between polymer molecules.

This makes plasticized polymer considerably softer than the pure polymer. This type of plasticizer will slowly leach out of the polymer resulting in the hardening of the polymer, e.g. Dibutyl phthalate.

Internal Plasticizers

Plasticizers can be added to the polymer by co-polymerization with a suitable comonomer. In this case, the plasticizer is a part of the polymer.

Dibutyl phthalate

This type of plasticizer does not leach out and the material remains more flexible, e.g. butyl methacrylate added as an internal plasticizer to methyl methacrylates.

SUGGESTED READING

1. Antonucci JM, Toth EE. Extent of polymerization of dental resin by differential scanning colorimetry. J Dent Res. 1983;62:121.
2. Cook WD. Rheological studies of the polymerization of elastomeric impression materials. J Biomed Mater Res. 1982;16:331.
3. Chun J, Pae A, Kim S. Polymerization shrinkage strain of interocclusal recording materials. Dent Mater. 2009;25:115-20.
4. Darr AN, Jacobsen PH. Conversion of dual cure luting cements. J Oral Rehabil. 1995;22:43.
5. Harashima I, Nomata T, Hirasawa T. Degree of Conversion of dual cured composite luting agents. Dent Mater. 1991;10:8.
6. Williams JR, Craig RG. Physical Properties of addition silicones as a function of composition. J Oral Rehabil. 1988;15:639.

Physical Metallurgy

5

In dentistry, metal represents one of the four major classes of materials used for the reconstruction of decayed, damaged or missing teeth. Other three classes are ceramics, polymers, and composites.

A metal is an element that forms positive ions in solution [tend to sacrifice their valence electrons to become positive ions in solution (ionizes positively in solution)].

"The metal handbook (1992)" defines a metal as 'an opaque lustrous chemical substance that is a good conductor of heat and electricity and when polished is a good reflector of light.'

CHARACTERISTIC PROPERTIES OF METALS

1. Metals are generally electropositive elements.
2. Metals are good conductors of heat and electricity due to the nature of metallic bonding.
3. Metals are malleable and ductile; i.e. they can hammer into sheets and can be drawn into wires.
4. Metals are opaque since the free electrons absorb electromagnetic energy of light.
5. Metals have high melting and boiling points.

    Exceptions are Gallium: 38°C
                   Cerium: 28°C
                   Rubidium: 30°C
                   Mercury: –39°C

These metals exist as liquid metals at room temperature.

6. Metals possess a peculiar shine on their surface called "metallic luster" and take good polish.
7. Metals have high density and are hard substances because the atoms are closely packed together in a crystalline lattice structure.
8. Metals can withstand very high stresses.
9. Metals form solid solutions with each other easily. These solutions are called alloys also possess metallic properties.
10. Metals generally are resistant to chemical attack, but some metals require alloying elements to resist tarnish and corrosion in the oral environment. Noble metals are highly resistant to chemical corrosion and oxidation and do not require alloying elements for this purpose.
11. When a metal is struck a metallic ring is usually generated.

METALLOID

Metalloid is an element such as carbon, silicone that does not ionize positively in solution to positive charges but is a good conductor of heat and electricity similar to metals and combines with other metals to form useful alloys.

METALLIC BOND

In addition to covalent bond and ionic bond, matter can also be held together by a primary atomic interaction known as "metallic bond" that occurs between valence electrons (see Fig. 3.1). It is nondirectional. The electrons are able to move

Table 5.1 Periodic chart of the elements

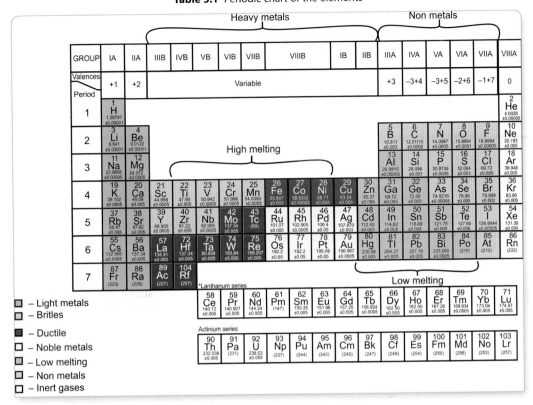

about in the space lattice to form an electron cloud. The electrostatic attraction between this electron cloud and the positive ions in the space lattice provides the force that bonds the metal atoms together as a solid.

SOLIDIFICATION AND MICROSTRUCTURE OF METALS

The process of conversion of liquid metal to a solid metal is known as "solidification".

If a metal is melted and then allowed to cool, and if its temperature during cooling is plotted as a function of the time, a cooling curve graph results (Figs 5.1A and B).

Pure metals often give a cooling curve in which super cooling of the liquid below the true freezing temperature may be experienced before crystallization of the metal begins (Fig. 5.1B).

Mechanism of Crystallization

In a metal, in the liquid state the atoms have sufficient energy to move about freely. But as the temperature falls the atomic movement becomes more sluggish.

The horizontal straight-line portion of the temperature curve (cd) in Figure 5.1B denotes the fusion temperature (T_f). All temperatures above T_f are associated with a molten metal and all temperatures below T_f are associated with a solid metal (Figs 5.1A and B).

The initial drop in temperature below the fusion temperature is called "supercooling" (b)

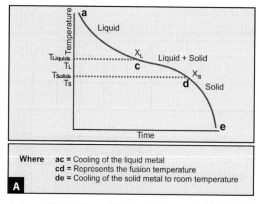

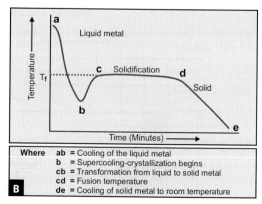

Where ac = Cooling of the liquid metal
        cd = Represents the fusion temperature
        de = Cooling of the solid metal to room temperature
A

Where ab = Cooling of the liquid metal
        b = Supercooling-crystallization begins
        cb = Transformation from liquid to solid metal
        cd = Fusion temperature
        de = Cooling of solid metal to room temperature
B

Figs 5.1A and B Cooling curve (A) Solidification cooling curve (B) Supercooling, solidification

at this stage crystallization begins (Fig. 5.1B). Tin normally exhibits supercooling and other metals commonly behave in the similar manner.

Solidification of metals is considered to take place in two stages, namely:

Nucleation: Formation of the smallest particle of a new phase that is stable in the existing phase.

Grain growth: Increase in the size of the nuclei.

Nucleation

As the temperature decreases down to b (supercooling), the internal energy of the metal atoms decreases and forms crystal nuclei. These crystal nuclei are called as "embryos". At higher temperatures, the embryos are few in number and small in size. Thus they are readily dissolved back into the matrix of random atoms (i.e. solution). On approaching solidification temperature these embryos increase in density and get larger but they still are unstable and tend to dissolve into the matrix (may be due to the transfer of thermal energy from metal atoms on collision or due to reheating).

Once the supercooled region is reached there is a tendency for some of these embryos to survive and thus form a 'solidification nucleus' or 'nucleus of crystallization', which is the first permanent solid phase. This general method of solidification is called "homogeneous nucleation" since the formation of nuclei in the molten metal is a random process and has

equal probability of occurring at any point in the metal.

Nuclei of crystallization can also be formed when the molten metal contacts some surface or particle, which it can wet. Such a process is also known as "heterogeneous nucleation", because a foreign body is seeded the nucleus. For heterogeneous nucleation supercooling is not necessary.

Grain Growth

Growth of crystals from nuclei of crystallization occurs in three dimensions in the form of dendrites or branched structures (Fig. 5.2A).

The crystals begin to grow toward each other and two or more adjacent growing crystals colloid; it stops growth in that direction. Thus a solid metal consists of large number of crystals and is therefore polycrystalline in nature (Fig. 5.2B). These crystals are referred to as 'grains'. The junction or union between the grains or crystals is known as 'grain boundary'.

As the nucleation and grain growth occurs the molten metal changes from liquid to solid state. During this transformation latent heat of solidification is evolved. Which raises the temperature where it remains constant until the crystallization is completed. It is equal to the latent heat of fusion.

Latent heat of solidification is defined as the number of calories of heat liberated from 1 g of a substance when it changes from liquid to solid.

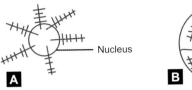

Figs 5.2A and B (A) Dendritic growth from nucleus (tree-like appearance) (B) Dendrites in polycrystals

Once the crystallization is completed, after d, the temperature decreases steadily to room temperature.

GRAIN SIZE AND SHAPE

The size of the grain depends on the number and location of the grains during crystallization.

In general, smaller the grain sizes better the physical properties of a metal. Rapid cooling of a metal from molten state to solid state gives rise to larger number of nuclei of crystallization in a given area and results in smaller grain size (Fig. 5.3A).

In slow cooling, rate of crystallization is faster than the nucleus formation and results in larger grains (Fig. 5.3B). The grains may have dendritic, lamellar needle type or acicular structures. The grains those are equal in diameter in all dimensions are known as 'equiaxed grains'.

Grain Boundary

The region of transition between the differently oriented crystal lattices of two neighboring grains is known as 'grain boundary' (Fig. 5.3C). The structure is nearly noncrystalline and is of high energy. This region is more readily attacked by chemicals and is more susceptible to corrosion.

DEFORMATION OF METALS

CRYSTAL GEOMETRY

Liquid metals nucleate crystals upon cooling. The atoms joining the crystals form a unique packing arrangement in space that is characteristic of that metal or alloy at equilibrium. The smallest division of the crystalline metal that defines the unique packing is called the unit cell.

Six different crystal systems have been recognized (cubic, tetragonal, orthorhombic, monoclinic, triclinic, and hexagonal) in which atoms can be arranged in 14 different arrays. They are simple cubic, fcc, bcc, simple tetragonal, body centered tetragonal (bct), rhombohedric, simple orthorhombic, base centered orthorhombic, face centered orthorhombic, body centered orthorhombic, simple monoclinic, base centered monoclinic, triclinic and hexagonal. Three most common arrays for the metals used in dentistry are (see Fig. 3.2):
1. Body centered cubic (bcc)
2. Face centered cubic (fcc)
3. Hexagonal close packed.

The atoms within each grain are arranged in a regular 3-dimensional lattice. Each crystal system can be defined in terms of distances between the atoms in all 3-dimensions as well as the angles formed by the three axes.

LATTICE IMPERFECTIONS

When a molten metal is solidified, crystallization from nucleus does not occur in a regular fashion, lattice plane by plane. Instead the growth is likely to be more random with lattice discontinuities and imperfections.

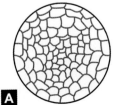
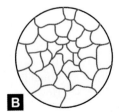
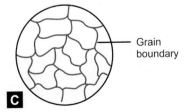

Grain boundary

Figs 5.3A to C (A) Rapid cooling results in small grains (B) Slow cooling results in larger grains (C) Grain boundary

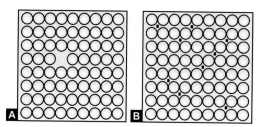

Figs 5.4A and B (A) Vacancy (One atom is missing) (B) Interstitial (Extra atom)

The imperfections in real crystals can be classified according to their geometry into four types:
1. Point defects
2. Line defects or dislocations
3. Surface defects
4. Volume defects.

Point Defects

A point defect can be defined as a pin point defect, which has occurred due to missing or misplacement or substitution of one atom by another. These defects weaken the structure.

For example, vacancy, interstitial, (Figs 5.4A and B) Schottky and Frenkel defects.

Line Defects or Dislocations

Dislocations are of two types:
  i. Edge dislocation
 ii. Screw dislocation.

Edge dislocation: An edge dislocation may be described as an edge of an extra plane of atoms in a crystal structure.

The crystal lattice is almost regular except for the one plane of atoms that is discontinuous forming a dislocation line at the edge of the half plane (Fig. 5.5A).

Dislocation Motion

If the shear force is applied to the crystal, the atoms in the plane above the dislocation easily break old bonds and establish new bonds with the lower atoms. This results in shifting of dislocation by one lattice spacing. A continued application of shear stress causes successive slipping

until finally the dislocation reaches the boundary of the crystal and disappears, leaving one unit of slip at the surface of the crystal. The plane along which dislocation moves is known as dislocation plane or slip plane (Figs 5.5B to D).

STRAIN HARDENING OR WORK HARDENING (METHOD OF STRENGTHENING METALS)

Metals show an increase in strength and hardness when plastically deformed at temperatures lower than the recrystallization temperature. This phenomenon is known as 'strain hardening' or 'work hardening'. It is also called as 'cold working' since the process is carried out at a lower temperature.

Mechanism

The mechanism of plastic deformation is called dislocation motion. When a shear force is applied dislocation moves in one plane. If this dislocation during translation meets some other type of discontinuity such as point defect, another type of dislocation, a foreign atom, or grain boundaries, its gliding movement under stress might be inhibited. In a polycrystalline metal, the dislocations tend to build up at the grain boundaries. Once all the dislocations are piled up at grain boundaries a great stress is required to produce further slip and metal becomes harder and stronger. Further increase in cold working results in fracture of metal.

Effects of Cold Working

• Work hardening introduces internal stresses in a material. These stresses are undesirable and can be removed by suitable heat treatment.
• Work hardening modifies the grain structure from equiaxed structure to fibrous structure.
• The surface hardness, strength, and proportional limit of the metal are increased.
• However modulus of elasticity is not changed appreciably.
• Ductility, malleability and resistance to corrosion are decreased.

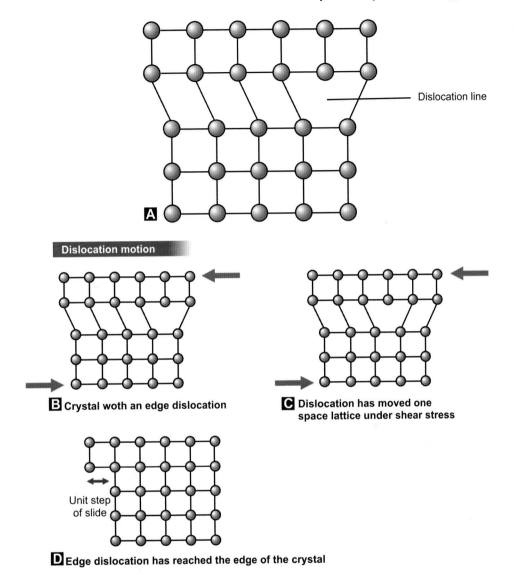

Figs 5.5A to D A: Line dislocation (B to D) Dislocation motion

Applications

- The formation of orthodontic wires, in which an alloy is forced through a series of circular dies of decreasing diameter.
- The bending of wires or clasps during the construction and alteration of appliances.
- The swaging of stainless steel denture bases.
- Compaction of gold foil.

ANNEALING (STRESS RELIEVING HEAT TREATMENT)

The effects associated with cold working, e.g. strain hardening lowered ductility and distorted grains; can be eliminated by simply heating the metal called annealing. It is a relatively low temperature heat treatment for removing

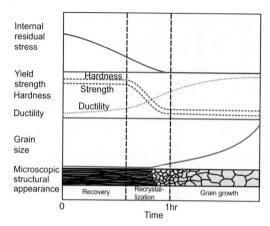

Fig. 5.6 Annealing decreases strength increases ductility and also modifies grain structure

residual stresses. It allows the dislocations and atomic vacancies to move and realign to lower the internal residual stress fields. The more the cold working, the more readily does annealing occur. Annealing is usually carried out at one half of the absolute melting temperature (in Kelvin) of the metal.

Annealing in general comprises three stages—recovery, recrystallization and grain growth (Fig. 5.6).

Recovery

Stress relief annealing takes place at relatively low temperature, when compared with recrystallization temperature. In stress relief anneal sufficient heat energy is applied for the dislocations to group into lower energy configurations, i.e. dislocation density decreases. The stresses that are produced due to cold working are relieved but there is no change in the grain structure. During this period there is slight decrease in the tensile strength and no change in ductility.

Recrystallization

Recrystallization is the process of nucleation and growth of new crystals, which replace all the deformed crystals of cold worked material. It occurs on heating to a temperature above the recovery range, usually half of the

melting point of the metal. The temperature at which recrystallization takes place is called 'recrystallization temperature'.

During recrystallization, the increased thermal vibration of atoms is sufficient to allow them to move to less strained position. The number of dislocations decreases and the distorted or strained grains are replaced by new smaller stress free ones.

After recrystallization, the metal possesses a lower tensile strength and hardness than the cold worked material but has improved ductility, malleability and better resistance to corrosion. Greater the amount of strain hardening, lower the recrystallization temperature.

Grain Growth

If annealing is prolonged at a higher temperature, there is a diffusion of atoms across the grain boundaries and eventually one large grain replaces several smaller ones. The resulting coarse-grained structure will have inferior mechanical properties to that of materials with a fine recrystallized structure. But the ductility and malleability will be increased.

Practical Significance

Orthodontic appliances fabricated by bending wires are often subjected to a stress relief anneal/ recovery anneal prior to their placement. Such a process stabilizes the configuration of the appliance and allows accurate determination of the force the appliance will deliver in the mouth.

Since both the recrystallization and grain growth decreases mechanical properties of the cold worked material, dental appliances should never be recrystallized. They should only be heat treated to recovery state. Recrystallization of orthodontic wire should be avoided during soldering operation because it may lead to the production of a wire of high ductility with a low proportional limit.

CAST STRUCTURE

A typical cast structure in dentistry is an inlay, bridge restoration which is not given further mechanical treatment except for polishing or marginal adaptation by hand operations. This limited treatment does not modify significantly the major internal structure of the casting.

The internal structure is equiaxed structure. Mechanical properties are inferior, for example; tensile strength and hardness of a cast gold inlay is 517 MPa and 160 BHN respectively.

WROUGHT STRUCTURE

Many dental appliances such as orthodontic wires and bands are formed by cold working operations. The finished product is often described as a wrought structure to denote that it has been formed by severe cold working procedures.

The internal structure is fibrous structure. Mechanical properties are superior, for example, tensile strength and hardness of a wrought gold inlay is 690 MPa and 175 BHN respectively.

CONSTITUTION OF ALLOYS

An alloy is a mixture of two or more metals in all-possible combinations, or an alloy is a mixture of two or more metallic elements. Sometimes an important constituent may be a metalloid or even a nonmetal provided the mixture of elements displays metallic properties.

In making an alloy a parent or basic metal is selected which possesses the most suitable properties and other metals (alloying elements) are added because a pure metal, in general, is not sufficiently strong to withstand the forces applied to it in the mouth.

An alloy system is an aggregate of two or more metals in all-possible combinations, e.g. The gold-silver system means that all of the possible concentrations of gold with silver and vice versa (100% Au and 100% Ag) are being considered.

CLASSIFICATION OF ALLOYS

According to the number of alloying elements, alloys are classified as, Binary alloys (2 metals/elements), Ternary alloys (3 metals/elements), and quaternary alloys (4 metals/elements).

According to the miscibility of the atoms in the solid state, alloys are classified into solid solutions, eutectic alloys, peritectic alloys, and intermetallic compounds.

According to the nobility, alloys are classified as high noble ($\geq$ 60 wt% of noble metals), Noble ($\geq$ 25 wt% of noble metals), and predominantly base metal alloys (< 25 wt% of noble metals).

According to their uses in dentistry, alloys are classified as alloys used for all metal inlays, crown and bridge, metal-ceramic restorations, removable partial dentures and implants.

SOLID SOLUTIONS

Metals, which are completely soluble in both liquid and solid states, are called as solid solutions.

When two metals are completely miscible in the liquid state and they remain completely mixed on solidification, the alloy formed is called as a '*solid solution*'.

A solid solution in a single phase, as it is chemically homogeneous and the component atoms cannot be distinguished physically or separated mechanically by ordinary means, e.g. the copper and gold combination crystallizes in such a manner that the atoms of copper are scattered randomly throughout the crystal structure (space lattice) of gold, resulting in a single phase system such a combination is called solid solution because it is a solid but has the properties of a solution.

Solute and Solvent

When two metals are soluble in one another in solid state the solvent is that metal whose space lattice persists or the metal whose atoms occupy more than half the total number of positions in the space lattice and the solute is the other metal. Solid solutions are of two types:
1. Substitutional solid solutions
   a. Ordered substitutional solid solutions
   b. Disordered or random substitutional solid solutions.
2. Interstitial solid solutions.

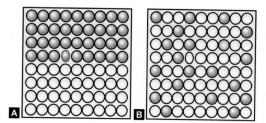

Figs 5.7A and B (A) Ordered substitutional solid solutions (B) Random substitutional solid solutions

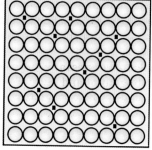

Fig. 5.8 Interstitial solid solutions

Substitutional Solid Solutions

In these solid solutions, the atoms of the solute occupy the space lattice positions that normally are occupied by the solvent atoms in the pure metal.

Atoms of one kind segregate to one site of atomic position and leaving the other atoms to occupy the remaining sites (Fig. 5.7A), e.g. Au-Cu at 50.2: 49.8 composition is said to be ordered.

If the atoms of the added metal take up positions at random in the parent lattice, then the solid solution is said to be disordered or random (Fig. 5.7B), e.g. Au-Cu at higher temperatures.

Interstitial Solid Solutions

In this type, the solute atoms are present in positions between the solvent atoms (the interstices between regular lattice positions). This type of solid solution requires that the solute atoms be much smaller in size than solvent atoms and are limited to small concentrations of solute atoms, e.g. an alloy of Fe and C (carbon occupies interstitial positions) (Fig. 5.8).

Conditions for Solid Solubility (Hume-Rothery Rules)

There are at least four factors, which determine the extent of solid solubility of two or more metals. They are:

Atomic Size

If the sizes of two metallic atoms differ less than 15%, they are said to possess a favorable factor for solid solubility.

Valence

Metals of same valance and size are more likely to form extensive solid solutions than are the metals of different valencies.

Chemical Affinity

It must be same or less for both metals otherwise they tend to form intermetallic compound rather than a solid solution.

Lattice Type

Only metals with same type of crystal lattice can form a complete series of solid solutions.

The size factor is possibly first consideration and there are exceptions to these rules.

Properties of Solid Solutions

In a solid solution, the solute atoms either substitute the solvent metal or occupy the interstitial positions. This results in a localized distortion or strained condition of the lattice (either expansion or contraction depending on the size difference between the solute and solvent atoms). This distortion interferes with the movement of dislocations and thereby slip becomes difficult. This results in increase in strength, proportional limit, and hardness but decreases ductility. This type of strengthening of an alloy is called as solution hardening or solid solution strengthening.

An increase in number of alloying atoms causes greater distortion and gives greater strength to the alloy. For example, pure gold in the cast condition is too weak and ductile. But, alloyed with 5% of copper can increase strength and hardness.

Solid solutions possess a melting range rather than a melting point and always melt below the melting point of the high fusing metal and sometimes below the melting points of both metals.

Solid solutions have better corrosion resistance. For example, in Cr-Co alloys chromium improves strength and hardness by solution hardening and also improves corrosion resistance by passivating effect (from chromic oxide layer).

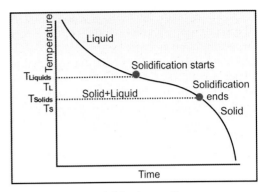

Fig. 5.9 Solidification cooling curve

CONSTITUTIONAL PHASE DIAGRAMS/THERMAL EQUILIBRIUM PHASE DIAGRAMS

An alloy system is an aggregate of two more metals in all-possible combinations.

A phase is a homogeneous portion of matter that is physically distinct and mechanically separable.

A phase diagram is a graphical method of showing the phases present in an alloy system of different temperatures and different compositions. The X-axis describes the composition of elements in either weight percentage (wt %) or atomic percentage. The Y-axis describes the temperature of the alloy system. Phase diagram shows the composition and types of phases present at a given temperature and at equilibrium (Fig. 5.9).

In this method, a mixture of metals (A and B) of different known compositions is prepared (Fig. 5.10). The alloy is cooled slowly from the liquid state and its temperature is recorded at frequent regular intervals of time. With alloys, solidification occurs over a temperature range on contrast to a pure metal and hence starts

and completion of solidification takes place at different temperatures.

Cooling curve experiments like the one discussed previously are now performed on a series of alloys from the A to B system.

Every phase diagram divides an alloy system into at least three areas namely, the liquid phase, the liquid + solid phase, and the solid phase (Fig. 5.9).

As shown in the graph (Fig. 5.10), the upper line (liquids T_L), is developed by drawing a continuous line through all points (T_L) representing the initiation of solidification process. This upper temperature for an alloy is called liquidus temperature because the alloys are entirely liquid above this temperature or the temperature at which the first solid begins to form on cooling.

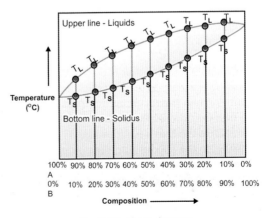

Fig. 5.10 Phase diagram

The bottom line (solidus T$_S$) is generated by connecting the points representing completion of the solidification process (T$_S$), this temperature is called as solidification temperature because the alloys are entirely solid below this line or the temperature at which the last liquid solidifies on cooling or the first liquid is formed on heating.

All the compositions above the liquidus temperature are in liquid state. All compositions below the solidus temperature are in solid state. Any compositions between the two lines are in both liquid and solid state.

Importance

Constitutional diagrams or phase diagrams can be used for the following purposes:
- For determining the solidification and liquefaction temperature of all alloy phases.
- For identifying the presence of various phases and their chemical compositions.
- For selecting various compositions for potential use as new alloys.
- For determining solubility of one metal in the other.
- For selecting heat-hardenable compositions.

SOLID SOLUTIONS PHASE DIAGRAMS

From the Figure 5.11 phase diagram, liquidus line is "AQC", and solidus line is "ARC".

At 0% B, a single phase (of 100%) exists that has a single melting point,1000°C. At 100% B, a single phase exists that has a single melting point, 500°C. At any composition between these extremes, the alloy will exist in two phases, i.e. liquid and solid, and the alloy will have a melting range.

Consider an alloy that is 60% A and 40% B, this alloy at a temperature of 1100°C is all liquid, point P. When the temperature drops to 930°C, the first portion of alloy solidifies. If a parallel line (1,2) to the X-axis (solidus line) is projected at 930°C to the solidus line the composition of the solid can be determined by projecting down to the X-axis (1,8). In this case, the solid will be 97% A and 3%B.

As the alloy is cooled further, more crystallization occurs and between 930°C–600°C (QYR)

a mixture of solid and liquid exists. At 800°C, the composition of both solid and liquid can be determined by drawing a parallel line to intersect both the solidus and liquidus lines called tie line (3,4,5).

To know the composition of solid, the alloy becomes completely solid at a temperature of 660°C. The composition of last liquid to solidify or crystallize can be determined by intersecting the liquidus line (6 and 7). The first portion of alloy solidifies at 660°C has a composition of 18% A and 82% B (7).

CORING OR NONEQUILIBRIUM SOLIDIFICATION

When two or more metals are heated to a liquid state they form alloys because of their miscibility in each other.

From the Figure 5.11, the composition of solid

at 930°C = 60% A and 40% B
at 800°C = 30% A and 70% B
at 660°C = 18% A and 82% B

This confirms that for solid solution alloys a cored structure exists in which the first material to crystallize is rich in the metal with higher melting point, while the last material to solidify is rich in the other metal.

Coring is a condition related to the inhomogeneity of component atoms in a last structure. If the cooling of alloy is rapid, there will be insufficient time for the composition of the separated solid to change by diffusion. Then the composition of dendrite or grain is not uniform. This difference in composition between the first and last formed portions of a crystal grain is called as coring.

During coring, the higher melting metal being concentrated close to the nucleus and the lower melting metal close to the grain boundaries. The longer the temperature difference between solidus and liquidus, the greater is the tendency towards coring.

Coring reduces the corrosion resistance since some portions of the alloy may have too little of the corrosion resisting component, and dissimilar alloys present may form a galvanic couple or galvanic cell.

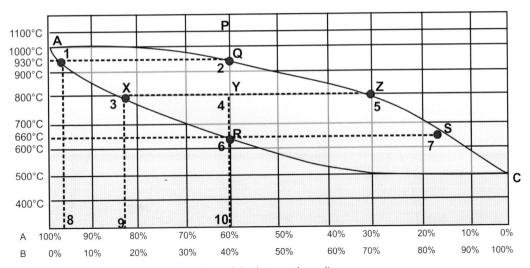

Fig. 5.11 Solid solutions phase diagram

HOMOGENIZATION OR HOMOGENIZING ANNEAL

Coring that results from rapid cooling of an alloy can be relieved or eliminated by a heat-treating process. This heat treatment, which is used to produce grains of same composition throughout the alloy is called as homogenization.

It is carried out by heating the cast alloy at a temperature just below the solidus temperature for a period of time (6–8 hours) to allow diffusion of atoms and the establishment of homogeneous structure. The alloy is then quenched in order to prevent grain growth from occurring. It takes place more rapidly in a grain structure, which has been cold worked. A homogenized solid solution alloy shows a microscopic structure identical with that of a pure metal.

EUTECTIC ALLOYS

Metals, which are completely soluble in liquid state and insoluble in the solid state (partially may be soluble) are called as eutectic alloys.

In a series of alloys of this type, the addition of increasing amount of one metal to other metal markedly reduces the melting point, until at a certain composition at which the lowest melting alloy is found. This particular alloy is called the eutectic alloy; from the Greek word 'Eutektos' means as 'easily melted'.

To be perfectly correct, the term eutectic alloy should be applied only to the one alloy of eutectic composition but it is applied loosely to describe alloys between metals, which combine to give an eutectiferous system.

Characteristics of Eutectic Alloys

For example, silver-copper system.

- No solidification range – Identified as E in the diagram (Fig. 5.12). The eutectic alloy has a solidification or melting point. The composition on each side of the eutectic alloy possesses melting range.
- Eutectic horizontal: The solidus temperature is constant for a wide range of compositions.
- Eutectic point: The solidification of eutectic composition occurs at a lower temperature than either metal ingredients and is the temperature at which any alloy composition of silver and copper is entirely liquid.

  Eutectic composition – 28.1% Cu and 71.9% Ag.

  Eutectic temperature – 779.4°C.

- Solid solutions: The two regions of solid solutions are located on each side of the phase diagram. The solution of copper in

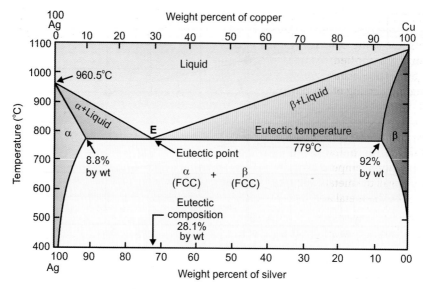

Fig. 5.12 Eutectic system

silver (silver rich) is called α-solid solution (hypoeutectic alloy). The solution of silver in copper (copper rich) is called β-solid solution (hypereutectic alloy).
- During solidification of eutectic alloys, constituent metals segregate to form regions of nearly pure parent metals. This results in the formation of a layered structure composed of alternating layers of α and β-solid solutions.

Eutectic Reaction

Liquid → α-solid solution + β-solid solution

It is referred as invariant transformation since it occurs at one temperature and one composition only.

Properties

1. Solders and low fusing materials, which are usually eutectic mixtures.
2. The silver and copper eutectic alloy (71.9% Ag and 28.1% Cu) is used in admixed high copper amalgam alloys. Here they act as strong fillers.
3. They are composed of two separate and dissimilar metals and their corrosion resistance is poor.
4. Stronger and brittle.

INTERMETALLIC COMPOUNDS

Intermetallic compounds are metals in solution in the liquid state that have a tendency to unite and form definite chemical compounds on solidification. These compounds frequently occur when the electrochemical characteristics of the two metals are markedly different. They are hard, brittle and have high melting points, e.g. Ag_3Sn in dental amalgam alloys.

PERITECTIC ALLOYS

Metals, which are soluble in the liquid state, insoluble in the solid state and which form a compound by a peritectic reaction.

Liquid + α → β

SOLID STATE REACTIONS

Metals can be strengthened by:
1. Reducing the grain size or grain refining.
2. Strain hardening or work hardening or cold working.
3. Solution hardening or solid solution strengthening.
4. Order hardening.
5. Precipitation hardening or age hardening.

HEAT TREATMENT

Heat treatment is the controlled heating and cooling process applied to the materials in order to get certain desirable properties, or it is the thermal processing of an alloy for a length of time above room temperature but below the solidus temperature.

All heat treatment processes consist of:
1. Heating the metal or alloy at a predetermined temperature.
2. Soaking of the metal at that temperature.
3. Cooling the metal at a specified rate.

Heat treatment may harden a metal or soften a metal or change its grain size or corrosion resistance. The effects of such a treatment depend entirely on the temperature, the metal and its previous history.

QUENCHING

The term quenching means that a metal is rapidly cooled from an elevated temperature or below. This is usually done for one of the two reasons.
1. To preserve at room temperature a phase ordinarily stable only at elevated temperatures.
2. To rapidly terminate the process that only occurs at elevated temperatures.

The rapid cooling is often accomplished by immersing the hot metal in a liquid such as water.

ORDER HARDENING (ORDER-DISORDER TRANSFORMATION)

An important mechanism responsible for major changes in hardness is the order-disorder transformation, which involves conversion from one crystal structure to another. One of the common examples in dental alloys is the Gold-Copper system in which fcc structure is converted to a tetragonal structure.

According to the phase diagram (Fig. 5.13)
- The melting range is very narrow for all compositions.

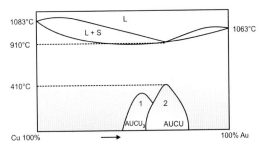

Fig. 5.13 AU-CU phase diagram

- Addition of copper to the gold lowers the liquidus temperature substantially.
- At temperatures below solidus and above 410°C, Gold-Copper exhibits completed solid solubility.

Below 410°C, there are two new solid phases designated as 1 and 2. These are the regions in which alloys are capable of undergoing a solid-solid transition to form an ordered rather than disordered lattice.

The ordered lattice in which gold and copper take up specific lattice sites often referred to as a super lattice. Formation of super lattice requires an atomic rearrangement by diffusion of atoms (thermal energy is required).

If an alloy of 50% gold and 50% copper is cooled rapidly from 450°C, the lattice structure is random or disordered (fcc). But slow cooling permits the formation of an ordered substitutional solid solution. Such an ordered structure is termed as super lattice. The formation of certain volume of a tetragonal lattice within a cubic structure involves contraction of one of the crystal axes. This sets up strains, which interfere with the movement of dislocations (since the atomic size of gold and copper are different, the crystal lattice becomes distorted). Hence the yield stress, UTS and hardness are raised and this is termed as order hardening heat treatment.

PRECIPITATION HARDENING OR AGE HARDENING

The precipitation hardening mechanism relies on the ability of an alloy to be converted from a solid solution to one that exhibits two phases. These two phases form individual crystal structures within the grain.

To carry out precipitation hardening, the alloy is heat treated at a temperature that the phase diagram indicates will produce precipitation.

For example, in case of gold alloys when heated at reduced temperature of 350°C, a diffusion of atoms occurs. The dissimilar atoms that previously were located randomly on the lattice sites are now forced to segregate and diffuse to specific positions. Localized areas of segregations within the crystal (precipitate) result in a lattice that is highly strained or deformed or distorted. The strain produced by the coherent precipitate within the lattice efficiently prevents slip and therefore hardens and strengthens the alloy.

Further growth of the precipitate during heat treatment results in the formation of a precipitate as a separate phase with a decrease in strength.

HEAT TREATMENT OF GOLD ALLOYS

Gold alloys can be significantly hardened if the alloy contains a sufficient amount of copper. Type-I and -II alloys do not harden or harden to a lesser degree than do the type-III and IV alloys.

The actual mechanism of hardening is probably the result of several different solid-solid transformations.

The heat treatment of dental gold alloys consists primarily of either a softening (solution heat treatment) or a hardening operation (age hardening), depending on the temperature to which the solid alloy is heated.

Softening Heat Treatment

In the metallurgical terminology, the softening heat-treatment is referred to as solution heat treatment. The casting is placed in an electric furnace for 10 minutes at 700°C and then is quenched in water. During this period, all intermediate phases are presumably changed to a disorder solid solution and the rapid quenching prevents ordering from occurring

during cooling at temperature between 450°C to 250°C (hardening process).

The tensile strength, proportional limit and hardness are reduced by such a treatment but the ductility is increased.

This is indicated for structures that are to be ground, shaped or cold worked either in or out of the mouth. In this condition they are soft enough to carry out mechanical work.

Hardening Heat Treatment

In metallurgical terminology the hardening heat treatment referred to as age hardening.

The hardening heat treatment of gold alloys can be accomplished by soaking or aging the casting at a specific temperature for a definite time usually 15–30 minutes before it is quenched in water.

By cooling from 450–250°C, an ordered phase of gold copper alloy is formed. The rate at which the alloy is cooled is very important, longer the time, within limits, the greater the amount of transformation of gold copper ordered phases that will take place, and harder the alloy is.

SUGGESTED READING

1. Clark GCF, Williams DF. The effects of proteins on metallic corrosion. J Biomed Mater Res. 1982;16:125.
2. German RM, Wright DC, Gallant RF. In vitro tarnish measurements on fixed prosthodontics alloys. J Prosthet Dent. 1982;47: 399.
3. Gülþen Can, Gül Akpýnar, Ahmet Aydýn. The release of elements from dental casting alloy into cell-culture medium and artificial saliva. Eur J Dent. 2007;1:86-90.
4. Hashimoto T, Zhou X, Luo C, Kawano K, Thompson GE, Hughes AE, et al. Nanotomography for understanding materials degradation. Scripta Materialia. 2010;63:835-8. eScholarID: 110631.
5. Iijima M, Yuasa T, Endo K, Muguruma T, Ohno H, Mizoguchi I. Corrosion behavior of ion implanted nickel-titanium orthodontic wire in fluoride mouth rinse solutions. Dent Mater J. 2010;29(1): 53-8.
6. Kikuchi M. Dental alloy sorting by the thermoelectric method. Eur J Dent. 2010;4:66-70.

7. Leinfelder KF. An evaluation of casting alloys used for restorative procedures. J Am Dent Assoc. 1997;128:37.

8. Lucas LC, Lemons JE. Biodegradation of restorative metal systems. Adv Dent Res. 1992;65:32.

9. Ma Y, Zhou X, Thompson GE, Curioni M, Zhong X, Koroleva E, et al. "Discontinuities in the Porous Anodic Film Formed on AA 2099-T8 Aluminium Alloy". Corrosion Science. 2011.

10. Malhotra ML. Dental gold casting alloys: A Review. Trends Tech Contemp Dent Lab. 1991;8:73.

11. Malhotra ML. New generation of palladium-indium-silver dental cast alloys: a review. Trends Tech Contemp Dent Lab. 1992;9: 65.

12. Mezger PR, Stolls ALH, Vrijhoef MMA, et al. Metallurgical aspects and corrosion behaviour of yellow low-gold alloys. Dent Mater. 1989;5:530.

13. Mistakidis I, Gkantidis N, Topouzelis N. Review of properties and clinical applications of orthodontic wires. Hellenic Orthodontic Review. 2011;14(1):45-66.

14. Pekkan G, Pekkan K, Hatipoglu MG, Tuna SH. Comparative radiopacity of ceramics and metals with human and bovine dental tissues. J Prosthet Dent. 2011;106:109-17.

15. Vallittu PK, Kokkonen M. Deflection fatigue of cobalt-chromium, titanium and gold alloy cast denture clasps. J Prosthet Dent. 1995; 74:412.

16. Wang Y, Xia M, Fang Z, Zhou X, Thompson GE. Effect of Al8Mn5 Intermetallic Particles on Grain Size of as-cast Mg-Al-Zn AZ91D alloy. Intermetallics. 2010;18:1683-9. eScholarID: 110634.

17. Wostmann B, Blober T, Gouentenoudis M, Balkenhol M, Ferger P. Influence of margin design on the fit of high-precious alloy restorations in patients. J Dent. 2005;33:611-8.

18. Wostmann B, Blober T, Gouentenoudis M, Markus Balkenhol, Paul Ferger. Influence of margin design on the fit of high-precious alloy restorations in patients. J Dent. 2005;33:611-8.

SECTION | 2

Clinical Dental Materials

- **Restorative Materials**
- **Impression Materials**
- **Orthodontic Wires**
- **Implant Materials**

Restorative Materials

6

Restoration is defined as a material so placed in the prepared cavity of a tooth so that the physiologic and mechanical functions, anatomic focus, occlusion contact point and esthetic appearance are properly restored or preserved and the tooth in the area of the restoration is protected as far as possible from recurrence of dental caries.

Restorative materials are those which are used to replace or restore the damaged, decayed, missing or lost tooth structure.

Loss of tooth structure arises due to:
- Caries
- Incisal edges break off
- Attrition and wear.

Objectives

The main objectives to be attained in the restoring operations are:
- Arrest of the loss of tooth structure or substance from caries and other causes.
- Prevention of recurrence of caries.
- Restoration or maintenance of normal interproximal spaces and contact points.
- Establishment of proper occlusion.
- Esthetic overall effect.
- Resistance against the stresses of mastication.

Desirable Properties of Restorative Materials

Biological
- Should be biocompatible with the pulp and other soft tissues.
- Should be bacteriostatic that means resist the growth of bacteria.
- Should have obtundent and promote healing effect.
- Should have anticariogenic properties.

Chemical
- Should be chemically inert.
- Should not be acidic or alkaline.
- Should not dissolve or disintegrate in oral fluids.
- Should be able to bond chemically with the tooth structure.

Rheological
- Should have good flow property during manipulation.
- Should have adequate working and setting times.
- Should have suitable film thickness (<25 for luting and about 40 for base consistency).

Mechanical

- Should have adequate strength to withstand large masticatory forces.
- Should have high proportional limit, elastic limit, and yield strength to resist permanent deformation.
- Should have high modulus of elasticity.
- Should have high abrasion resistance.
- Should have high fatigue strength.

Thermal

- Should be good insulator.
- Should have low thermal diffusivity.
- COTE should be equal to that of the natural tooth.

Esthetic

- The color of the material should match with the natural tooth structure.
- Should have same refractive index as tooth material.
- The color parameters should not change or undergo discoloration.

Minor Requirements

- Should be inexpensive.
- Should have longer shelf-life.
- Should be easy to manipulate.
- Should be radiopaque.

Classifications of Restorative Materials

1. According to nature of materials:
   a. *Metallic:* Dental amalgam, direct filling gold, miracle mix, casting gold and base metal alloys.
   b. *Nonmetallic:* Dental cements, composites, and ceramics.
2. According to life span:
   a. *Permanent restorative materials:* Dental amalgam, direct filling gold, miracle mix, casting gold and base metal alloys, composites, ceramics, and modified glass ionomer cement.
   b. *Semipermanent/intermediate:* Life span is weeks to months. Modified zinc

oxide eugenol cements, zinc phosphate cements, zinc polycarboxylate cement.
   c. *Temporary:* Life span is days to weeks. Acrylic resins, zinc oxide eugenol cement.
3. According to placement:
   a. *Anterior restorations:* Glass ionomer cement, silicate cement, composites and ceramics.
   b. *Posterior restorations:* Dental amalgam, posterior composites, metal modified glass ionomer cement, base metal alloys, and metal-ceramics.
4. According to the technique:
   a. *Direct restorations:* Dental cements, dental amalgam, direct filling gold, composites.
   b. *Indirect restorations:* Ceramics, casting gold and base metal alloys.
5. According to hardening:
   a. *Acid-base reactions:* Dental cements except resin cements.
   b. *Polymerization:* Composites, resin cements, compomers.
   c. *Solidification:* Casting gold and base metal alloys, ceramics.

Dental amalgam, cements, composite resins and direct filling gold were discussed in this section. Dental ceramics and casting alloys have been discussed in section III of this book.

DENTAL AMALGAM

Because of congenial properties dental amalgam is widely used as 'direct posterior restorative material' and at places where esthetics are not required dental amalgam is a restorative material made by mixing a finely divided alloy of silver, tin, and copper with mercury to form a paste. Since mercury is liquid at room temperature, it will combine with many metals to form alloys without the application of heat. The restoration is formed by compacting the plastic mix directly into the prepared tooth and hand carving with instruments to reproduce lost tooth anatomy. The paste sets by complex reactions among mercury, silver, tin, and copper to give a brittle composite alloy. The microstructure of the set material consists of the unreacted centers of the alloy particles bonded together by a matrix composed of the intermetallic compounds formed in the reaction.

AMALGAM

An alloy that contains mercury as one of its constituents.

Dental Amalgam

An alloy of mercury, silver, tin, and copper that may also contain zinc, palladium, and other elements to improve handling characteristics and clinical performance.

Dental Amalgam Alloy

An alloy of silver, copper, tin and other elements that is formulated and processed in the form of powder particles or as a compressed pellet.

HISTORY

- 659 AD—by Chinese "Sukung".
- 1579—by "Lishihchan".
- 1601—by German doctor "Tobias Dorn".
- 17th century—Introduced by "D Arcets" as mineral cement.
- 1810—by "Sir Regnart", called as "Father of Amalgam".
- 1826—by French scientist; "Taveall".
- But in 1845, American Society of Dental Surgeons considered amalgam filling as malpractice and accepted in 1850.
- 1845-1850—Amalgam War – the period of controversy over amalgam.

- In 1895—"GV Block"; 'Father of Operative Dentistry'; found a final formula which is successful.
- In 1937—"Gayles et al." Showed the chemical reactions.
- In 1900—First commercial amalgam alloy was marketed by "SS White" (Dent alloy).

Various alloying elements have been used with silver since centuries. Different generations of amalgam and their compositions are given in Table 6.1.

CLASSIFICATIONS OF AMALGAM

a. Based on copper content:
   i. Low copper alloys (copper < 6%) – traditional or conventional alloys (Fig. 6.1A).
   ii. High copper alloys (Copper > 6%)
      - Admixed alloys
         - Spherical eutectic high copper alloy + lathe cut low copper alloy (Fig. 6.1C).
      - Single composition or uni composition alloys (Fig. 6.1B)
b. Based on zinc content
   i. Zinc containing alloys – Zinc is greater than or equal to 0.01%.
   ii. Zinc-free alloys – Zinc is lesser than or equal to 0.01%.
c. Based on shape of particle
   i. Lathe cut (Fig. 6.1A)
   ii. Spherical (Fig. 6.1B)
   iii. Spheroidal.
d. Based on size of alloy powder
   i. Microcut (small)
   ii. Macrocut (big).

Table 6.1 Generations of amalgam

Generation	Composition
First generation alloy recommended by GV Block	Silver-Tin: 3:1 ratio
Second generation alloy	Copper – 4%, Zinc – 1%, Silver – 3%, Tin – 1%.
Third generation admixed alloy	Ag-Eu eutectic alloy + Low copper lathe cut alloy
Fourth generation alloy	Copper – 24%
Fifth generation alloy	Indium is added
Sixth generation alloy	Palladium – 10%, Silver – 62%, Copper – 28%

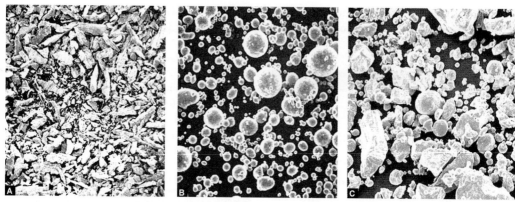

Figs 6.1A to C (A) Irregular or lathe cut alloy particle (B) Spherical alloy (C) High-Cu admixed alloy

e. Based on number of alloying elements
    i.   Binary: Two metals – Silver and tin.
    ii. Ternary: Three metals – Silver, tin and copper.
    iii. Quarternary: Four metals – Silver, tin, copper and indium.
f. Based on noble metal content
    i.   Nonnoble metals
    ii. Noble metal alloys.

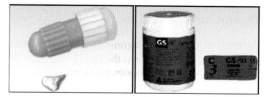

Fig. 6.2A Amalgam capsules and pellets

DISPENSION

Amalgam alloy is dispensed in the form of finely divided powder or disposable capsules or pellets and mercury is available in the form of liquid (Figs 6.2A and B).

Composition

Composition of low copper and high copper amalgam alloys has been given in the Table 6.2 and functions of each ingredient have been discussed in the Table 6.3.

MANUFACTURING OF ALLOY POWDER

Manufacturing of alloy powder includes three main stages.

For Lathe Cut Powder

Stage I: An annealed ingot of alloy is placed in a milling machine or in a lathe and is fed into a

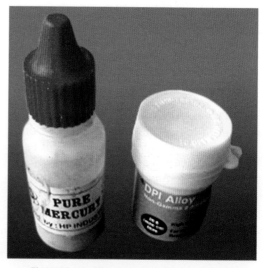

Fig. 6.2B Amalgam powder and liquid form

cutting tool as bit, and finally the chip size can be reduced by ball milling.

Stage II—Homogenizing anneal: Because of rapid cooling of alloy, it has a cored structure

Table 6.2 Composition of different amalgam alloys

Ingredients	Low copper alloys (Wt%)	Admix alloy (Wt%)	Single composition alloy (Wt%)
Silver	67–70	50–65	45–60
Tin	26–28	20–25	15–25
Copper	2–5	13–30	13–30
Zinc	1–2	0–2	0
Indium and Palladium	Traces	Traces	Traces

Table 6.3 Functions of each metal in an amalgam alloy

Components	Functions
Silver	• Major component. • Whitens the alloy. • Decreases the creep. • Increases the strength. • Increases resistance to tarnish.
Tin	• Controls the reaction between silver and mercury. • Decreases setting expansion. • Decreases strength and hardness. • Decreases resistance to tarnish.
Copper	• Increases strength and hardness along with silver. • Decreases brittleness of alloy. • Increases setting expansion.
Zinc	• Acts as a scavenger and prevents oxidation of silver. • Zinc less alloys are more brittle. • Zinc leads to delayed expansion if contaminated with moisture during manipulation.
Platinum and Palladium	• Increases the hardness and whitens the alloy.

and contains nonhomogeneous grains of varying size and composition.

The homogenizing heat treatment is performed to reach homogeneity. For which the ingot is placed in an oven and heated at a temperature below the solidus temperature for sufficient time and cooled to room temperature.

Stage III—Particle treatment: This includes acid treatment for surface components to dissolve so that alloy becomes more reactive.

Particle treatment is followed by annealing; this is done to relieve residual stresses carried out for several hours at approximately 100° C. Annealing increases shelf-life of alloy.

Atomized Powder for Spherical Particles

The desired elements are melted together and passed through a small crevice in an atomizer. If they solidify before hitting the base they retain their spherical shape. This is followed by heat treatment and acid wash.

Chemistry

When the alloy powder and mercury are mixed together, which forms a plastic mass; this process is called as 'trituration' or 'amalgamation'. During this process the mercury comes in contact with alloy powder and dissolves silver-tin in the outer portion of the particles and diffuses into alloy particles. But due to limited solubility of silver (0.035 wt%) and tin (0.6 wt%); in some time; two binary metallic compounds precipitate into the mercury.

- Body centered cubic – Ag_2Hg_3 (γ_1)
- Hexagonal – $Sn_{7-8}Hg$ (γ_2)

γ_1 is being first to form as silver has high solubility. γ_1 and γ_2 crystals grow as the remaining mercury dissolves into the alloy powder. With the disappearance of mercury the alloy hardens. The final phase consists of the unreacted centers of the alloy particles bonded together by a matrix composed of the intermetallic compounds formed in the reaction such as γ_1 and γ_2.

This basic reaction changes from alloy to alloy and forms various phases (Table 6.4).

CHEMICAL REACTIONS FOR INDIVIDUAL ALLOY MIXTURES

Low Copper Alloys

It includes γ and β phases. After mixing γ_1 phase precipitates first followed by γ_2 phase, which grows and binds the unreacted $(\beta + \gamma)$ core (Figs 6.3A to D).

Table 6.4 Different amalgam phases and their functions

Phases	Functions	Formula
γ (Gamma)	Basic constituent increases strength	Ag_3Sn
γ_1 (Gamma 1)	• Binds the alloy • Increases corrosion resistance	Ag_2Hg_3
γ_2 (Gamma 2)	• Weakest phase • Decreases resistance to tarnish and corrosion. Increases creep	$Sn_{7-8}Hg$
ϵ (Epsilon)	• Increases strength and hardness of the alloy	Cu_3Sn Cu: 4–5%
η (Eta)		Cu_6Sn_5
Silver-Copper eutectic	• Acts as filler	Ag – Cu
β (Beta)	• Forms core and strengthens the alloy	AgSn

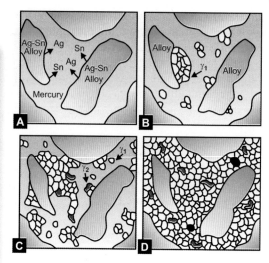

Figs 6.3A to D (A) Microstructure during trituration (B and C) Condensable and carvable state (D) Microstructure after setting that is not workable

and reacts with the Cu to form the η phase (Cu_6Sn_5) and eliminates the weakest γ_2 phase to improve the strength.

First,

Ag_3Sn + Ag-Cu + Hg $\rightarrow$ Ag_2Hg_3 + $Sn_{7-8}Hg$ + Unreacted (Ag_3Sn + Ag-Cu)

Later,

γ_2 phase gets eliminated by Ag-Cu particles forming η, γ and Cu core.

$Sn_{7-8}Hg$ + Ag-Cu $\rightarrow$ Cu_6Sn_5 + Ag_2Hg_3

Microstructure

γ_1 and η phases formed separately act as binders, binding the unreacted hard core, which include $\beta + \gamma + Ag_3Sn$ and traces of γ_2 may also be found.

Single Composition High Copper Alloys

It contains γ, ϵ, η and γ_1.

In uni compositional alloys, the difference in solubility of mercury in Sn, Cu, and Ag plays an important role.

Solubility of Hg is 170 times greater than Sn followed by Cu and Ag due to which Sn reacts first forming γ_2 phase followed by Cu due to its limited reactivity. Due to which particles of uni compositional alloys in the very early stages

$\beta + \gamma$ + Hg $\rightarrow$ $\gamma_1 + \gamma_2$ + unreacted $\beta + \gamma$

Ag – Sn + Ag_3Sn + Hg $\rightarrow$ Ag_2Hg_3 + $Sn_{7-8}Hg$ + Unreacted (Ag – Sn + Ag_3Sn)

Microstructure

A typical low-copper amalgam is a composite in which the unconsumed particles are embedded in γ_1 and γ_2 phases (Fig. 6.3D).

High Copper Amalgam Alloys

It includes γ_1, η + ($\gamma + \epsilon$).

Admix Alloy

Ag-Cu, eutectic spherical alloy are added to lathe cut low copper alloy in ratio of 1:2. This Ag-Cu alloy increases the strength.

On mixing, the Ag-Sn particles react first to form γ_1 and γ_2 phase, but later Sn in solution diffuses to the surface of Ag-Cu alloy particles are covered by γ_1 and γ_2 phases and Ag-Cu at periphery. But due to Ag-Cu phase the γ_2 phase is eliminated forming η and γ_1.

The difference in the elimination of the γ_2 in admixed and unicomposition alloy is that in the admixed type the γ_2 forms around the Ag-Sn particles and is eliminated around the Ag-Cu.

But in single composition alloy these particles at first formation like Ag-Sn particles of admixed type and later the same particles function like the Ag-Cu particles of admixed type to eliminate γ_2 type. Hence, there is only one reaction.

$$Ag_3Sn + Ag\text{-}Cu + Hg \rightarrow Cu_6Sn_5 + Ag_2Hg_3$$

$$(\gamma + \varepsilon + Hg \rightarrow \eta + \gamma_1)$$

Microstructure

η phase prismatic crystals grow and intermesh with γ_1 crystals, which lead to superior properties.

PHYSICAL AND MECHANICAL PROPERTIES

Strength

As it is a posterior restorative material compressive strength plays an important role (as it is subjected to masticatory forces) (Table 6.5).

Strength Measurement (as per ADA)

A cylindrical sample of height 8 mm and diameter 4 mm is prepared keeping variable parameters constant and preserved at 37°C for 7 days and tested by straining machines at 0.5 mm, 0.2, 0.05 mm/min.

Surface hardness – 100 to 120 KHN.

Factors Affecting Strength

Constituent Phases

The following order shows the decreasing order in strength.

$$\gamma > \gamma_1 > \eta > \gamma_2 \text{ and voids.}$$

- γ phase has high strength and whereas γ_2 phase is least.

Time

Strength increases with increase in time as the matrix continues to form which binds unreacted mass.

- After 20 minutes – 6% of maximum strength (i.e. 25–30 Mpa).
- After 7 days – 95% of maximum strength is attained.

The compressive strength and tensile strength of amalgam alloys at the end of first hour and after seven days respectively were given in Table 6.5.

In practice, a minimum of 8 hrs time should be allowed for amalgam to set during which taking solid food is contraindicated.

Composition

Depending on alloy type the strength changes, as there is alteration in constituent phase.

Type	Strength (Mpa)	Reason
High copper single composition alloy	250–290 Mpa at 1 hr	Due to interlocking of γ_1 with γ and due to lack of γ_2 phase.

Table 6.5 Strength and creep properties of amalgam

Types	Compressive strength 1 hr.	(Mpa) 7 days	Tensile strength (Mpa) 24 hrs	Creep (%)
Low copper	145	343	60	1-2
Admixed	137	431	48	0.5-1
Single composition	262	516	64	0.05-0.1

Mercury Alloy Ratio

An increase in mercury leads to increase in γ_2 and γ_1 phases, hence strength decreases. Decrease in mercury content leads to improper wetting of particles, which becomes more brittle and results in decrease in compressive strength and poor bonding.

Amount of mercury required is determined by surface area. Smaller the surface area, lesser is the mercury required and higher the strength.

For example, Spherical alloys.

Effect of Particle Size

As mentioned earlier, decrease in particle size increase in strength.

Effect of Trituration

Prolonged trituration decreases strength due to increase in γ_1 and γ_2 phases and hence decreases strength.

Undertrituration does not form adequate matrix to bind core and hence the mix becomes brittle leading to porosities and voids.

Condensation Pressure

Larger condensation force causes better adaptation, cohesion and increases strength. Larger condensation forces also lead to exclude excess mercury that in turn increases strength.

Dimensional Changes

Dimensional changes include either expansion or contraction. Expansion leads to amalgam fracture or dislodgement from cavity, hyperocclusion, and pulpal pain. Contraction leads to marginal leakage and secondary caries.

Expansion

After amalgamation, initially the γ_1 crystals formed will start to grow in due time which push each other and cause expansion and this continues until the mass becomes rigid.

Contraction

Due to inadequate mercury, which required for later reaction, i.e. growth of crystals and condensation.

Factors Increasing Setting Expansion

- Increase mercury – alloy ratio.
- Larger surface area of alloy particle.
- Spherical particles.
- Slow mixing speed.
- Prolonged trituration.
- Low condensation pressures.
- Moisture contamination.

Measurement

A sample cylinder of 4×8 mm is placed at 37° C and change is measured by dial gauge as interferometer.

According to ADA specification number 1 the dimensional change should be less than 0.2% at 37°C under normal pressures.

Delayed Expansion

Delayed expansion is a 4% as more expansion as taking place in zinc containing alloys after a period of 3–7 days due to moisture contamination during manipulation.

$$Zn + H_2O \rightarrow ZnO + H_2$$

The produced H_2 gas gets accumulated and leads to:
- Protrusion of restoration.
- Increases creep.
- Microleakage.
- Pitted surface and corrosion.
- Dental pain.
- Recurrence of caries.
- Fracture of restoration.

Prevention

Creating dry conditions by using gloves, rubber dams, and using nonzinc containing alloys.

Creep

Creep is a time dependent plastic deformation taking place in viscoelastic materials by static or dynamic forces.

Mechanism

As the amalgam restoration is constantly subjected to masticatory forces it undergoes creep which leads to elevated thin margins (Fig. 6.4) and fracture of these elevated thin margins leading to microleakage and caries.

According to ADA specification number 1 the creep should be less than 3%. But low copper alloys have a creep value of 0.8–8%, and high copper alloys have a creep value between 0.1–0.4%.

Determination of Creep

A cylindrical sample of 4 mm diameter and 8 mm height is prepared, preserved for 7 days at 37°C and then subjected to a static load of 36 N. The percentage decrease in the height in 3 hrs, in between the ends of 1 hour and 4 hours is taken as creep.

Factors Minimizing Creep

- Composition.
  For example, single composition high copper alloys.
- Minimum mercury-alloy ratio.
- Optimum trituration.
- Large condensation pressure.

- Homogeneous condensation.
- Proper cavity design.
- Good finishing.

Tarnish and Corrosion

Tarnish is surface discoloration and corrosion is loss of surface caused by chemical and electrochemical attack (see Fig. 3.23).

Influences of Tarnish and Corrosion on Amalgam

- Unesthetic restoration.
- Pitting and breakdown.
- Marginal leakage.
- Decrease in tensile strength by 3%.
- Surface particles leading to plaque accumulation.

Mechanism of Corrosion

It is mainly due to γ_2 phase, which acts as anode due to more active electrochemical nature and other phases act as cathode and saliva acts as a medium. Corrosion products will be released into the interfacial space between restoration and tooth structure that prevents the microleakage, called as self-sealing ability of amalgam (Fig. 6.5).

Factors Leading to Tarnish and Corrosion

- Improper polishing.
- Improper condensation.
- Two opposite different metallic restorations.

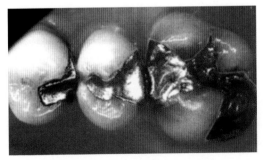

Fig. 6.4 Creep in amalgam restoration

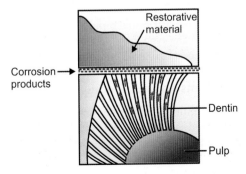

Fig. 6.5 Corrosion products preventing microleakage

For example, gold and amalgam restorations in opposing teeth.

THERMAL PROPERTIES

Thermal Diffusivity

Amalgam is good conductor of heat. Care should be taken in case of large amalgam restorations by lining cement to protect pulp.

Thermal Expansion

Coefficient of thermal expansion (α = 25 ppm) is double that of tooth, may lead to marginal leakage. But this leakage decreases with time due to accumulation of corrosion products.

MERCURY TOXICITY

Mercury toxicity is the reason which led to amalgam war and was responsible for its ban in many countries. The main property leading to its toxicity is vapor pressure (20 mg/m^3 at 25°C) and melting point (-39°C).

Mechanism of Intoxication as Contact

It mainly occurs by the inhalation of mercury vapor during manipulation, such as:
- Trituration
- Condensation
- Polishing and burnishing
- During removal of old restorative material
- By accidental spillage.

Other routes, which are minor, include skin, and methyl mercury though is considered as fatal. The elemental vapors inhaled reach blood via lungs and distributed rapidly throughout the body. Crossing even the blood-brain barrier and placental barrier.

Symptoms on Dose Dependent Manner

The maximum level of occupational exposure considered safe is 50 μg/m^3 of air per day as per ADA and OSHA (Occupational Safety and Health Administration).

$\geq$ 1 mg/kg Ataxia

$\geq$ 2 mg/kg Joint pains

$\geq$ 4 mg/kg Death.

Other Symptoms

Other symptoms with mercury toxicity include fatigue, weakness, headache, dizziness, paresthesia, and renal disorder.

Recommendations in Mercury Hygiene

1. Store Hg in unbreakable, tightly sealed containers.
2. Confine and facilitate the recovery of spilled Hg or amalgam.
3. Clean up any spilled Hg immediately.
4. Use tightly closed capsules during amalgamation.
5. Use a no-touch technique for handling the amalgam.
6. Salvage all amalgam scrap and store it under water that contains sodium thiosulfate.
7. Work in well-ventilated spaces.
8. Avoid carpeting dental office.
9. Eliminate the use of Hg-containing solutions.
10. Avoid heating Hg or amalgam.
11. Use water spray and suction when grinding dental amalgam.
12. Use conventional dental amalgam condensing procedures.
13. Perform yearly Hg checks.
14. Check Hg vapor levels periodically.
15. Alert all personnel who handle Hg of the potential hazard of Hg vapor and the necessity for observing good Hg and amalgam hygiene practice.

TECHNICAL CONSIDERATIONS IN MANIPULATION OF AMALGAM

During restoration, amalgam needs a thorough step-by-step procedure to attain the superior restoration. The main advantage of amalgam is it can be placed in cavity in a plastic form, which later hardens and allows ease for placement. The manipulation of amalgam involves the following steps:

Selection of Materials

This plays an important role and it varies depending on the condition of the patient and the desired properties, e.g.
- In case of sialorrhea patient – Indium containing and zinc free alloys.
- When hardness is desired–Cu containing alloys.
- When fast setting is required–Spherical alloy powders.

Apart from the above, the alloy should meet ADA Specification No. 1 standards for
- Creep: Less than or equal to 3%
- Compressive strength: 0.25 mm/min, i.e. 80 MPa.
- Dimensional change: ± 20 μm/cm.

Mercury-Alloy Ratio (Proportioning)

It is the ratio of the amount (by weight) of alloy to mercury used for a particular technique. Mercury-alloy ratio plays an important role on determining the properties of mix.

Ideal Proportioning

- Lathe cut – 1:1 (50:50)
- Spherical alloy – 40:60

  In general, older alloys contain large amount of mercury because of large particle size and hand mixing techniques to obtain a plastic mix (8:5 or 8:10). But due to introduction of mechanical trituration and other modifications on particle size it made possible to decrease the mercury content in mix.

  As per ADA specification the final set amalgam should contain less than or equal to 50% of mercury and it should not decrease less than or equal to 40%. So to get the mercury content low, the final mix is either subjected any one of the followings.

1. *Squeeze dried technique:* In this technique a gauge cloth is taken and the mix is placed on it and squeezed to remove excess mercury.
2. *Eame's technique or minimum mercury technique:* In this technique the actual volume of mercury taken is regulated, i.e. in the ratio of 1:1.

3. *Condensation technique or increasing dryness technique:* The mix is condensed to remove excess mercury, which comes to surface.

Other methods for proper proportioning and dispensing are as follows:
  i. Weigh the mercury and alloy using a balance.
  ii. *By using volume dispensers:* A dispenser is a glass bottle with a plastic screw top cap. The cap has a spring-loaded plunger, which releases a known volume of either mercury or alloy when dispensed. But for powder as the amount of alloy to be delivered depends on density of powder and hence not indicated, but it is suitable for mercury.
  iii. *Preproportioned alloy and powder:* Powder pre- weighted in a small sachet or tablet form and mercury in preweighed sachets.
  iv. *Disposable capsules:* The capsules contain both mercury and powder preweighed being separated by a membrane, which breaks before mixing, allowing both to mix.

Effect of Mercury-Alloy Ratio on Properties

- *Low mercury-alloy ratio*
  — The mix is dry, difficult to condense.
  — Subjected to marginal fracture.
  — Subjected to tarnish and corrosion.
- *High mercury-alloy ratio*
  — Mix is wet.
  — Prolongs setting.
  — Physical properties are inferior.
  — More toxic due to vapor release.

Trituration

Objective

The objective is to remove the oxide layer formed on the particles so that mercury can react with powder.

  Trituration is done in an amalgamator or triturator, it is a process in which both mercury and alloy powders are mixed to get a plastic mix.

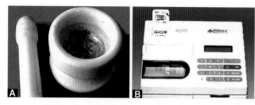

Figs 6.6A and B (A) Mortar and pestle
(B) Amalgamator

Hand Trituration

Hand trituration is done with mortar and pestle (Fig. 6.6A). The inner surface of mortar is roughened to increase friction and can be done by intentional grinding with Carborundum paste. A pestle is a glass rod with a round end.

The factors to obtain a good mix are as follows:

- Number of rotations (for 25-45 seconds).
- The speed of rotations.
- The magnitude of pressure placed on the pestle.

Mechanical Trituration

Mechanical amalgamators (Fig. 6.6B) are used into which a capsule is fitted. The amalgamators are devices with two arms covered by a hood and include an automatic controlled timer and speed control device and work by either vibratory or oscillatory movements.

The capsules are either disposable or nondisposable. The capsule serves as a mortar to hold alloy, a cylindrical metal or plastic piston is placed in the capsule that serves as a pestle. Reusable capsules are provided with cups that are either friction fit as screw.

Precautions

- Lid should be fitted tightly to prevent mercury mist to escape.
- Place hood to amalgamator.
- Follow proper mixing time and procedure.

Advantages of Mechanical Trituration

- Shortens mixing time.
- Most standardized and accurate procedure.

Mixing Time

Mixing time is 25-30 seconds but varies depending on alloy and amalgamator or recommended by manufacturer.

- *Under triturated mix*
  - Rough, grainy and may crumble.
  - Strength decreases.
  - Rough surface leads to tarnish and corrosion.
  - Mix hardens too rapidly and excess mercury will remain.
- *Normal mix*
  - Has shiny surface with smooth and soft consistency.
  - High resistance to tarnish and corrosion.
  - Make luster after polishing.
  - Mix is warm when removed from capsule.
- *Over triturated mix*
  - Soupy, too plastic hence difficult to remove from capsule.
  - Weight is reduced.
  - Results in high concentration of mercury.
  - Lathe cut alloys increases strength and high copper alloys decreases strength.
  - Creep is increased.

Mulling

Mulling is done to improve homogeneity of mix to get a single consistency. Mulling is done in two ways.

1. The mix is enveloped in a dry piece of a rubber dam and vigorously rubbed between first finger and thumb or thumb of one hand and palm of other hand for 2-5 seconds.
2. The piston or rod of capsule is removed and triturated for 2-5 seconds.

Condensation

Condensation is a process of inserting a plastic mass of amalgam into a prepared cavity by force under pressure.

Aims

- Good marginal adaptability.
- Good bonding between incremental layers of amalgam.

- Removal of excess mercury.
- To increase the density of mix hence optimum mechanical properties and also decrease porosities and voids.

Condensers

These are devices by which condensation is carried out. These are steel hand instruments with their ends with flat or serrated tips of different shapes and sizes. The shapes can be oval, round, parallelogram, diamond, trapezoidal and straight.

These are selected as per the area and shape of the cavity. Smaller is the condenser greater is the pressure exerted per unit area. Other condensers used are ultrasonic condensers, etc.

Procedure

It must always be accomplished within four walls and a floor. If one or two walls are missing they can be replaced by a thin strip of stainless steel sheet called matrix band (Fig. 6.7A). Condensation is of two types:
a. Hand condensation.
b. Mechanical condensation.

Hand Condensation

The plastic mix is carried in increments to the cavity using an amalgam carrier (Fig. 6.8) (mix should never be touched with bare hands) and condensed with suitable condensers. The selection depends on the type of alloy used. If alloy is lathe cut; small increments with small condenser tips of 1–2 mm high forces. If alloy is spherical the condenser punches through the alloy. So larger condensers with less force are used.

The placed alloy should be condensed in a stepwise manner from center to periphery without leaving adjacent areas. If left, it may lead to voids, which decrease strength. So care should be taken then all areas are condensed. Before adding next increment additional mercury is removed and is left which facilitates bonding with next increment and procedure is carried out until cavity is over filled. Condensing pressures are 66.7 N or 15 lb (range from 13.3 N to 17.8 N in reality).

Mechanical Condensation

Condensation is done by an automatic device either by impact type of force or by using rapid vibration.

Advantages
- More accurate.
- Time saving.
- Easy method.

Effect of Delay on Condensation

Condensation should occur immediately after trituration, usually within 3–3½ minutes. If delayed, it leads to cracks in formed matrix leading to fracture, corrosion and micro-leakage. So, if delay has occurred, the operator must discard old mix and prepare new mix.

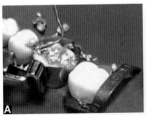 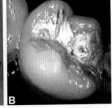

Figs 6.7A and B (A) Condensation of plastic mass-tooth is isolated by using matrix band (B) Condensed restoration

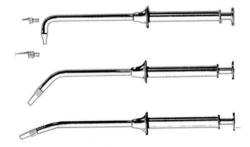

Fig. 6.8 Amalgam carriers used for carrying plastic mix to the tooth cavity

Burnishing

Burnishing is the rubbing of surface to make it smooth, since amalgam restoration has slightly uneven surface after condensation as shown in Figure 6.7B.

Aim

- To remove excess material.
- Better marginal adaptability.
- Increase resistance to tarnish and corrosion.

Burnishing is of two types:
a. Precarve burnishing.
b. Postcarve burnishing.

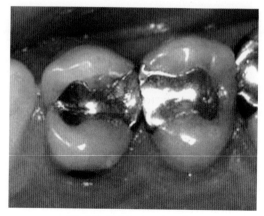

Fig. 6.9 Finished restoration

Precarve Burnishing

Precarve burnishing is a form of condensation. Over packed amalgam is burnished with a large ball burnisher. This procedure is used to remove excess material and better marginal adaptation.

Procedure

Using heavy strokes on all four sides of margin.

Postcarve Burnishing

This is done after carving to make surface smooth.

Precautions

- Proper pressure without generating heat. Heat generated greater than 60°C may lead to elevation of mercury vapor, which alter properties.
- *Time of burnishing:* Before carving, i.e. after hearing amalgam cry.

Carving

Carving is done to reproduce tooth anatomy for occlusal benefits. Carving is done after hearing amalgam cry, i.e. scrapping or ringing sound which indicates initial set. Over- carving and under-carving should be avoided.

Finishing and Polishing

Finishing and polishing is done after 24 hours by using wet abrasives such as pumice. Care should be taken to avoid high temperatures. As shown in Figure 6.9, the finished restorations have smoother surfaces.

Indications of Amalgam

- Class I, class II restorations.
- Nonesthetic class V restorations.
- Core-build up.
- Root canal filling.
- Amalgam pins.
- Crowns build up.

Contraindications

- In esthetic areas.
- Where isolation is difficult (no moisture contamination as in sialorrhea).
- In allergic patients.

Advantages

- Easy to use.
- High tensile strength
- Excellent wear resistance.
- Long-term results.
- Inexpensive.

Disadvantages

- Poor insulator.
- Nonesthetic.
- Less conservative (more removal of tooth structure)
- Weakens tooth structure.
- Initial marginal leakage.
- Discolors of tooth.
- Postoperative sensitivity.

MODIFIED AMALGAMS

Galloy

Galloy is mercury-free amalgam alloy. It contains silver, tin, copper, indium and gallium. Studies of gallium alloys have reported problems with corrosion, durability, tooth fracture and tooth sensitivity.

Bonded Amalgams

In bonded amalgams the bonding is achieved with the help of "4-methacryloxyethyl trimellitic acid." Amalgam bond (Fig. 6.10) is one of the commercial products available for bonded amalgams.

Advantages

- Less microleakage.
- Less interfacial staining.
- Increase strength of remaining tooth structure.
- Minimal postoperative sensitivity.
- Some retention benefits.
- Esthetic benefit by sealing.

DENTAL CEMENTS

Dental cements used as restorative materials have low strengths compared with those of resin-based composites and amalgams, but they can be used for low stress areas.

Cements are widely used in dentistry for a variety of applications. In general, cements are employed for two primary purposes:

1. To serve as a restorative filling material either alone or with other materials.
2. To retain restorations or appliances in a fixed position within the mouth.

However, cements are used for specialized purposes in the restorative, endodontic, orthodontic, periodontic and surgical fields of the dentistry.

General applications of dental cements include, temporary and permanent cementation of indirect restorations and orthodontics bands, temporary, intermediate and permanent restorations, surgical dressing materials, root canal sealers, pit and fissure sealants, core build-up material, cavity liners, low strength and high strength bases.

Some dental cements exhibit anticariogenic properties, anodyne and obtundent effect, bacteriostatic properties, and can directly bond to the tooth structure and some are highly acidic and irritant to the pulp cavity if used in deep cavities.

CLASSIFICATION

1. Based on their chemical name
   Zinc oxide eugenol cement, zinc phosphate cement, silicate cement, glass ionomer

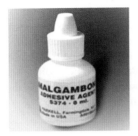
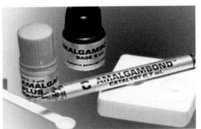

Fig. 6.10 Amalgam bonding agents

cement, zinc polycarboxylate cement, and resin cements.

2. Based on adhesion to tooth structure
   a. Direct bonding or chemical bonding to the tooth
      For example, zinc polycarboxylate cement and glass ionomer cement.
   b. Cements having mechanical retention
      For example, zinc oxide eugenol cement, zinc phosphate cement, silicate cement, etc.

3. Based on composition of powder
   a. Cements possessing zinc oxide in powders:
      For example, zinc oxide eugenol, zinc phosphate, zinc silico phosphate, ethoxy benzoic acid cement, and zinc polycarboxylate.
   b. Cements possess ion leachable glasses in powder:
      For example, silicate, glass ionomer, and copper phosphate.

4. Based on functions (Craig's classification)

Craig's classification	
Cements	Functions
Zinc phosphate, zinc silico-phosphate, reinforced ZOE, zinc polycarboxylate, and glass ionomer cements	Final cementation of completed restorations
Zinc oxide eugenol, and non- eugenol zinc oxide	Temporary cement-ation of completed restorations
Zinc phosphate, reinforced ZOE, zinc polycarboxylate, and glass ionomer cements	High strength bases
Zinc oxide eugenol, reinforced ZOE, zinc polycarboxylate cements	Temporary filling
Zinc oxide eugenol, calcium hydroxide cements	Low strength bases and liners
Resin in solvent	Varnish

Special applications	
Zinc oxide eugenol, and zinc poly- carboxylate cements	Root canal sealer
Zinc oxide eugenol	Gingival tissue pack
Zinc oxide eugenol and zinc oxide preparations	Cementation of orthodontic bands
Zinc oxide eugenol and zinc phosphate cements	Surgical dressing
Resin cements	Orthodontic direct bonding

5. Based on chemistry/setting reaction (EC Coomb's classification)
   The materials may be classified as follows:
   a. Acid-base reactions
      For example, zinc oxide eugenol, cement, zinc phosphate cement, zinc polycarboxylate cement, glass ionomer cement.
   b. Polymerizing materials
      For example, cyanoacrylates, dime-thacrylate polymers, and polymerceramic composites.
   c. Other materials
      For example, calcium hydroxide, gutta-percha, and varnishes.

IDEAL REQUIREMENTS OF RESTORATIVE CEMENT

1. Should be nonirritant to the pulp and gingiva.
2. Should not cause any systemic reactions.
3. Should be cariostatic thus preventing secondary caries formation.
4. Should possess enough abrasion resistance to dentifrices and food.
5. Solubility of the cement in oral fluids should be negligible. Maximum allowable solubility of cements in oral conditions is 0.2%.

6. Ideal cement should bond to the enamel and dentin to avoid marginal leakage.
7. Should possess a COTE to that of enamel and dentin.
8. Cement should have adequate working time.
9. Should exhibit minimum dimensional changes on setting.
10. Restoration should take and retain a smooth surface finish.
11. Should have adequate radiopacity to enable—
    a. Detection of secondary caries.
    b. Detection of incompletely filled cavities due to trapped air.

ZINC OXIDE EUGENOL CEMENT

Zinc oxide eugenol (ZOE) cement was introduced into dentistry in 1890's. They have been widely employed for various purposes in dentistry especially as temporary and intermediate restorative material, cavity liners, thermal insulating bases, root canal sealant, periodontal dressings, luting cement for restorations and possess a sedative effect on exposed dentin.

Their pH is approximately 7 at the time they are inserted into the tooth. ZOE cement is one of the least irritating materials among all dental materials and provides an excellent seal against leakage.

Commercial Names

1. Unmodified
   Tempac—Type III
   Cavitic—Type IV
   Temp bond—Type I
2. EBA alumina modified
   Opotow
   Alumina EBA—Type II
3. Polymer modified
   Fynal—Type II
   IRM—Type III
4. Noneugenol
   Nogenol—Type I
   Freegenol—Type I

ADA specification number: 30

Classification

According to ADA Specification Number 30

Type I ZOE: Temporary luting cement
Type II ZOE: Long-term luting cement
Type III ZOE: Temporary restoration and thermal insulating base.
Type IV ZOE: Intermediate restoration, cavity liner and chemical insulator.

Dispension

This cement is dispensed in two forms:
a. Powder and liquid (Fig. 6.11A).
b. Two paste system.

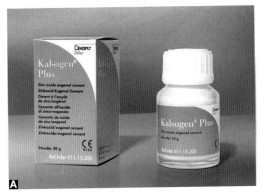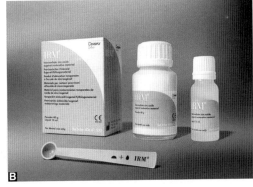

Figs 6.11A and B (A) Zinc oxide eugenol cement (B) Intermediate restorative material

Composition

Powder		
Ingredient	*Wt (%)*	*Functions*
Zinc oxide	69%	Primary reactive ingredient, takes part in the setting reaction.
White rosin	29.3%	1. To reduce brittleness of set cement. 2. Improves consistency and provides smoother mixing.
Zinc stearate	1%	Acts as a plasticizer.
Zinc acetate	0.7%	1. Acts as an accelerator. 2. Improves strength of the cement.
Magnesium oxide		It is added in some powders. It acts with eugenol in similar manner as zinc oxide.
Liquid		
Ingredient	*Wt (%)*	*Functions*
Eugenol	85%	Primary reactive ingredient. Reacts with zinc oxide
Olive oil	15%	Acts as a plasticizer – controls the viscosity.
Glacial acetic acid		Acts as an accelerator

Chemistry of Setting

The chemistry of setting of the ZOE cements is similar to the ZOE impression materials. The reaction is measurably exothermic and the presence of moisture is essential for setting to occur. The setting reaction is a typical acid-base reaction.

The relative proportions of powder and liquid are not normally measured accurately, although some manufacturers provide a scoop, which gives a known volume of powder to which a given number of drops of liquid are added. Then mix the powder with liquid. The setting reaction involves in two steps.

a. **Hydrolysis**

Zinc oxide reacts with water to form zinc hydroxide. Water is an essential for the reaction to proceed (dehydrated zinc oxide will not react with dehydrated eugenol).

$$ZnO + H_2O \longleftrightarrow Zn(OH)_2$$

b. **Acid-base reaction**

Zinc hydroxide reacts with eugenolic acid and forms zinc eugenolate.

Eugenolic acid   Zinc eugenolate

Acid base reaction ZOE cement

Structure of Set Cement

Thus the set cement consists of particles of zinc oxide embedded in a matrix of particles of zinc eugenolate.

Properties

Biological Properties

- **Effect on pulp:** Least irritating. Pulpal response is mild.
- **Bacteriostatic and obtundent properties:** They inhibit the growth of bacteria and have an anodyne or soothing effect on the pulp in deep cavities, reduce pain when it is present.

Chemical Properties (pH is around 6.6-8)

Their pH is approximately 7 at the time they are inserted into the tooth. ZOE cement is one of the least irritating materials in dental materials and provides an excellent seal against leakage.

Solubility

Eugenol is released from the set cement by the hydrolytic decomposition of the zinc eugenolate. The cement disintegrates rapidly when exposed to oral conditions. According to ADA specification number 30 the maximum allowable solubility is 2.5% for type I and II cements and 1.5% for type III and IV cements. But the actual solubility of ZOE cement is 0.04%.

The test used is the amount of solubility and disintegration, measured by weight loss that occurs in a disk of the cement immersed in distilled water for 24 hours.

Rheological Properties

Setting Time

The setting time is the time elapsed between the end of mixing and the time of setting as measured by resistance to a standard indenter. Setting time is around 4–10 minutes.

Control of Setting Time

- *Particle size:* Cements prepared from smaller particles of zinc oxide powder set more rapidly than those prepared with larger particles.
- *Accelerators:* Alcohol, glacial acetic acid, and small amounts of water accelerate the reaction.
- *Temperature:* If the temperature is below the dew point the setting reaction will increase. Below the dew point, condensate that is incorporated into the mix and setting reaction is accelerated.
- *Powder/liquid ratio:* The higher the P/L ratio, the faster the set. Cooling the mixing slab slows the setting reaction.

Film thickness: The film thickness of zinc oxide eugenol is higher than other cements, i.e. 25 μm for luting consistency. The film thickness is an important factor in the complete sealing of restorations at the time of cementation. Some of the early ZOE cements had a greater film thickness than desirable. But the products dispensed currently to the dentist have the film thickness is not more than 25 μm, as determined by the specification test. This requirement is not applied to cement used for purposes other than cementation.

The particle size of the ZnO and viscosity of the mix govern the film thickness. Using a fluid mix gives values of about 40 μm.

Mechanical Properties

- Compressive strength, tensile strength and modulus of elasticity (MOE) of ZOE cement were given in Table 6.6. These cements are weakest among luting agents.
- *Adhesion:* These cements do not adhere chemically to enamel or dentin.

Thermal Properties

- *Thermal conductivity:* Thermal insulating properties of ZOE cements are excellent and are approximately same as for human dentin.
- *Coefficient of thermal expansion:* $35 \times 10^{-6}/°C$.
- Very high compared to the natural tooth.

Optical Properties

The set cement is opaque.

Table 6.6 Mechanical properties of ZOE cement

Property	Values
Compressive strength	They are relatively weak cements. It ranges from a low value of 3–4 Mpa up to 50–55 Mpa.
Tensile strength	Ranges from 0.32–5.8 Mpa.
Modulus of elasticity	Ranges from 0.22–5.4 GPa or 0.03–0.79 Psi.

Manipulation

Selection of Materials

Dry and cool glass slab, stainless steel spatula, required amount of powder and liquid.

Powder-Liquid ratio: 4:1–6:1 by weight.

Mixing

Measured quantity of powder and liquid is dispensed onto a cool slab. The bulk of the powder is incorporated into the liquid and spatulated thoroughly in a circular motion with a stiff bladed stainless steel spatula. Smaller increments are then added and mixed using folding technique or in sweeping and stopping motion until a smooth and creamy mix is obtained.

Oil of orange can be used to clean eugenol cements from instruments.

Two paste system: Equal lengths of each paste are dispensed and mixed until a uniform color is observed.

Applications

- Bases
- Temporary restorations
- Intermediate restorations
- Temporary and permanent cementation
- Endodontic sealers.

Advantages

- Obtundent effect on pulp
- Good sealing ability
- Postoperative sensitivity is virtually eliminated
- Prevents penetration of acid into the pulp.

Disadvantages

- Difficult to manipulate
- Low strength
- Low abrasion resistance
- Solubility and disintegration in oral fluids
- Poorer retention than zinc phosphate cement
- Reparative dentin formation is variable
- Burning sensation.

Modifications

1. Ethyl benzoic acid – Alumina modified cement.
2. Polymer reinforced ZOE.
3. Cements containing vanillate esters.
4. Special ZOE product.

EBA-Alumina Modified Cements

In order to further improve on the basic ZOE system many researchers have investigated mixtures of zinc and other oxides with various liquid chelating agents. The only system that has received extensive commercial exploration for luting and lining is that containing orthoethoxy benzoic acid (EBA).

Recently, cements for luting and intermediate restorations based on vanillic acid (4-hydroxy-3 methoxy benzoic acid) have studied extensively. These cements have no odor, higher strength, and lower solubility.

In these cements, alumina is added to the powder and EBA is added to the liquid. These cements improve the mechanical properties compared to ZOE.

Dispension

Powder and liquid system.

Composition

Powder		
Ingredient	*Wt %*	*Functions*
Zinc oxide	64–73%	Principle ingredient
Alumina	25–32%	Increases strength
Hydrogenated resin	0–6%	Increases strength, reduces brittleness and improves mixing qualities.
Copolymers	0–2%	
Liquid		
Orthoethoxy benzoic acid	62.5–87.5%	Main reactive ingredient
Eugenol	0–37.5%	Reacts with ZnO.
n-hexyl vanillate	0–12.5%	

Setting Reaction

The setting mechanism has not been fully understood. It appears to involve chelate salt formation between the EBA, eugenol and zinc oxide.

Manipulation

Desired amount of the powder and liquid (3.5 g/ml for cementation and 5-6 g/ml for lining and base) are dispensed onto the glass slab. Powder is incorporated onto the liquid in bulk and kneaded for 30 seconds followed by strapping for another 60 seconds with broad strokes of the spatula to obtain creamy consistency.

Setting Time

These possess greater setting time compared to unmodified ZOE cement, i.e. 9.5 minutes.

Properties

As given in Table 6.7, the compressive strength, tensile strength of EBA-Alumina cements were improved significantly. Solubility and disintegration has been reduced compared to conventional ZOE cement.

Uses

- For the cementation of inlays, crowns and bridges.
- For temporary fillings.
- As a base or lining material.

Table 6.7 Properties of EBA-Alumina cements

Property	Values
Compressive strength	55–70 Mpa
Tensile strength	4.1 Mpa
Modulus of elasticity	2.5 GPa (0.36 Psi $\times$ 10^6)
Film thickness	25 μm
Solubility and disintegration in water	0.05% wt
Setting time	9.5 minutes

Advantages

- Easy to manipulate.
- Long working time.
- Good flow characteristics.
- Low irritation to the pulp.
- Strength and film thickness can be comparable to that of zinc phosphate cement.

Disadvantages

- The critical proportioning.
- Hydrolytic breakdown in oral fluids.
- Liability to plastic deformation.
- Poorer retention.

Polymer Reinforced ZOE or Intermediate Restorative Material (IRM)

This cement possesses improved mechanical properties than unmodified ZOE.

Dispension

Dispensed in the powder and liquid form (Fig. 6.11B).

Composition

Powder		
Ingredient	*Wt%*	*Functions*
Zinc oxide	10-80%	Main reactive ingredient.
Finely divided natural or synthetic resins, e.g. Colophony (pine resin), PMMA, polystyrene or polycarbonate.	20%	These resins may react with the ZnO and improve the strength of the matrix.
Acetic acid or Zn acetate.		Acts as an accelerator.
Liquid		
Eugenol	85%	Main reactive ingredient, which reacts with ZnO to form Zn eugenolate.

Dissolved resins, e.g. Pine resin, PMMA, polystyrene, and polycarbonate.	Gives more strength.
Acetic acid	Acts as an accelerator.
Thymol or 8-hydroxyl-quinone	Plasticizer.
Olive oil 15%	

Setting Reaction

The setting reaction is similar to the setting mechanism of conventional zinc oxide eugenol cement. Acidic resins such as colophony (abietic acid) may react with zinc oxide and strengthening the mix.

Properties

These cements do not exhibit better compressive strength and modulus of elasticity (MOE) compared to conventional ZOE cement (Table 6.8)

Manipulation

Desired quantity of powder and liquid is dispensed onto the glass slab. The powder is mixed into the liquid in small portion with vigorous spatulation.

Both powder and liquid containers should be kept closed and stored under dry conditions.

Table 6.8 Properties of polymer reinforced zinc oxide eugenol cement

Property	Values
Compressive strength	35–55 Mpa
Tensile strength	5–8 Mpa
Modulus of elasticity	2.5 GPa
Film thickness	35–75 µm
Solubility and disintegration	0.03% Wt
Pulpal response	Moderate pulpal response
Setting time	6–10 minutes

Advantages

- The minimum biologic effects.
- Good initial sealing properties.
- Adequate strength for final cementation of restorations, compared with unmodified ZOE.

Disadvantages

- Lower strength compared to zinc phosphate cement.
- Higher solubility and disintegration.
- Hydrolytic instability.
- High film thickness.
- May cause softening and discoloration of some resin restorative materials when they are used with resin restorative materials.

Cements Containing Vanillate Esters

Recently, cements have been developed with hexyl vanillate and orthoethoxy benzoic acid as a substitute for eugenol. This liquid is mixed with ZnO powder. This shows high strength and low solubility.

Special ZOE Products

ZOE materials contain antibiotics such as tetracycline and steroids as anti-inflammatory agents. Their principal use is in Pulpal capping, and root canal therapy. Another product also contains $BaSO_4$, which is radiopaque.

Endodontic Sealers

Endodontic ZOE preparations have been used as a root canal sealer alone and with gutta-percha and silver points. There are two major groups of products based on ZOE cements–Conventional and therapeutic sealers.

- ADA specification number: 57

Types

Type I: Core and auxiliary points.
Type II: Sealer cements used with cores.
Type III: Filling materials used without cores (therapeutic).

Composition

The conventional sealers generally are based on the formulas of Grossman's and Rickets'.

Rickets formula

Powder

Ingredient	Wt%
Zinc oxide	41%
Silver	30%
White rosin	17%
Thymol iodide	12%

Liquid

Oil of cloves	78%
Canada balsam	22%

Grossman's formula

Powder

Ingredient	Wt%
Zinc oxide	42%
Staybilite resin	27%
Bismuth subcarbonate	15%
Barium sulfate	15%
Sodium borate anhydrate	1%

Liquid

Eugenol	100%

Therapeutic Formula

Powder	Liquid
Zinc oxide	Eugenol
Bismuth subnitrate	Creosote
Iodoform	Thymol
Rosin	

Properties: Table 6.9

ZINC PHOSPHATE CEMENT

A group of widely used cements is based on the vigorous reaction, which occurs between

Table 6.9 Properties of endodontic sealers

Property	Values
Solubility	0.10%-3.5%
Viscosity	$8\text{-}680 \times 10^3$ Cp
Setting time	15 minutes–12 hours at mouth temperatures
Film thickness	80-500 μm (depending on the testing load).
Compressive strength	8-50 Mpa.

Radiopacity
  Silver points
  Gutta-percha points
	
	0.34
	0.78

Dimensional change	0.7%-5.0% (volume loss after 90 days in a capillary tube)

certain basic oxides and phosphoric acid to form phosphate salts of low solubility. The three products considered in this selection are the zinc phosphate, silicophosphate and copper phosphate cements.

Zinc phosphate is the oldest (1878) of the cementation agents and thus is the one that has the longest track record. It serves as a standard by which newer systems can be compared. The terms "crown and bridge", "zincoxy phosphate" have also been used for this cement.

Commercial Names

1. Confit
2. Harvard
3. Zinc cement improved
4. Modern tenascin.
• ADA specification number: 8

Classification

ADA specification number 8 designates them as—

Type I: Fine grained for luting (Film thickness - 25 μm or less).

Type II: Medium grain for luting and filling (Film thickness not more than 40 μm).

Dispension

It is available as:
- Powder and liquid system.
- Capsules of preproportioned powder and liquid.

   A variety of shades are available like yellow, gray, golden brown, pink and white.

Composition

Powder		
Ingredient	*Wt%*	*Functions*
Zinc oxide	90.2%	Main reactive ingredient. It provides Zn ions for the reaction
Magnesium oxide	8.2%	It is added to the ZnO to reduce the temperature of the calcination process
Other oxides (Bismuth trioxide, Calcium oxide, and Barium oxide)	0.2%	Improves smoothness of mix. In large amounts it may also lengthen the setting time
Silica	1.4%	It is an inactive filler and during manufacture aids in the calcination process

Liquid		
Ingredient	*Wt%*	*Functions*
Aqueous solution of phosphoric acid	38.2%	Main reactive ingredient. It reacts with ZnO to form zinc phosphate salt
Water	36%	Controls the rate of setting reaction
Aluminum phosphate or zinc phosphate	16.2%	Acts as a buffer. Partial neutralization of the phosphoric acid by aluminum
Aluminum	2.5%	Provides additional aluminum ions Improves cohesiveness
Zinc	7.1%	Provides additional zinc ions for the reaction

Manufacture

Powder

The powder is manufactured by a process called sintering. The ingredients of the powder are mixed and heated at temperatures between 1000°C and 1400°C for 4–8 hours. The cake formed is then grounded into a fine powder.

Liquid

The liquid is produced by adding aluminum and sometimes zinc or their compounds into orthophosphoric acid solution.

Setting Reaction

When the powder is mixed with the liquid, the phosphoric acid attacks the surface of the particles, dissolving the ZnO forming acid zinc phosphate.

   The aluminum of the liquid is essential for cement formation. The aluminum complexes with the phosphoric acid to form zinc aluminophosphate gel (without aluminum, a noncohesive, crystalline structure matrix of hopeite, i.e. $Zn_3(PO_4)_2 \cdot 4H_2O$ would be formed). The reaction is exothermic.

Structure of Set Cement

The set cement is a cored structure consisting primarily of unreacted zinc oxide particles embedded in a cohesive amorphous matrix of zinc aluminophosphate (Fig. 6.12).

Properties

Biological Properties

Zinc phosphate cement causes prolonged pulpal irritation, especially in deep cavities that necessitate some form of pulpal protection, which may be associated with the extended duration of low pH of the set material. This is minimized by high P/L ratio, rapid setting, lining the cavity with $Ca(OH)_2$ and cavity varnishes.

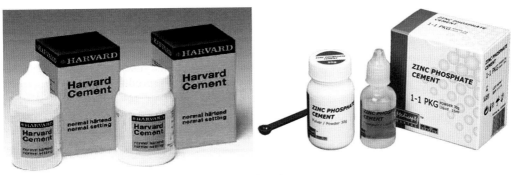

Fig. 6.12 Zinc phosphate cement

Table 6.10 pH of zinc phosphate cement at different time intervals

Time in minutes/ hours	3 minutes	1 hour	24 hours	48 hours	7 days
pH	3.5	5.9	6.6	6.8	6.9

Chemical Properties

The freshly mixed zinc phosphate is highly acidic with a pH between 1 and 2 after mixing. After 24 hours the pH is usually 6–7. The pH of zinc phosphate cement at different time intervals was given in Table 6.10.

Pain on cementing is not only due to free acidity of the mix but also to osmotic pressure movement of fluid through the dentinal tubules.

The damage to the pulp from acid attack by zinc phosphate cement probably occurs during the first few hours after insertion. So, the underlying dentin should be protected against the infiltration of acid via the dentinal tubules, otherwise pulpal injury may occur.

Rheological Properties

- **Mixing time:** 60–90 seconds.
- **Working time:** It is the time measured from the start of the mixing during which the viscosity (consistency) of the mix is low enough to flow readily under pressure to form a thin film.

The working time of a luting consistency at room temperature for most of the brands is around 3–6 minutes.

- **Setting time:** It is the time elapsed between the end of the mixing and the time of setting as measured by a resistance to a standard indenter.
- **Test:** Setting time can be measured with a 4.5 N (1 pound) Gillmore needle at a temperature of 37°C and relative humidity of 100%. It is defined as the time elapsed from the start of mixing until the point of the needle no longer penetrates the cement as the needle is lowered onto the surface. Practically, it is the time at which the zinc phosphate cement flash (excess cement) should be removed from the margins of the restoration.

A reasonable setting time for zinc phosphate cement is between 5–9 minutes.

Control of Setting Time

- *Factors under control of manufacturer*
  a. *Sintering temperature:* The higher the temperature, more slowly the cement sets.
  b. *Particle size:* Finer particles react more quickly as a greater surface area is exposed to the liquid.
  c. *Water content of liquid:* Presence of excess water accelerates the reaction, whereas insufficient water retards the reaction.

d. *Buffering agents:* The added buffering agents slow down the reaction.

- *Factors under control of operator*
  a. *Mixing temperature:* The most effective method of controlling the working and setting times is to regulate the temperature of the mixing slab. Cooling the glass slab markedly retards the chemical reaction between the powder and liquid so that matrix formation is retarded. This permits incorporation of the optimum amount of powder into the liquid without the mix developing an unduly high viscosity. High temperature accelerates the reaction.
  b. *Powder/Liquid ratio:* More liquid employed, slower the reaction.
  c. *Rate of addition of powder to liquid:* The reaction is slower if the powder is incorporated into the liquid slowly.
  d. *Mixing time:* The longer the mixing time, the slower is the rate of setting reaction.

Film Thickness

According to ADA Specification number 8, for
   Type I: Fine grained for luting (Film thickness - 25 μm or less).
   Type II: Medium grain for luting and filling (Film thickness not more than 40 μm).

Consistency

- **Luting consistency:** Forms a string of 1 inch height and springs back into the mix, when lifted with a spatula (Fig. 6.13).
- **Base consistency:** When lifted, the string breaks up to form a hook-like structure (Fig. 6.13).

Mechanical Properties

- *Compressive strength:* Zinc phosphate cements are stronger than zinc oxide eugenol cements but not as strong as silicophosphate cements. Seventy-five percent of maximum strength is obtained in the first one hour. Maximum strength is attained in the first day.
  Compressive strength: 103.5 Mpa.

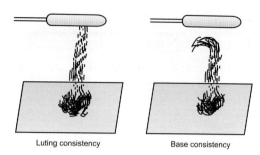

Luting consistency   Base consistency

Fig. 6.13 Luting consistency and base consistencies of zinc phosphate cement

- *Tensile strength:* This cement is weaker in tension, thus making it brittle.
  Tensile strength: 5.5 Mpa.
- *Modulus of elasticity:* It is comparatively high. This makes it stiff and resistant to elastic deformation even when it is employed as a luting agent for restorations that are subjected to high masticatory stress.
  MOE: 13.5 GPa (1.96×10^6 Psi)
- *Adhesion:* These cements do not form a chemical bond with enamel or dentin. However, there is undoubtedly a mechanical interlocking, which provides a certain amount of retention of restoration. Whenever a cast is seated in the prepared cavity, the surfaces of both the casting and the tooth structure have slightly roughness and irregularities into which the plastic cement is forced. After the cement hardens such extensions, many of which are undercut, assist in providing retention for the inlay. For this reason highly polished surfaces do not exhibit as great retention when they are united with dental cement as do slightly roughened surfaces.

Thermal Properties

These cements are good insulators and may be effective in reducing galvanic effects.

Optical Properties

The set cement is opaque.

Manipulation

Selection of Materials

Cool and dry glass slab, cement spatula, required amount of powder and liquid.

Proportioning

1.4 g of powder to 0.5 ml of liquid.

Mixing

On a cool dry glass slab, the required amount of powder is taken first and liquid should be dispensed just before mixing. Spatulation is carried out in a circular motion followed by folding technique with stainless steel spatula. A large area is covered during mixing in order to dissipate the exothermic heat. It is advised to add little amount of powder to the liquid initially in order to delay the rate of setting reaction.

Cementation or Restoration

As soon as the mix is reached to the required consistency it should be used for suitable purpose such as either for cementation of base application or as a temporary restoration.

Uses

- Luting of indirect restoration.
- Luting of orthodontic bands and brackets.
- Temporary restorations.
- Cavity liners or high strength bases to protect the pulp from mechanical, thermal or electrical stimuli.

Advantages

- Easy to mix.
- Sharp and well-defined set.
- Good compressive strength. So it can be used as a strong base under amalgam restorations.

Disadvantages

- Potential for pulp irritation.
- Very brittle.
- Do not adhere chemically to the tooth.

- Susceptible for acid attacks (solubility in oral fluids).
- Lack of antibacterial action.

MODIFICATIONS OF ZINC PHOSPHATE CEMENT

Modifications

1. Cu and Ag cements
2. Fluoride cements
3. Water settable zinc phosphate cements.

Copper and Silver Cements

Silver salts or Cu oxides are sometimes added to the powder of the zinc phosphate cement supposedly to increase their antibacterial properties.

Black Cu cements contain – CuO (cupric oxide).

Red Cu cements contain – Cu_2O (cuprous oxide).

Others may contain cuprous iodide or silicate.

Since a much lower P/L ratio is necessary to obtain satisfactory manipulative characteristics with these cements, the mix is highly acidic, resulting in much greater pulpal irritation. Their solubility is higher and their strength is lower than the zinc phosphate cements. Their bacteriostatic or anticariogenic properties seem to be slight. Ag cements generally contain a few percent of a salt such as Ag phosphate.

Their advantages over zinc phosphate cement have not been substantiated. The disadvantage of the Ag phosphate is discoloration with respect to light.

Fluoride Cements

These modified cements contain 1–3% of stannous fluoride in addition to the regular components of zinc phosphate cement.

The use of adding fluoride content is for anticariogenic property. Particularly, used for orthodontic cementation.

These cements have a higher solubility, 0.7% due to the fluoride leaching, lower strength than the zinc phosphate cements. Fluoride uptake by enamel from such cements results in reduced enamel solubility.

Water-Settable Zinc Phosphate Cement or Hydrous Phosphate Cement

Zinc phosphate cement has been developed that uses water as the liquid rather than a buffered phosphoric acid solution. The composition varies from one brand to another.

General Composition

a. ZnO
b. Monozine or mono Mn phosphate
c. 3° zinc phosphates
d. Some contain monocalcium phosphate.

Cements may result in improved properties. Physical properties of the currently available water-settable cements are generally somewhat inferior to those of conventional zinc phosphate cement. Neither do they appear to afford biological advantage. Since they contain acid phosphate salts, both the pH level and the pattern of pH change is same as with the conventional type of zinc phosphate cement.

These cements are mainly used for luting and base purposes.

SILICATE CEMENTS

Silicates were the earliest of the direct tooth colored filling materials. They have been available since the beginning of the 20th century (1903). The durability of a silicate restoration depends critically on the care taken in handling the material and on the oral hygiene of the patient. Thus, silicate restorations may have a life time of only a few months or less or on the other hand, may last 20 years or more.

Composition of Silicate Cements

Powder		
Ingredient	Wt %	Functions
Silica (SiO_2) (acid soluble glass)	40%	1. It reacts with alumina to form alumino silicate network of the fused glass. 2. Acts as filler. 3. It provides more translucency to the set product.
Alumina (Al_2O_3)	30%	1. It reacts with silica to form aluminosilicate network. 2. When attacked by H^+ ions of the liquid it releases Al^{3+} ions into the medium to form the hydrated Al phosphate of the set matrix. 3. Acts as filler. 4. More amount of alumina will lengthen the setting time.
Sodium fluoride or calcium fluoride	4%	1. Acts as flux. 2. Gives the opacity to the glass. 3. Fluorides act as anticariogenic agents. 4. Can also alter the physical properties.
Hydrated Ca biphosphate [$CaH_2 (PO_4)_2$. H_2O or Na Phosphate or CaO (Lime)] Al Phosphate	7%	
Liquid		
Phosphoric acid	42%	Main reactive ingredient, which releases H^+ ions on dissociation that attacks the fused glass powder, which in turn, releases its cations to form their respective phosphates.
Al phosphate	10%	Acts as a buffering agent, which neutralizes the phosphoric acid partially.
Zn and Mg phosphate	8%	Also acts as a buffering agent.
Water	40%	It serves as a reaction medium initially. It facilitates the release of protons from the phosphoric acid.

The silicates may be considered as precursors of more modern products such as composite resin and glass ionomer cements.

ADA specification number: 9.

Australian standard specification number: T8.

British standard specification number: 3365.

FDI standard specification number: 1961.

Dispension

Silicate cement is available as powder and liquid. The powder is finely ground ceramic that is essentially an acid-soluble glass.

Composition

(see Table on previous page).

Manufacture

The powder ingredients are fused at approximately 1400°C to form an acid-soluble glass and cooled quickly. This causes the glass to crack which helps in grinding of the material to a fine powder. This process is known as fritting.

Setting Reaction

The reaction, which occurs when powder and liquid are mixed together is fairly complex. In simplified terms it may be regarded as a series of acid base reactions in which metal ions in the glass react with phosphoric acid to form a series of phosphate salts.

$$Al^{3+} + H_3PO_4 \longrightarrow AlPO_4 + 3H^+$$
$$Ca^{2+} + H_3PO_4 \longrightarrow CaHPO_4 + 2H^+$$
$$Na^{2+} + H_3PO_4 \longrightarrow NaH_2PO_4 + 2H^+$$

The H^+ ions of the H_3PO_4 attack the glass displacing Al^{3+}, Na^{3+}, Ca^{2+} ions. The silicon is not removed, nor do the phosphates transfer to the glass. The displaced ions collect in the semiliquid phase together with phosphate and other metal ions contained in the cement liquid.

The mechanism of the reaction is depicted as follows:

a. Formation of protons

$$H_3PO_4 \rightleftharpoons H^+ + H_2PO_4^-$$

b. Protons enter the outer layers of glass particles, displacing cations.

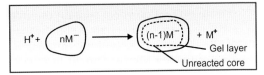

c. Cations react with phosphate ions to form a matrix of metallic phosphates.

$$M^+ + H_2PO_4^- \longrightarrow MH_2PO_4$$
Where M^+ represents Al^{3+}, Ca^{2+} and Na^+

Hydrated protons (H_3O^+) from the liquid disrupt the aluminosilicate network by attacking the Al sites. Other cations (Na^{3+} and Ca^{2+}) are displaced by hydrated protons; as a result there is degradation of the glass network to form a "hydrated siliceous gel".

The powder is "amphoteric", i.e. it can react chemically as an acid in the presence of strong bases, and as a base towards strong acids.

Structure of the Set Cement

A core of unreacted glass particles is present. Hydrated aluminosilicate gel, which covers the surface of the glass particles, is present. An amorphous matrix of hydrated aluminum phosphate gel, which contains some crystals of $Al_2(OH)_3 PO_4$ is seen.

Properties

Biological Properties

Related to pulpal response, it is classified as a severe irritant and often serves as the reference material to judge the potential of other materials to elicit a relatively severe reaction. Thus, a silicate cement restoration requires a greater need for pulp protection than other cements.

• *Acidity:* The pH value of freshly mixed cement is around 2.8. The pulp must be protected from the possible harmful effects of such an acidic material by using a cavity base, normally calcium hydroxide product. The pH of the cement rises to a value of about 5 after 24 hours and it remains below 7 after one month.

- *Anticariogenic property:* Most commercial silicate cement powders contain fluoride salts up to 15%. The clinical significance of the fluoride is extremely important. Thus, although silicate cement has many weaknesses, its anticariogenic potential has been impressive.

    The release of fluoride is small, but significant amounts for an indefinite period from the silicate cements contribute to caries inhibition in the oral environment by means of both physicochemical and biologic mechanisms.

Physicochemical concept of caries inhibition: Fluoride ions released from the restorative material during setting reaction and become incorporated in hydroxyapatite crystals of adjacent tooth, to form an acid resistant structure called "fluorapatite"; which is slightly more resistant to acid mediated decalcification this prevents caries.

$$F + \text{Hydroxyapatite of } Ca_3(PO_4)_2 \rightarrow \text{Fluorapatite}$$

Biological mechanism: The fluoride ions released from the silicate restoration can enter bacterial cells present in the plaque and inhibit the carbohydrate metabolism thus preventing the production of acids. This prevents the caries formation.

Chemical Properties

- *Solubility and Disintegration:* The silicate restorations have high solubility and disintegrate in oral fluids. Some of the constituents of matrix dissolve. Particles of unreacted silicate powder are washed away. Solubility of silicate cement is affected by—
    - Lower the powder/liquid ratio, higher the solubility.
    - Water content of liquid.

Rheological Properties

- *Setting time:* Setting time is the time elapsed between end of the mixing and the time of setting as measured by resistance to a standard indenter.
    The setting time is about 3–8 minutes.
- *Factors affecting setting time*
    a. Manufacture: Controls the composition and particle size of material. Finer the particles the more rapid is setting.
    b. Slower setting time is by:
        - Longer mixing time.
        - Lower temperature.
        - Loss of water from liquid.
        - Lower powder/liquid ratio.
- *Drying out:* After setting, the surface of the material must not be allowed to dry out since it desiccates, becomes opaque and cracks. This may be a problem in anterior restorations of mouth breathing patients for whom the silicate materials cannot be recommended.
    Silicate restorations should be coated with varnish before carrying out such procedures.

Mechanical Properties

- *Compressive strength:* Silicate is the strongest of all the dental cements. The powder/liquid ratio and the water content of the liquid affect the strength. The compressive strength of silicate cements is about 180 Mpa or 27000 PSI.
- *Tensile strength:* Silicate cements are weak under tension. The tensile strength of these cements is 3.5 Mpa or 500 PSI.
- *Hardness:* The hardness of silicate cements is similar to that of the dentin (70 KHN).
- *Adhesion:* There is no adhesive bond between silicate and enamel. Adhesion is mechanical adhesion.
- *Erosion:* A major drawback of silicates is their potential to undergo erosion. They erode very slowly at neutral pH but are less stable if the pH drops much below a value of 5. Plaque

pH values are commonly around 4 and under these conditions silicates may erode quite rapidly. Restorations produced with a high P/L ratio are less susceptible to erosion than those with a low P/L ratio. This indicates that the matrix phase of the set material is most vulnerable to erosion.

Another mechanism of erosion involves the formation of soluble complexes of cement cations with certain anions, particularly citrates. Silicate fillings erode quite rapidly in patients who consume large quantities of fruit juices.

Thermal Properties

Thermal properties of silicate cements match those of tooth substance more closely than those of most other materials.

Thus silicate cements are good thermal insulators, expand and contract at about the same rate as tooth substance. Thermal properties of silicate cements and natural tooth are compared in Table 6.11.

Esthetic Properties

The initial esthetics are excellent. The refractive index is similar to that of enamel and dentin. The surface is difficult to polish satisfactorily.

Manipulation

Dry field is required during manipulation. The liquid is dispensed just prior to the mixing in order to preserve the acid water balance.

Table 6.11 Comparison of thermal properties of silicate cement with tooth

Material	COTE	Thermal diffusivity
Silicate materials	10×10^{-6} /°C	3.4×10^{-3} cms^{-1}
Enamel	11.4×10^{-6} /°C	4.7×10^{-3} cms^{-1}
Dentin	8.0×10^{-6} /°C	2.0×10^{-3} cms^{-1}

Selection of Materials

Dry cool glass slab and agate or plastic or cobalt-chromium spatula, a cellulose acetate strip, varnish.

Proportioning

Powder/liquid ratio is about 16 g/4 ml.

Mixing (Folding and Tapping Technique)

The powder is dispensed on a thick, cool, dry glass slab and divided into two or three large increments. The increments are then rapidly folded into the liquid over a small area with an agate spatula, in order to preserve the gel structure. A thick mix produces crumbly mass. Too much of liquid increases the setting time, reduces pH and strength, increases solubility and makes it more prone to staining.

Cementation/Restoration

- Luting consistency is placed in the indirect restoration and fixed on the prepared tooth.
- Restorative consistency is directly placed in the prepared tooth cavity.
  A cellulose strip is held against the setting material in the cavity. The strip is removed after the material sets.
  The restoration is painted by water insoluble varnish to protect it from contact with oral fluids.

Precautions

- Liquid bottle should be kept closed when not in use.
- Cloudy liquid should be discarded.
- Last portion of the liquid should be discarded because it will be contaminated due to repeated use.
- Steel spatula should not be used for mixing.

Uses

- Anterior esthetic material.
- Sometimes as intermediate restorative material in high carious risk patients.

Advantages

- Translucent material so good esthetics.
- Adequate strength.
- Anticariogenic property because of fluoride release.
- Good thermal insulator.

Disadvantages

- Highly acidic – so severe irritant to the pulp.
- Highly soluble.
- Contraindicated in mouth breathers.
- Cannot be used in patients consuming highly acidic food because erosion may take place.
- Low tensile strength and highly brittle in nature.
- Low impact strength.
- Highly susceptible to moisture contamination.
- No proper adhesion to the tooth structure.

ZINC SILICOPHOSPHATE CEMENT

Zinc silicophosphate cement is resulted from the combination of zinc phosphate cement and silicate powders. It is sometimes called as zinc silicate, silicate zinc cement or simply silicophosphate cement. These cements are also called as synthetic porcelain.

The presence of the silicate glass provides a degree of translucency, improved strength and fluoride release. Esthetically, it is superior to the opaque zinc phosphate cement for cementation of ceramic restorations.

- ADA specification number: 21

Classification

Type I – Cementation of fixed restorations and Orthodontic bands.
Type II – Temporary posterior filling material.
Type III – Used as a dual purpose cement (as both a cementing medium and a temporary posterior filling material).

Dispension

These cements are available in the form of powder and liquid.

Composition

Powder

Ingredient	Wt %	Functions
Zinc oxide		It is the main reactive ingredient.
Silicate glass SiO_2 Al_2O_3 $Ca_3(PO_4)_2$, Na_3PO_4	10–20%	Provides Al^{+3} ions into the reactive medium. Which later forms "Zn aluminophosphate gel" as the set product.
Fluorides like CaF_2 or NaF	12–25%	Acts as flux. This also decreases fusion temperature.
Al PO_4		Also acts as a flux. Provides additional Al^{+3} ions to the glass powder.
Ag or Hg compounds	Trace	Acts as germicidal agent.
MgO		It is added to ZnO to reduce the sintering temperature of calcination process of ZnO.

Liquid

H_3PO_4	42%	Main reactive ingredient, releases H^+ ions into the reaction medium, which attacks the cations to form respective phosphates.
Al PO_4, Zinc phosphate	18%	Buffering agent.
Water	40%	Serves as reaction medium. Plays an important role in strength properties of the set cement.

Setting Reaction

The setting reaction has not been fully investigated but may be represented as follows:

ZnO/aluminosilicate glass + $H_3PO_4 \rightarrow$ Zinc aluminosilicate phosphate gel.

The set cement consists of unreacted core of ZnO glass particles bonded together by the "aluminosilicophosphate gel matrix gel".

Properties

Biological Properties

a. Toxicity: Nontoxic to the oral tissues.
b. *Acidity:* High initial acidity and prolonged low pH (4-5) after setting.
c. *Anticariogenic action:* Exhibits anticariogenic property due to leaching of fluoride ions and other ions from set cement.
d. *Germicidal effect:* Presence of silver and mercury compounds provides a germicidal action.
e. *Solubility and disintegration:* 0.9% by weight.

Rheological Properties

a. Working time: 4 minutes for type I.
b. Setting time: Type I: 5-9 minutes.
   Type II: 3-8 minutes.
c. Consistency: Type I: 25 ± 1 mm.
   Type II: 25 ± 1 mm.
d. Film thickness: 25 μm.

Mechanical Properties

a. Compressive strength
   Type I: > 140 Mpa.
   Type II: 170 Mpa.
b. Tensile strength: 7 Mpa.
c. Diametral tensile strength: 7.6 Mpa.
d. Surface hardness: Type I: 70 KHN.

Manipulation

The powder and liquid are dispensed on a cool glass slab. The powder is incorporated into liquid in 2-3 large increments. Mix it in a circular motion (mixing time—1 minute) to obtain required consistency.

Uses

- Luting agent for porcelain restorations.
- Intermediate restorations.
- Luting agent for orthodontic appliances.
- As a die material.
- Temporary posterior restorations.
- Restoration in deciduous teeth.

Advantages

- Better strength, toughness, and abrasion resistance than zinc phosphate cement.
- Good anticariogenic property.
- Lower solubility and better bonding properties.
- These are translucent unlike zinc phosphate.

Disadvantages

- High initial pH and total acidity greater than zinc phosphate cement.
- Pulpal sensitivity may be of longer duration than zinc phosphate cements.
- Manipulation is more critical than with the zinc phosphate cement.
- Stainless steel spatula should not be used for mixing.

ZINC POLYCARBOXYLATE CEMENTS

Smith discovered zinc polycarboxylate cements. It was the first cement system developed with a potential for adhesion to tooth structure. It is primarily used for cementation of restoration and thermal insulating base. It is also used as an intermediate restoration and luting agent for orthodontic purposes. These cements are also called as "Polyacrylate cements".

- ADA specification number: 61

Dispension

These cements are available as powder and liquid (Fig. 6.14).

- Powder, which is mixed with water (water settable cements).
- Precapsulated powder, liquid system.

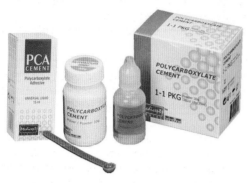

Fig. 6.14 Zinc polycarboxylate cement

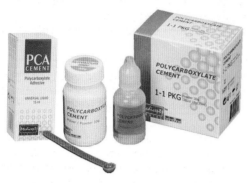

Fig. 6.15A Cross-linking of polyacid chains with Zn^{+2} ions

Composition

Powder		
Ingredient	Wt %	Functions
Zinc oxide	90%	Main reactive ingredient.
Magnesium oxide	1–5%	• Acts as modifier and aids in sintering. • Reduces the reactivity of ZnO.
Stannous oxide (part of MgO is replaced)		Decreases the reactivity of ZnO and adjusts the working time.
Stannous fluoride		• Helps in sintering by acting as a flux. • Increases the strength. • Anticariogenic effect.
Alumina, Silica, Bismuth, Stainless steel fibers	2–4%	Reinforcing fillers

Liquid	
Polyacrylic acid	• Main reactive ingredient. • Helps in bonding the material to tooth.
Water	Provides the reaction medium.
Tartaric acid	Decreases the setting time and increases the working time.
Copolymers like itaconic acid, maleic acid, and acrylic acid	Decreases the viscosity.

Manufacturing of Powder

The ingredients of the powder are sintered at temperature between 1000°C and 1400°C into a cake. The ingredients melt due to the presence of the fluoride, which acts as a fusing agent to form an ion leachable glass mass. The fused mass is then pulverized to form a powder and sieved to obtain the desired particle size.

Setting Reaction

The setting reaction of zinc polycarboxylate cement involves powder particles dissolution by the polyacrylic acid of liquid that releases Zn, Mg, Sn ions. These ions bind to the polymer chain via the carboxyl groups. These ions react with carboxyl group of adjacent polyacid chains. So that a cross-linked salt is formed as cement sets as shown the Figure 6.15A.

Structure of Set Cement

The set cement composes of an amorphous zinc polycarboxylate ionic gel matrix in which unreacted zinc oxide particles are dispersed.

Properties

Biological Properties

Biocompatibility A major factor in the popularity of this cement system is its excellent biocompatibility to the pulp. The chief reasons for this property are:

1. The rapid rise of the cement pH towards neutrality.
2. Localization of the polyacrylic acid and limitation of diffusion by its molecular size and ion bonding to dentinal fluids and proteins.
3. The minimal movement of fluid in the dentinal tubules in response to the cement.
4. Contains fluoride releasing agents and releases fluoride ions, which are taken up by neighboring enamel and which presumably will exert anticariogenic effect.

Toxicity This cement is nonirritant and nontoxic to the dental tissues. The effect of these cements on the pulp is less than that of ZOE cement. Polyacrylate cements induce the formation of reparative dentin in exposed pulp. It has good compatibility with the pulp.

Acidity The pH of the liquid cement is approximately 1.7 when the cement is first mixed. However, the liquid is rapidly neutralized by the powder. Thus, the pH of the mix rises rapidly as the setting proceeds.

Rheological Properties

Viscosity Initial viscosity is higher than zinc phosphate cement and a delay of 2 minutes in cementation increases the viscosity considerably.

Film thickness Film thickness (25–48 µm) of this cement is higher than that of zinc phosphate cement. It acts as pseudoplastic material and undergoes thinning at an increased shear rate.

Working and setting time Working time is shorter than zinc phosphate cement, lowering the temperature of the reaction can increase the working time.

    Mixing time – 30-45 seconds.
    Working time – 1-1½ minutes.
    Setting time – 7 to 9 minutes.

Factors affecting setting time
1. Sintering temperature: Increase in the temperature decreases the rate of setting reaction.
2. Particle size: Finer particles react quickly.

3. Tartaric acid: Increases the working time and decreases the setting time.
4. Setting time increases by using cool glass slab.
5. Presence of additives: Additives such as stannous fluoride act as fusing agents. Increasing the concentration of fluorides will prolong the working and setting time.
6. Molecular weight and concentration of polyacrylic acid: Increase the molecular weight and concentration of polyacrylic acid longer the setting time because polyacrylic acid is a weak acid and hence undergoes feeble dissociation, further the molecular weight inhibits the mobility of its ions and reacts with the constituents of the powder, thereby lengthening the setting time.
7. P/L ratio: Increases the P/L ratio decreases the setting time and vice-versa.
8. Reactivity of ZnO: Greater the reactivity of ZnO, faster is the rate of setting reaction and shorter is the setting time.

Mechanical Properties

Compressive strength: Compressive strength of luting cement is 55 to 85 MPa and for the base cement it is around 70-90 MPa. The cement gains strength rapidly after the initial setting period, the strength at 1 hour is about 80% of the 24 hours value.

Tensile strength: It is 40% higher than strength of zinc phosphate cement. The tensile strength is 8-12 MPa for luting and for base is around 9-14 MPa.

Modulus of elasticity: It is about 1/3rd of that of zinc phosphate cement, mixed to a luting consistency. The MOE is 5-6 GPa for luting and for base is 4-5 GPa.

Adhesion and bond strength: Bond strength is highest of the cements as it chemically bonds to the enamel and dentin of the tooth. Polyacrylic acid reacts with Ca^{+2} ions via carboxyl groups on the surface of enamel or dentin as shown in the Figure 6.15B. The bonding mechanism with dentin collagen can be explained by two

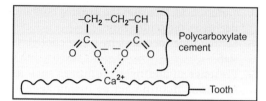

Fig. 6.15B Polyacid ions reacting with Ca^{+2} ions of tooth

methods, such as hydrogen bonding and ion diffusion. Hydrogen bond is formed between the carboxylic group (COO^-) of poly acrylic acid and NH_2 groups of dentin collagen. In case of latter method, Mg^{+2} ions are diffused and form cation bridges between the carboxylic groups (COO^-) of polyacrylic acid and collagen. The bond strength to enamel is greater than dentin. It is about 3.45–13.1 MNm^{-2} to enamel and 2.07 MNm^{-2} to that of dentin.

Dimensional stability This cement shows a linear contraction when setting takes place at 37°C. The amount of contraction varies from 1% for wet specimen in one day to 6% for a dry specimen in 14 days.

Surface hardness Surface hardness for these cements is 60 KHN.

Optical Properties

They are very opaque due to large quantities of unreacted zinc oxide.

Thermal Properties

They are good thermal insulators.

Manipulation

Surface Preparation

Clean surfaces are essential for promoting adhesion. Commonly used method is etching with polyacrylic acid for 10–20 seconds, followed by washed with water for 20 seconds.

Selection of Materials

Cool and thick glass slab or nonabsorbing paper pad, stainless steel spatula.

Proportioning

Luting consistency: 1.5 g/1 ml.
Base consistency: 2–3 g/1 ml.

Mixing

Glass slab or plastic coated paper pad is recommended for mixing in order to avoid absorption of liquid.

Liquid is dispensed just before mixing onto the slab. Half of the powder is incorporated into the liquid and mixed for the prescribed time; next increment of the powder is incorporated into the liquid and mixed until a creamy consistency is reached. The mix should have a shiny glossy appearance.

Mixed cement is thixotropic; viscosity decreases as the shear rate increases. The correct consistency of the cement is indicated by a viscous mix that will flow back under its own weight, when lifted with spatula.

Mixing time: 45 seconds.
Setting time: 7–9 minutes.

Cementation

The mix is applied to the seating surfaces of indirect restoration as well as on the prepared tooth structure. The cost restoration is then placed on the prepared tooth and is firmly held under pressure until the cement sets.

Precautions

- A meticulously clean surface is necessary in order to provide intimate contact between the cement and the tooth.
- The cavity should be isolated after cleansing to prevent further contamination from the oral fluids.
- Polyacrylic acid liquid should not be stored in refrigerator, because the viscosity of the liquid increases with decrease in temperature (the intramolecular bonding will form to make it gel).
- Liquid should not be dispensed until just before the mixing is to be started.
- Cementation should be done before the cement loses its glossy appearance or before cob-webbing occurs.

- Instruments should be cleaned before cement sets on them.

Advantages

1. Excellent biocompatibility to the pulp.
2. Anticariogenic property.
3. Adhesion to the tooth substance and some alloys.
4. Freshly mixed cement exhibits pseudoplastic property.
5. Adequate tensile strength, film thickness and solubility.
6. Easy to manipulate.

Disadvantages

1. Accurate proportioning is required for optimum properties.
2. Need for clean surfaces to utilize adhesion property.
3. Shorter mixing and working time.
4. Lower compressive strength than zinc phosphate cement.
5. Anticariogenic property is not as good as silicate cement.
6. Poor bonding to the metallic restoration unless a rough surface is created at the metal-cement interface.
7. Removal of excess material is difficult after set.

Uses

- Used for luting of indirect restorations.
- For cementation of orthodontic bands.
- As bases and liners.
- Rarely for temporary restorations.

Water Settable Cement

The powder composition is same as the conventional zinc polycarboxylate cement with slight changes. Polyacrylic acid is freezed, dried and added to powder. The cement powder, i.e. mixed with water contains 15–18% polyacrylic acid coated on the oxide particles.

The water-mix materials tend to give slightly longer setting times as with other cements, working time can be substantially increased by mixing the material on a cool glass slab and by refrigerating the powder. The liquid should not be chilled as this encourages gelation due to hydrogen bonding.

GLASS IONOMER CEMENTS

Wilson and Kent developed Glass Ionomer Cements in 1969. Glass ionomer is the generic name of a group of materials that use silicate glass powder and an aqueous solution of polyacrylic acid. This material acquires its name from its formulation of glass powder and an ionomeric acid. That contains COOH groups.

Glass ionomer cements are also referred to as poly- alkanoate cements or ASPA (Aluminosilicate polyacrylic acid) cement.

Glass ionomer cements were developed in an attempt to capitalize on the favorable properties of both silicate and polycarboxylate cements.

These cements contain an ion leachable glass, which is mainly composed of fluoro-aluminosilicate glass and a polyelectrolyte (polyacrylic acid) as liquid. The ion leachable glass can react with water-soluble polymer acid to yield cement. A polyelectrolyte is an electrolyte where either the cation or the anion is a polymer bearing a multiplicity of electrical charges. Polyacrylic acid is an example for anionic polyelectrolyte.

Originally, the cement was designated for the esthetic restoration of anterior teeth and it was recommended for use in restoring teeth with class III and V cavity preparations. Also, because the cement produces a truly adhesive bond to tooth structure, it is particularly useful for the conservative restoration of eroded areas. The need for mechanical retention via a cavity preparation is eliminated or reduced. Thus, it has one advantage over composite resins when used for this purpose.

Development

1969	First developed by AD Wilson and BE Kent.
1973	First material marketed (ASPA IV)

1975	First luting material.
1978	Cermet ionomer cements
1982	Water activated cements
1986	Resin modified cements
1988-89	First commercial product from 3M (Vitrebond)
1990-93	Resin-ionomer hybrid, liners and restoratives were introduced
1994	Resin-glass ionomer hybrids officially named – Resin modified glass ionomer cements at the International Symposium on Glass Ionomer cements.
1995	Present: Introduction of compomers and packable glass ionomers.

Commercial Names

Aquacem	Type I
Fuji I	Type I
Chem Film	Type II
Logo Film	Type II
Ketac Bond	Type III
Vitra Bond	Light cure glass ionomer

- ADA specification number: 66

Classifications

Type I	Luting
Type II	Restorative
Type III	Liners and bases
Fuji IV	Pit and fissure sealants
Fuji V	Orthodontic purpose
Fuji VI	Core build up

Fuji VII	Caries stabilization and protection
Fuji VIII	Atraumatic restorative treatment
Fuji IX	Geriatric patients

Modes of Supply/Dispension

- Powder and liquid form (Figs 6.16A and B).
- Preproportioned powder/liquid in capsules (Fig. 6.16C).
- Light cure system.
- Powder and distilled water or water-settable cement.

Manufacture of Powder

The components of powder are fused together at a temperature of 1100°C–1500°C. The fused glass is then grounded to particle size of 20–50 μ.

Setting Reaction

The setting reaction is an acid-base reaction between the acidic polyelectrolyte and the aluminosilicate glass.

When the powder and liquid are mixed together, the acid liquid attacks the surface of the glass particles. Thus calcium, aluminum, sodium and fluoride ions are leached into the aqueous medium, probably in the form of complexes as shown in Figure 6.17.

The salts hydrate to form a gel matrix and the unreacted glass particles are sheathed by silica gel, which arises from removal of cations from the surface of the particles .

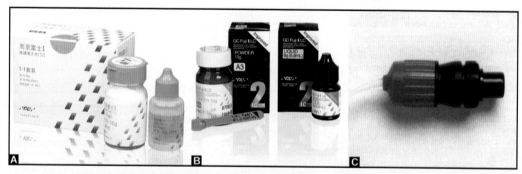

Figs 6.16A to C Glass ionomer cement (A) Type I; (B) Type II; (C) Glass ionomer cement capsule

Composition

Powder		
Ingredient	*Wt %*	*Functions*
SiO_2	29%	Reacts with Al_2O_3 to form the aluminosilicate network of the Ca aluminofluorosilicate glass powder.
Al_2O_3	16.6%	• Acts as filler. • Regulates the setting reaction of the cement.
CaF_2	34.3%	• Acts as a flux. • Reduces fusion temperature of the glass powder. • Produces opacity to the mix.
Na_3AlF_6	5.0%	• Acts as flux. • F^- acts as anticariogenic agent. • Provides opacity to the mix.
AlF_3	5.3%	Acts as flux.
$AlPO_4$	9.8%	Also acts as flux and also furnishes additional Al ions to the set matrix.
Liquid		
Polyacrylic acid in the form of copolymers	50%	Increases the reactivity of liquid. Decreases viscosity and gelation tendency.
Tartaric acid	5%	Improves the handling characteristics.
Water	45%	Serves as a reaction medium initially and then slowly hydrates the cross-linked matrix.

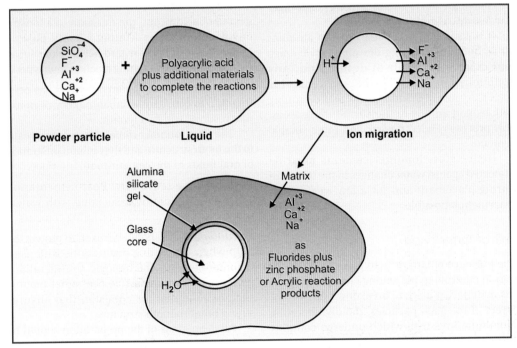

Fig. 6.17 Setting mechanism of glass ionomer cement

Structure of Set Cement

The structure of set cement comprises unreacted glass particles surrounded by silica gel in a matrix of polyanions cross-linked by ionic bridges.

Role of Water

Water present in the liquid is an important ingredient.

- Acts as a reaction medium during the initial reaction phase. During this phase water can be readily removed by desiccation and is called as loosely bound water.
- As the reaction continues the same water hydrates the matrix and cannot be removed by desiccation and is then called as tightly bound water.
- Hydrates the cross-linked matrix, increasing the strength of the cement and results in a stable gel structure.

If freshly mixed cements are kept isolated from ambient air, the loosely held water will slowly become tightly bound water over time. This phenomenon results in cement, i.e. stronger and less susceptible to moisture.

If the same matrix is exposed to ambient air without any covering the surface will craze and crack as a result of desiccation. Any contamination by water that occurs at this stage can cause dissolution of the matrix forming cations and anions to the surrounding areas. This process results in weak and more soluble cement.

Hence glass ionomer cements must be protected against water changes in the structure during placement and for a few weeks after placement if possible.

Role of Tartaric Acid

The presence of tartaric acid plays a significant part in controlling the setting characteristics of the materials. It helps to breakdown the surface layers of the glass particles, rapidly liberating aluminum ions with which undergo complex formation. Hence the aluminum ions are not immediately available for reaction with the poly acid. So the working time of the cement is prolonged. The initial onset of setting is further inhibited by the tartaric acid preventing unwinding and ionization of the poly acid chains.

Water-Settable Cements

The polyacrylic acid copolymer may be frozen, dried and then mixed with glass ionomer powder. In this case, the liquid is water or water with tartaric acid. These cements are known as water-settable cements and they set faster than those with polyacrylic acid.

Properties

Biological Properties

Biocompatibility: Many histological studies indicate that type-II glass ionomers are relatively biocompatible. They elicit a greater pulpal reaction than ZOE but generally less than that from zinc phosphate cements. Poly acids are relatively weak acids.

However, the P/L ratio influences the degree of acidity and the duration of a low pH environment. Type-I luting cement poses a greater hazard in this regard because of a lower P/L ratio and slower setting reaction than type-II.

Effect on pulp: Glass ionomer cement has been reported to cause some inflammatory response that resolves within a month.

The glass ionomer cements bond chemically to the tooth structure and they inhibit infiltration of oral fluids at the cement-tooth interface.

Postoperative sensitivity: Post-cementation sensitivity frequently associated with water-settable cements and various luting cements.

Precautions: Care should be taken to protect the pulp when cementing restorations with glass ionomer cement. The biologic considerations take a more important role over other matters such as potential for adhesion that ensures strong bond to tooth structure.

All deep areas of the preparation should be protected by a thin layer of hard setting calcium hydroxide cement.

Table 6.12 pH of poly acid liquid and water settable cements at different time

Type of cement	2 min.	5 min.	10 min	15 min	20 min	30 min	60 min	24 hrs
Polyacid liquid	2.33	3.26	3.78	3.91	3.98	4.18	4.55	5.67
Water-settable	1.76	1.98	3.36	3.88	4.19	4.46	4.84	5.98

Acidity: One of the factors for pulp irritation is the pH and the length of the time that this acidity persists. The pH values of water settable and traditional powder poly acid cement over time were mentioned in the Table 6.12.

Although, the pH values of the two formulations are virtually same at 10 minutes, the pH water-settable cement is considerably lower than that of poly acid powder mix at 2 and 5 minutes. This low initial pH contributes to the moderate pulpal sensitivity.

Anticariogenic Property

Glass ionomer cements possess the same anticariogenic properties as does silicate cement. Type-II glass ionomers release fluoride in considerable amounts for an extended period. Anticariogenic property is discussed in detail in silicate cements of this book.

Chemical Properties

Solubility and disintegration: Like silicates, the initial solubility is high due to leaching of intermediate products or those not involved in matrix formation.

Rheological Properties

Working time: Working time is the time elapsed from the start of the mixing during which the consistency of the mix is low enough to flow readily under pressure to form a thin film.

Setting time
    Type I – 4 to 5 minutes.
    Type II – 7 minutes.

Film thickness: Film thickness should not exceed 20 µm for luting agents.

Table 6.13 Comparison of mechanical properties of type II glass ionomer cement with small hybrid composite

Property	Type II glass ionomer	Typical small hybrid composite
Compressive	Up to 200 MPa	350–500 MPa strength
Tensile strength	15 MPa	34–62 MPa
MOE	20,000 MPa	13,500–18,000 Mpa
COTE	$10.2–11.4 \times 10^{-6}/°C$	$25–38 \times 10^{-6}/°C$
Thermal diffusivity	$0.198 \text{ mm}^2/ \text{sec.}$	$0.675 \text{ mm}^2/ \text{sec.}$

Mechanical Properties

Compressive strength: Compressive strength is less than that of silicate cement. The compressive strength of glass ionomer cements is 150 MPa.

Tensile strength: Higher tensile strength when compared to silicates. The tensile strength of glass ionomer cements is 6.6 MPa or 960 PSI.

Hardness: Wear resistance of glass ionomer cement is also less when compared to composites. The hardness of glass ionomer cements is 48 KHN.

Adhesion: Glass ionomer cement has good adhesion to enamel and dentin. The bond strength is around 225 MN/m² after 7 days.

Glass ionomer bonds chemically to tooth structure. The bonding is due to the reaction between the carboxyl groups of the poly acids and the calcium in the apatite of the enamel and dentin. Comparison of mechanical properties of Type II glass ionomer cement with small hybrid composites were given in Table 6.13.

Other Mechanical Properties

- COTE is similar to dentin
- Low flexural strength (type I – 12 MPa)
- Low shear strength
- Dimensional change (slightly expands). Also undergoes shrinkage on setting, expands with water sorption
- Brittle in nature
- Lacks translucency
- Rough surface texture.

Optical Properties

Glass ionomers are inferior to silicates and composites in this respect. They lack translucency and have a rough surface texture.

Manipulation

For a successful restoration of glass ionomer cement, the rules to be followed are:
- Conditioning of the tooth surface.
- Proper manipulation.
- Protection of cement during setting.
- Finishing.

Preparation of Tooth Surface

The smear layer present after the cavity preparation tends to block off the tooth surface. This can be eliminated by—
a. Pumice wash.
b. Polyacrylic acid solution.

Proportioning

Powder/liquid ratio is generally 3:1 by weight. However, the manufacturer's recommendation should be followed.

Mixing

Mixing can be done either of two mixing techniques depends on the kind of material being used.

a. *Hand mixing*
- The powder and liquid is dispensed onto a paper pad or glass slab, just prior to mixing. A cool dry glass slab is used (Fig. 6.18A).
- The powder is divided into two equal increments (Fig. 6.18A).
- Mixing is done with an agate spatula. Mixing time is 45 sec (Fig. 6.18B).
- As soon as the mix reached to the required consistency as shown in Figure 6.18C, the mix is immediately used for cementation or packed into the cavity with a plastic instrument.

b. *Mechanical mixing:* This method is used for cements supplied in capsule form, which contains preproportioned powder and liquid and is mixed in an amalgamator.

Advantages
- Better properties due to controlled P/L ratio.
- Less mixing time involved.
- Convenient delivery system.

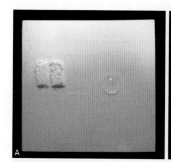 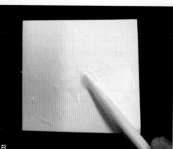 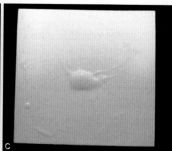

Figs 6.18A to C Stages in GIC mixing. (A) Dispension of powder and liquid on paper mixing pad; (B) Mixing; (C) Consistency for cementation

Disadvantages
- Amount of cement needed is limited by the manufacturer.
- Number of shades provided is limited.

Protection of Cement during Setting

A preshaped matrix is applied.
- Protect the cement from the environment during initial set.
- Provide maximum contour.

Finishing

Excess material should be trimmed from the margins. Failure to protect the cement surface results in a chalky or crazed surface.
- Due to lack of protection with matrix.
- Low P/L ratio.
- Improper manipulation.

Precautions
- Tooth should be clean for effective adhesion.
- The surface should be kept free from saliva or moisture, which interferes with bonding.
- Dispense the liquid just before mixing.
- Spatula used is either agate or plastic.
- Liquid should not be stored in refrigerator.
- Last portions of the liquid should be discarded.

Uses

- Cementation of cast and porcelain restorations and orthodontic bands.
- As cavity liners and base materials.
- As a restorative material.

Indication for use of Type II Glass Ionomer Cements

- Nonstress bearing areas.
- Class-I and II restorations in primary dentition.
- Class-III and V restorations in adults.
- Temporary or caries control restorations.
- Crown margin repairs.
- Cement base under amalgam, resin, ceramics, and direct and indirect gold.

- Core buildups when at least 3 walls of tooth are remaining (after crown preparation).

Contraindications

i. High stress applications.
ii. Class IV and II restorations.
iii. Cusp replacement.
iv. Core buildups with less than 3 sound walls remaining.

Advantages

- Biocompatible with tooth substance and surrounding tissues.
- Significant anticariogenic property.
- Bonds chemically with enamel and dentin.
- No marginal leakage.
- COTE is similar tooth structure.
- Low thermal conductivity.
- Good esthetics.
- Ten years of clinical studies (conventional glass ionomers).

Disadvantages

- Susceptible to acid attack.
- High initial solubility.
- Susceptible to attack by water during setting.
- Brittle and low tensile strength.
- Cannot be used to restore fractured incisal edges because of its brittleness.
- Poor abrasion resistance.
- Insufficient translucency and opacity is higher than resin.
- Less polishability than resin.
- Should not be used in high stress bearing areas.
- Poor longevity in xerostomic patients.

MODIFICATIONS

Metal Modified Glass Ionomer or Glass Cermet or Ketac Silver

Glass ionomer cements have been modified by the inclusion of metal filler particles in an attempt to improve the strength, fracture toughness and resistance to wear.

Two methods of modification have been employed.

1. The first approach is that of mixing spherical silver amalgam alloy powder with the type II glass ionomer powder. This cement is referred to as a "silver alloy admix".
2. The second system involves fusing glass powder to silver particles through high temperature sintering of a mixture of the two powders. This cement is commonly referred to as a "Cermet".

Manufacturing of Cermets

The cermet powder is manufactured by mixing and palletizing under pressure a mixture of metal or glass powder. The pellets are fused at around 800°C, and then grounded to fine powder. The powder particles consist of regions of metal firmly bonded to the glass.

Biological Properties

Biocompatibility: These properties are similar to that of the conventional glass ionomers. pH is around 6–7.

Anticariogenic property: The admixed cement release more fluoride ions than type-II glass ionomer cement. Less fluoride ions are released from cermet than type-II glass ionomer cement.

Mechanical Properties

- Strength and fracture toughness is same as conventional cement.
- Wear resistance increased slightly than conventional cements.
- Chemically bonds to the enamel and dentin.

Esthetics

Gray in color. So cannot be used as anterior restorative material.

Fissure Sealing

The use of glass ionomer in sealant therapy will increase, as formulations are developed that are less viscous and have good wear resistance.

Applications

- Core buildup material.
- Posterior restorative material.

Advantages

- Have greater value of compressive strength and fatigue limit than conventional glass ionomer cement.
- The rapid setting, which occurs with these materials is probably responsible for their marked improvement in erosion resistant when compared with most other glass ionomer cements.
- Wear resistance increased slightly than conventional cements.

Disadvantages

- Flexural strength and resistance to abrasive wear appear to be no better than values recorded for conventional glass ionomers.
- Poor esthetics.

Resin Modified Glass Ionomer Cement

To overcome the two inherent drawbacks such as moisture sensitivity and low early strength due to slow acid-base reaction, these resin modified glass ionomers were developed. Products are available as chemical curing and light curing.

These materials are known as:

- Light cure glass ionomer cements
- Dual cure
- Tricure
- Resin ionomers
- Hybrid ionomers.

Composition

Powder	
Powder	*Liquid*
Ion leachable glasses	Polyacrylic acid
Light or chemical cure initiators or both	Water
Polymerizable resin	Methacrylates monomer HEMA monomers

Properties

Mixing time: 30 seconds.
Working time: 2.5 minutes.
pH: 3–5 initially.

There is reduction in translucency due to the difference in refractive index between the powder and set matrix.

Strength: Tensile strength is higher than conventional glass ionomer cement due to greater plastic deformation. Compressive strength is 105 MPa.

Adhesion to tooth structure: They have less shear bond strength than conventional glass ionomer cements.

Adhesion to restorative materials: They are used primarily as liners and bases. Resin modified glass ionomer cements have higher bond strength to composite.

Marginal adaptation: They exhibit greater shrinkage on setting due to polymerization. More P:L ratio exhibits greater microleakage.

Water sensitivity: Liner versions of these glass ionomer cements are susceptible for dehydration and also absorb water.

Clinical Considerations

- Used as liners and bases
- As fissure sealants.
- As core buildup material.
- As luting medium for orthodontic brackets.
- Repair for damaged amalgam core and cusps and retrograde root canal fillings.

Packable or High Viscosity Glass Ionomers

These are also called as "high strength glass ionomer cements". These are developed for the atraumatic restorative technique (ART) for use in third world countries.

These are the strong caries control restorations they require no curing light. The setting reaction is similar to that of the conventional cement. These cements require high P:L ratios.

Properties

- Increased compressive and flexural strengths.
- Low solubility.
- Improved wear resistance.
- Increased surface hardness.
- More "Packable" than conventional glass ionomers.
- Radiopaque.

Atraumatic Restorative Technique

ART is an acronym for "Atraumatic Restorative Technique." This procedure was designed to combat rampant caries in second and third world regions around the globe where immediate dental care was not available. Patients with rampant caries were treated by nondental personnel or themselves by scooping out caries, mixing P/L components between their thumb and forefinger into a ball, and plugging the hole to create a temporary restoration. These materials release some fluoride but succeed mostly because they are capable of producing a good seal to tooth structure, are sufficiently tough to resist fracture, and can be easily repaired. They are simply a holding procedure to buy time (perhaps 12–18 months) until a patient can get to a normal dental clinic and receive professional care. The remarkable offshoot is that these materials perform better than expected and often provide 3–4 years of service. For that reason, pediatric dentists now consider ART materials as substitutes for both amalgam and composites. They can be easily placed and do not require special isolation techniques.

Low Viscosity Glass Ionomer Cements

These materials are also called as *flowable glass ionomer cements*. They require low P:L ratio to increase flow.

Clinical Applications

- Lining.
- Pit and fisure sealer.
- Endodontic sealer.
- Sealing hypersensitive cervical area.

Compomers

Compomers are also called as polyacid-modified composite resins. They were introduced to the profession in the early 1990s. These are a group of esthetic materials for the restoration of teeth damaged by dental caries. The trivial name was devised from the names of these two "parent" materials, the "comp" coming from composite, and "omer" from Ionomer. They were designed to combine the esthetics of traditional composite resins with the fluoride release and adhesion of glass-ionomer cements.

Composition

- Macro-monomers/Prepolymerized polymers: Main ingredient, e.g. Bis-GMA, and/ or UEDMA.
- Diluents: Added to reduce the viscosity of polymers, e.g. Triethylene glycol dimethacrylate (TEGDMA).
- Fillers: Improves strength, e.g. Quartz or a silicate glass.
- Coupling agents: Added to provide bonding between resin matrix and filler particles.
- Photo initiator: Initiates polymerization, e.g. camphorquinone
- Photo accelerator: Accelerates the polymerization reaction, e.g. Amine accelerator.
- Reactive glass powder, which is similar to the powder of conventional glass ionomer cements.
- In addition, compomers also contain *additional monomers* that differ from those in conventional composites, e.g. Acidic functional groups such as TCB, which is a *diester of 2-HEMA* with *butane tetracarboxylic acid*.

Clinical Applications

Compomers are designed for the same sort of clinical applications as conventional composites. These include Class II and Class V cavities, as fissure sealants, and as bonding agents for the retention of orthodontic bands.

Their fluoride release, however, is seen as a useful feature for use in pedodontics, and certain brands have been produced that are specifically aimed at children. Recently, a multicolored dual-cure compomer known as MagicFil produced by Zenith Dental of Englewood, New Jersey that is available in four bright colors with glitter inclusions.

Amino Acid Modified Glass Ionomer Cements

Fracture toughness of glass ionomer cement can be improved by modifying acrylic acid copolymers with *N-acryloyl- or N-methacryloyl-amino acids,* e.g. N-methacryloyl glutamic acid.

Nanoionomers

These are hybrids of a resin modified GIC and nano filled dental composites. These are designed to be quickly and easily mixed, e.g. Ketac nano light curing GIC.

Advantages

- Greater wear resistance.
- Esthetics and polish compared to conventional and RMGIC.

Ceramic Reinforced Posterior Glass Ionomer Cements

These are designed to match strength and durability of amalgam. It is available in white and a universal tooth shade. Dispensed in powder-liquid form and water settable form is also available, e.g. Amalgomer.

Advantages

- Excellent wear resistance.
- Superior radio opacity.
- High level of fluoride release.
- Good compatibility.
- Natural adhesion.
- Excellent for core build ups and posterior restorations.

Pit and Fissure Sealant

A cariostatic effect is a desirable property of any material used for patients who are highly likely to develop caries. Thus, glass ionomer cements are viable materials as fissure sealants. However, the traditional ionomer cement is somewhat viscous, which prevents penetration of depth of the fissure.

The use of glass ionomers in sealant therapy should increase as less viscous formulations are developed especially if they are marketed especially as sealant, e.g. light cured products.

The retention rate of glass ionomer sealant may be poor after one year, but no sign of caries can be observed.

RESIN CEMENTS

A variety of resin-based cements have now become available because of the development of the direct filling resins with improved properties, the acid-etch technique for attaching resins to enamel and molecules with a potential bond to dentin conditioned with organic or inorganic acid. Some are designed for general use and others for specific uses such as attachment of orthodontic brackets or resin-bonded bridges.

The majority of the materials in this group are polymethacrylates of two types:

Type I: Materials based on methyl methacrylate.

Type II: Materials based on aromatic dimethacrylate of BIS-GMA type.

The closely related cyanoacrylate monomers, notably ethyl and isobutyl, have found some limited use for the attachment of facings and for cementation. However, the hydrolytic stability and biologic effects in this situation is suspect and little use is made of them.

Acrylic Resin Cements

These cements are based on chemically activated methyl methacrylate (MMA).

Dispension

These cements are dispensed in the form of powder and liquid.

Composition

Powder
- Finely divided PMMA (low molecular weight polymer) or copolymer.
- Benzoyl peroxide – Initiator.
- Mineral filler.
- Color pigments – Gives characteristic color.

Liquid
- MMA monomer
- Accelerator – Amine (3° amine) – Dimethyl P-toluidine.
  Benzoyl peroxide reacts with the 3° amine under certain conditions to yield free radicals, which propagate the polymerization reaction.

Setting

The monomer dissolves and softens the polymer particles and concurrently polymerizes through the action of free-radicals from the peroxide-amine interaction (or by light activation also [Camphoroquinone-amine system]). Several systems use both mechanisms and are referred to as "dual-cure" systems.

Properties

Biological properties: These cements cause irritation to the pulp. Thus, pulp should be protected either with a Ca(OH)$_2$ or glass ionomer liners.

Obviously, if the bonding area involves only enamel, or if the dentin thickness is sufficient, the irritating properties of the monomers are not significant.

Other properties: The properties of those materials are comparable to those of cold curing acrylic resin filling materials. They are stronger and less soluble than other types of cements but display low rigidity and viscoelastic properties (Table 6.14). These have effective bond to tooth structure in the presence of moisture, and they may show better bonding than other cements to resin facings and polycarbonate crowns.

Table 6.14 Properties of acrylic resin cements

Setting time (Min.)	Film thickness (µm)	Compressive strength 24 hrs (Mpa)	MOE (GPa)	Solubility and Disintegration in water (%)	Pulpal response
2-4	< 25	70-172	2.1-3.1	0.0-0.01	Moderate

Manipulation

The two components are combined by mixing on a treated paper pad for 20–30 seconds. The liquid is added to the powder with minimum spatulation to avoid air incorporation. The mix must be used immediately because working time is short. Excess material must be removed at the final set hard stage and not when the material is in rubbery state, otherwise the cement may be pulled from beneath the margin of restoration leaving a void that increases the risk of plaque build up and secondary caries. Removal of the excess cement is difficult if it is delayed until the cement has polymerized. It is best to remove the excess cement immediately after the restoration is seated.

Uses

- Used for cementation of temporary crowns and conventional bridges.
- Also can be used for cementation of resin bridges and facings.

Advantages

- Relatively high strength and toughness.
- Low solubility.

Disadvantages

- Short working time.
- Deleterious effects on the pulp.
- Difficult in removal of excess cement from margins.
- Polymerization shrinkage.

Modified Acrylic Resin Cements

Uses

- Used primarily for the direct bonding of orthodontic brackets.
- Also used for crown and bridge cementation.

Dispension

Dispensed as powder and liquid system.

Type I: Methacryloxy ethyl phenyl phosphonate (Organophosphonate system).

Type II: 4-META system.

Type III: HEMA (Hydroxy ethyl methacrylate) system.

Composition

These cements are self-cured, P–L systems formulated as shown below:

System I: This phosphonate cement recently reformulated as a 2-paste system, contains Bis-GMA resin and silanized quartz filler.

The phosphonate is very sensitive to O_2, so a gel is provided to coat the margins of a restoration until setting occurs.

The phosphate end of the phosphonate reacts with Ca of the tooth or with a metal oxide.

System II: The 4-META cement is formulated with MMA monomer and acrylic resin filler and is catalyzed by tributyl boron, which is an additional initiator.

The double bonded ends of both phosphonate and 4-META cement react with other double bonds when available.

System III: HEMA is added to the monomer liquid.

These three systems are added to the monomer liquid, i.e. MMA. The powder is as usual, PMMA with silane-treated inorganic fillers. The fillers are those used in composites and colloidal silica.

Properties

Biological properties: Biological properties are almost similar that of the conventional acrylic resin cements.

Bond strength: The adhesive resin cements generally develop good bond strengths to dentin.

Table 6.15 Mechanical properties of modified acrylic resin cements

Compressive strength (MPa)	Tensile strength (MPa)	MOE (GPa)	Bond strength to dentin (MPa)
52–224	37–41	1.2–10.7	11–24 with bonding agent

The adhesive resin cements have superior bonding to sand blasted Ni-Cr-Be and type IV gold alloys.

Mechanical properties were given in Table 6.15.

Manipulation

Manipulation is similar to that of the conventional acrylic cement.

Dimethacrylate Cements

These materials are of more recent development usually based on the bis–GMA system. They are combinations of an aromatic dimethacrylate with other monomers.

These dimethacrylates are discussed in detail in composite resins.

Dispension

- As P/L system and paste system: Self-cure-chemically activated.
- Two paste-dual cure system.
- One paste (step) conventional composite resin cement.
- Single component: Single paste light cure system.

Composition

P/L system: The powder is finely divided borosilicate or silicate glass or colloidal silica particles. In highly filled composite resin cements the silanated inorganic filler particles are more than 60% by weight and about 13 μm in diameter. In slightly filled cement the concentration of colloidal silica is 28%.

The liquid is mixture of bis-GMA or similar aromatic dimethacrylate, which is divided with low viscosity, low molecular weight alkyl dimethacrylate monomer. An amine accelerator is also present.

The paste systems contain a mixture of bis-GMA and monomers with variable amounts of fillers according to brand and chemical or light curing initiator systems similar to composite resin restorative materials.

Two paste-dual cure system: The dual cure cements come in a base-catalyst form and must be mixed before use. They are radiopaque for use in posterior portion of the mouth.

Light cured system: The light cured systems are single component systems, photo initiated by camphoroquinone and visible light. These are not usually radiopaque but provide a wide selection of shades, tints and opaquers.

Applications

1. These cements are used for the cementation of etched cast restorations and orthodontic bands.
2. Duel-cure composite resin cements are ideal for bonding of cast or CAD/CAM ceramic restorations or composite inlays prepared by an indirect technique.
3. Light-cure composite resin cements are useful for bonding of thin porcelain veneers where achieving adequate depth of cure is not a problem.

Advantages

- High strength.
- Low solubility.

Disadvantages

- Critical manipulative procedures.
- Low film thickness.
- High pulpal irritation and sensitivity.
- Difficulty in removing excess cement.

CAVITY LINING AGENTS AND CEMENT BASES

Dentin is a vital cellular tissue whenever it is injured by caries, cavity preparation, chemical irritation from restorative materials or bacterial contamination, a response will be manifested in the pulp. Significant pulp protection and other benefits can be obtained by the proper selection and use of cavity varnishes and liners.

The metallic restorations, being excellent thermal conductors can cause thermal sensitivity during the intake of hot and cold foods, or beverages. The phosphoric acid containing cements (i.e. $ZnPO_4$, silicate and Zn silico-phosphate) and direct filling resins, and some instances GIC can produce chemical irritation. Also, microleakage or interfacial leakage as a result of setting contraction of amalgam and resin composite restorations may also cause pulpal irritation.

As shown in Figure 6.19 cavity varnishes, liners, and bases are designed as adjuncts to the restorative materials, to protect the pulp against chemical and thermal trauma. In addition to serving as barriers against thermal change, irritants within the material, and interfacial leakage with associated bacterial invasion, some of these agents may have beneficial effects on the pulp. For example: ZOE compounds have a palliative effect upon the pulp and can aid in reducing sensitivity. $Ca(OH)_2$ is particularly beneficial, since it accelerates the formation of

reparative dentin and is employed as a pulp-capping agent. Thus, in the situation where there is the slightest possibility of microscopic pulp exposure, a layer of $Ca(OH)_2$ is applied to the pulpal wall regardless of the type of restorative material that is to be employed.

Technically, both varnishes and liners are classified as cavity lining agents because both are used as protective coatings. On the other hand, bases also serve as thermal insulations for metallic restorations. Varnishes and liners usually form a coating by evaporation of solvent, whereas bases and some newly introduced liners set by chemical process.

Requirements

1. Should be nontoxic and nonirritant to the pulp and other tissues.
2. Should be able to protect the pulp from effects of other restorative materials.
   a. Thermal insulation: Cement is used under a large metallic restoration (amalgam) to protect the pulp from temperature changes.
   b. Chemical protection: Cement should be able to prevent penetration of harmful chemicals from the restorative materials into the pulp.
   c. Electrical insulation under a metallic restoration to minimize galvanic effects.
3. Should have an antibacterial effect.
4. Ideally there should be adhesion between the cement and tooth tissue and between the cement and the tooth filling materials.
5. Should be insoluble in saliva and in liquids taken into the mouth.
6. Must develop mechanical properties such as strength rapidly to permit packing of a filling material.
7. Should have low thermal diffusivity and low COTE.
8. Should have good flow characteristics and adequate working time.

Cavity Varnishes

A cavity varnish is used to provide a barrier against the passage of irritants from cements

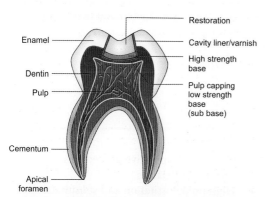

Fig. 6.19 Relative positions of cavity lining agents and cement bases in the prepared tooth cavity

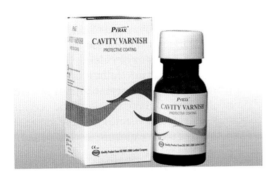

Fig. 6.20 Cavity varnish

or other restorative materials and to reduce the penetration of fluids at the tooth-restoration interface into the underlying dentin and pulp. They also reduce postoperative sensitivity.

As the thickness of the cavity varnish is very less they cannot be used as effective thermal insulators under metallic restorations.

Composition

Cavity varnishes are supplied as liquid in dark colored bottles (Fig. 6.20). Cavity varnish is a solution of one or more resins from natural gums (copal), synthetic resin or rosin (nitrated cellulose) which are dissolved in solvents like chloroform, acetone, benzene toluene, ethyl acetate and amyl acetate and also contains medicinal agents like chlorobutanol, thymol, and eugenol.

Properties and Indications

- Varnishes are insoluble and have a low resistance to abrasion.
- No antibacterial effects.
- Cavity varnishes neither possess mechanical strength nor provide thermal insulation because of the thin film thickness (2–40 μm).
- Protects the pulp from chemical and metallic irritants from the overlying restorations. For example, phosphoric acid is released into the underlying dentin and pulp from zinc phosphate, silicate and zinc silicophosphate cements and metallic irritants from amalgam or other metallic restorations.
- Prevents the discoloration of natural tooth by preventing the penetration of metallic ions from amalgam restoration into adjoining enamel and dentin.
- Reduces marginal leakage around amalgam restorations.
- Surface coating or protective agent for silicate cements to prevent desiccation.
- Surface coating agent over metallic restorations to prevent galvanic shocks by preventing the possible pathway of current generated.

Contraindications

- Acrylic or composite resins restoratives: The solvent of the varnish may react with resins and soften them.
- Glass ionomer cement: Varnish eliminates the potential for adhesion if applied between glass ionomer and the cavity walls.
- When therapeutic action is required from the overlying cement. For example: ZOE cement and calcium hydroxide cement.

Manipulation

Selection of varnish: Based on the characteristics of handling, flow and ability to be sealed when applied on the surface of the prepared cavity.

Painting (application) of varnish: The usual technique involves dipping a small cotton pledget (ball) held in pliers, into the varnish and then thoroughly painting all cavity walls. Brush or a wire loop may also be used for this purpose. The cotton pledget should not be dripping with excess varnish; the excess is removed by pressing the pledget against a bracket table cover.

1. Uniform and continuous coating should be made on all surfaces of prepared cavity.
2. Uneven coating or voids may produce erratic results.
3. Several thin layers should be applied.
4. When the first layer dries, small pinholes may develop which are filled up by second or third applications of the varnish and ensure a more continuous coating.

5. Approximately, 15–20 seconds should elapse between applications to allow the varnish to dry.
6. Varnish is applied in thin consistency. Thick varnishes will not wet the cavity wall and do not effectively inhibit marginal leakage.
7. The thick varnish is thinned with an appropriate solvent.

Precautions

1. Varnish solution should be tightly capped immediately after use to prevent loss of solvent by evaporation.
2. It should be applied in a thin consistency. Viscous varnish does not wet the cavity walls properly. It should be thinned with an appropriate solvent.
3. Excess varnish should not be left on the margins of the restorations as it prevents proper finishing of the margins of the restorations.
4. The cavity varnish must not be peeled from the cavity walls.

Cavity Liners

A cavity liner is used like a cavity varnish to provide barrier against the passage of irritants from cements or other restorative materials and to reduce the sensitivity of freshly cut dentin. Unlike a varnish, a liner may provide some therapeutic benefits to the tooth.

Ca(OH)₂ Liners

Composition

- One type of liner consists of a liquid in which calcium hydroxide or zinc oxide eugenol is suspended in a solution of natural or synthetic resin, methyl ethyl ketone or ethyl alcohol or in an aqueous solution of methyl cellulose. The methyl cellulose functions as a thickening agent. On evaporation of the volatile solvent, the liner forms a thin film on the prepared tooth surface.
- Two-paste systems (base and catalyst) form a fluid that flows readily over the cavity floor and hardens quickly into a solid mass.

- One paste with a solvent that evaporates and leaving a film of calcium hydroxide. The paste is an aqueous suspension of calcium hydroxide in methyl cellulose.
- Single paste system of calcium hydroxide and fillers of barium sulfate dispersed in a urethane dimethacrylate resin is also available. This contains initiators and accelerators, activated by visible light. The material polymerizes upon exposure to visible light.

Applications of Calcium Hydroxide Liners

- Accelerates the formation of reparative dentin.
- Which can neutralize or react with acid release from adjacent phosphoric acid containing cement since the pH of this is 11.
- As direct pulp-capping agent.
- As indirect pulp-capping agent.
- Some calcium hydroxide cements are too flexible and soluble to be used as sole bases or liners under amalgam restorations.
  When a calcium hydroxide liner contacts the pulp tissue a calcified bridge is formed that seals the vital tissue.

Zinc Oxide Eugenol Liners

Type-IV low viscosity zinc oxide eugenol cements are used as cavity liners.
- These liners are noted for their palliative effect upon pulp.
- These are considered as least irritating materials to the pulp of all materials used in cavity preparations.
- These materials are contraindicated under composite restorations because the eugenol interferes with polymerization and a defective restoration would result.

Glass-ionomer Liners

Two types of glass-ionomer liners are available. The first is a conventional P/L system. These materials tend to set little faster initially than do the restorative cements and are more free flowing.

The second type is light cured glass-ionomer cement. The liquid of at least one product contains hydroxy ethyl methacrylates (HEMA) and additional light activated accelerators. The material is placed in the prepared tooth and then exposed a resin curing light. With the light cure ionomer liners, conditioning of dentin surface is not required.

These liners are indicated in routine cases of composite resin restorations where there is no danger of pulp exposure.

In deep cavities the glass ionomer liner should be preceded by a calcium hydroxide liner covering the possible exposure site.

Sandwich Technique

In this technique, glass ionomer cement is sandwiched between the tooth and the composite resin restorative material as shown in Figure 6.21. Glass ionomer cement acts as bonding agent. This technique is recommended for the class-II composite restorations in particular.

Advantages of GIC Liners

- Anticariogenic property.
- Minimizes marginal leakage.
- Chemical bonding to the tooth structure.

Cement Bases

Cement bases are applied on the exposed dentin to protect the underlying pulp from external chemical, thermal, electrical and mechanical insults. The thickness of the base is usually 0.75–2 mm.

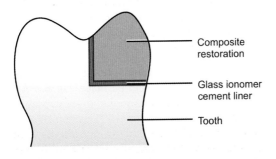

Fig. 6.21 Glass ionomer liner is sandwiched between the tooth and composite restoration

Classification of Cement Bases

According to its chemical nature

Acidic: Zinc phosphate, zinc polycarboxylate, glass ionomer cements

Neutral: ZOE cements

Alkaline: Calcium hydroxide cement.

According to the strength
a. Low strength bases
   For example, $Ca(OH)_2$ cements, ZOE cements.
b. High strength bases
   For example, zinc phosphate, zinc polycarboxylate, glass ionomer cements.

According to the dispension

Two-paste system: $Ca(OH)_2$ cements, ZOE cements

Powder-liquid system: Zinc phosphate, zinc polycarboxylate, $Ca(OH)_2$ cements, ZOE cements.

Single-paste system: Light activated $Ca(OH)_2$ cements.

Calcium Hydroxide Cements (Dycal)

Dispension

These materials are supplied in the form of powder-liquid, two-paste system (Fig. 6.22) and single-paste system.

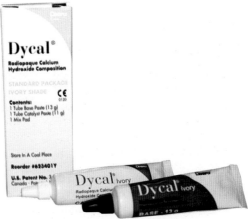

Fig. 6.22 Calcium hydroxide cement

Composition

Two-paste system

Base paste		
Ingredients	Wt %	Functions
Glycol salicylate	40	Main reactive ingredient
Calcium tungstate	16	Radiopacifiers
Calcium sulfate	30	Gives strength
TiO_2	14	Fillers
Reactor paste		
Ingredients	Wt %	Functions
$Ca(OH)_2$	50	Main reactive ingredient
ZnO	10	Reactive ingredient
Zn stearate	0.5	Provides strength

Properties

- These cements are alkaline in nature (pH is around 12).
- Setting time is 2.5–5.5 minutes.
- Compressive strength: 10–27 MPa.
- Tensile strength: <1.5 MPa.
- Good thermal insulator.

Uses

- Can be used as pulp capping agent (both direct and indirect).
- Can be used as a liner in deep cavities.
- Can be used as thermal insulating base.

Advantages

- Reparative dentin formation.
- Can neutralize strong acids.
- Easy to manipulate.
- Good sealing abilities.
- Rapid hardening in thin layers.

Disadvantages

- Strength is very less.
- Thermal insulation is not up to the mark.
- Dissolves in acidic conditions.
- Very weak when exposed to moisture.

COMPOSITE RESINS (TOOTH COLORED RESTORATIVE MATERIALS)

EVOLUTION

During 1st half of twentieth century – Silicates were widely used but because of severe erosion and lack of strength they were discontinued.

During late 1940 and 1950 – Resin was added to prevent this erosion led to the evolution of polymethyl methacrylate but due to curing shrinkage, lack of wear resistance, and thermal expansion led to the failure of these resins.

To overcome these drawbacks, inert filler called quartz was added which reduced curing shrinkage and thermal expansion, but due to the inability of the filler to bond to resin led to the failure, as it caused microleakage, staining and poor wear resistance.

But in 1962, Dr Ray L Bowen achieved bonding between filler particles and resin and designed a perfect composite. **Bowen's composite included** resin, filler and coupling agents.

DEFINITIONS

Composite

Composite is a mixture of two or more macromolecules, which are essentially insoluble with each other and produce properties superior or intermediate to those of the individual constituents.

Matrix

A plastic resin material that forms the continuous phase and binds the filler particles (Fig. 6.23A).

Fillers

The inorganic or organic particles that are designed to strengthen a composite, decrease

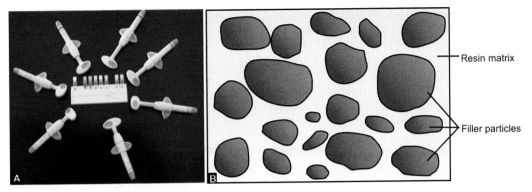

Figs 6.23A and B (A) Microstructure of composite (B) Light curing composite resin

thermal expansion, minimize polymerization shrinkage and decrease water sorption of the resin (Fig. 6.23A).

Coupling Agents

A bonding agent applied to filler particles to ensure chemical bonding to resin matrix.

CLASSIFICATIONS

a. *According to filler particles*
   - Macrofilled: 8–12 μm
   - Small particle: 1–5 μm
   - Microfilled: 0.04–0.4 μm
   - Hybrid: 0.6–1 μm.
   - Nanofilled: 1–100 nm
b. *According to method of activation*
   - Chemically activated composites
   - Light activated composites
     i. UV light activated composites
     ii. Visible light activated composites
c. *According to method of dispension*
   - Two-paste system: It includes base + reactor.
     For example, chemically activated composites.
   - Single paste and liquid
     For example, chemically activated composites.
   - Single paste system: Supplied in syringes
     For example, light activated composites.
   - Disposable capsules
     For example, compomers.

d. *Based on their applications*
   - Posterior composites, e.g. Hybrid and traditional composites.
   - Pit and fissure sealants, e.g. Bis-GMA resin.
   - Luting of orthodontic appliances.
   - Restoration of eroded areas.

Dispension

- Chemical cure composites: Two-paste system, single paste and catalyst liquid.
- Light cure composites single paste system (Fig. 6.23B).

COMPOSITION AND MICROSTRUCTURE

Dental composites mainly contain:
- Resin matrix
- Filler
- Coupling agents
- Activators and initiators
- Inhibitors
- Optical modifiers.

Resin Matrix

Most common resins used are:
- Bis GMA (Bis phenol A glycedyl dimethacrylate)
- Triethylene glycol dimethacrylate (TEGDMA)
- Urethane dimethacrylate (UDMA).

As the monomer (MMA) combines to form polymer the potential energy of monomer to polymer is less than 20% which led to volume contraction to resin and causes microleakage, staining and secondary caries. But in the case of Bis-GMA and UDMA the molecular weight is five times the methyl methacrylate, hence double bond strength is greater and more effective polymerization takes place. But it increases the viscosity, which makes it difficult to manipulate, hence to reduce viscosity diluent resins were added such as TEGDMA.

Fillers

Fillers are mainly aimed to substitute resin and decrease its content.

Classification of Fillers

a. Based on their nature:
   i. Organic fillers
   ii. Inorganic fillers.
b. Based on particle size:
   i. Microfillers
   ii. Macrofillers
   iii. Nanofillers.

Inorganic fillers: It includes inorganic components like ground quartz, pyrolytic silica, aluminum silicate, and barium glasses. These are present in 30–70 volume % or 50–58 wt%.

Pyrolytic/precipitated/colloidal silica: The term pyrolytic is derived from "pyrogen", which means, *"born in fire"*. These are obtained by precipitation of silicone present in low molecular weight compounds such as $SiCl_4$. The $SiCl_4$ is burned in oxygen and hydrogen atmosphere to form macromolecules. These macromolecules are of colloidal size and constitute the inorganic filler particles.

Organic fillers: Silane coated colloidal silica is mixed with resin monomer with chloroform at a slightly elevated temperature. Filler is thoroughly mixed with resin and the composite paste is heat cured using a conventional benzoyl peroxide initiator. The cured composite is then grounded into powder.

Macrofillers: The average particle size is 8–12 μm. These include colloidal silica in the form of silicic acid, barium, zinc, and yttrium.

Microfillers: The particle size is 0.04–0.4 μm. These include quartz, cristobalite, tridymite, fused silica, silicate glass, barium aluminum borosilicate.

Nanofillers: The average particle size of nanofillers is 1–100 nm.

Desirable Properties of Fillers

- It should be chemically inert.
- Refractive index should match with that of matrix.
- It should be hard enough to resist abrasion.
- It should be radiopaque.

Advantages of Fillers

- Reduces the volume of resin matrix and hence decreases the polymerization shrinkage.
- Improves the mechanical properties such as compressive strength, tensile strength, MOE, abrasive resistance, hardness, etc.
- Reduce the COTE.
- It gives radiopacity to the mix.
- Decreases the water sorption and softening of the resin.

Coupling Agents

Coupling agent bonds the resin to filler in order to improve the strength and durability of the composite. These act as stress absorbers at filler-resin interface. It provides hydrolytic stability by preventing water from penetrating along the filler-resin interface. The coupling agents are γ-methacryloxy propyl trimethoxy silane. In the presence of water the methoxy groups ($-OCH_3$) are hydrolyzed to silanol (Si-OH) groups that can bond with resin.

Initiators and activators

In the Table 6.16 different activator and initiator systems were given for various composites.

Table 6.16 Initiator and activator systems for various composite resins

Type of materials	Initiator	Activator
Chemically activated composites	Benzoyl peroxide	N,N–Dimethyl para toluidine 3° amine
UV light activated composites	Benzoin methyl ether	UV light (365 nm)
Visible light activated composite	Camphoroquinone (0.2 wt%) + tertiary amine (0.15 wt%)	Visible light (460–480 nm)

Table 6.17 Properties of composite restorative materials

Characteristic/property	Unfilled acrylic	Traditional	Small-particle	Hybrid	Microfilled
Size (μm)	—	8–12	0.5–3	0.4–1.0	0.04–0.4
Inorganic filler (vol%)	0	60–70	65–77	60–65	20–59
Inorganic filler (wt%)	0	70–80	80–90	75–80	35–67
Compressure strength (Mpa)	70	250–300	350–400	300–350	25–350
Tensile strength (Mpa)	24	50–65	75–90	40–50	30–50
MOE (GPa)	2.4	8–15	15–20	11–15	3–6
COTE (ppm/°C)	92.8	25–35	19–26	30–40	50–60
Water sorption (mg/cm^2)	1.7	0.5–0.7	0.5–0.6	0.5–0.7	1.4–1.7
Hardness (KHN)	15	55	50–60	50–60	25–35
Curing shrinkage (vol%)	8–10	—	2–3	2–3	2–3

Polymerization Inhibitors

These are added to prevent autopolymerization on storage.

For example, butylated hydroxytoluene (0.01 wt%).

Advantages

- Extend storage and stability of resin.
- Delays polymerization thereby providing working time.

Optical Modifiers

These optical modifiers improve esthetic properties by providing visual shading and translucency close to natural teeth. Metal oxides of minute quantity are used, e.g. TiO$_2$, aluminum oxide (0.001–0.007 wt%).

GENERAL PROPERTIES OF COMPOSITES

General properties of composites have been given in Table 6.17.

Biocompatibility

Properly polymerized composites are relatively biocompatible. However, monomer from unpolymerized materials can enter the dentinal tubules and cause pulpal inflammation.

Polymerization Shrinkage

The volumetric shrinkage during polymerization leads to marginal leakage and breach in bonding and this shrinkage increases with an increase in organic matrix. The volumetric shrinkage can be minimized by manipulation in increments and use of indirect composite restorations.

Water Sorption

Water sorption depends on the resin content and in the quality on bond between the resin and the filler. Water sorption increases when—

- Increase in resin matrix as it is high soluble fraction.
- Incomplete curing.
- Air voids.

Coefficient of Thermal Expansion (COTE)

COTE should be as close to the tooth as possible, i.e. $11.4 \times 10^{-6}/°C$ and this can be achieved by increase in the filler content using prepolymerized filler particles.

Thermal Conductivity

Thermal conductivity matches closely to enamel and dentin and does not pose any problem and acts as a good thermal insulator.

Compressive Strength

It increases with increase in the volume fraction of the filler and decreases with increase in the resin content.

Tensile Strength

The composites have very low tensile strength so they are more likely to fail under tension.

Modulus of Elasticity

It increases with an increase in the volume fraction of the filler.

CONVENTIONAL COMPOSITES (TRADITIONAL OR MACROFILLED COMPOSITES)

Composition

The composition discussed previously in this chapter was same for all the varieties of composites except in filler size, type and quantity.

- Type of filler: Quartz.
- Size: Average 8–12 μm
- Filler loading: 70–80 wt% or 50–60 vol%.

Properties

The properties are superior when compared to unfilled restorative resins characteristic properties of different composites are given in Table 6.17.

Advantage

- More strength and superior to unfilled resins.

Disadvantages

- Rough surface leading to staining.
- Poor resistance to occlusal wear.
- It is difficult for conventional composite to polish as it has high filler content leading to rough surface.

MICROFILLED COMPOSITES

These are smoother comparable to the unfilled resins but at the same time they are hard and durable (Fig. 6.24A).

Composition

The composition previously discussed in this chapter was same for all the varieties of composites except in filler size, type and quantity.

- Type of filler: Microfiller, colloidal silica.
- Size: 0.02–0.04 μm
- Filler loading: 80 wt% or 70 vol% (actual inorganic filler content is only 50 wt%).

Drawbacks

- Due to large surface area of the colloidal silica, more amount of resin is required which leads to more viscous mix. Hence, more amount of filler cannot be incorporated to obtain a workable mix.

Remedy

Methods of increasing filler loading:
- Reduce surface area by fusing colloidal particles with sintering procedure.
- Addition of prepolymerized filler or organic fillers.

Properties

High resin content of this composite led to inferior mechanical properties. Characteristic properties of microfilled composites were given in Table 6.17.

SMALL PARTICLE COMPOSITE

All the other components are similar but vary only in filler size, type and quantity (Fig. 6.24B).
- Type of filler: Glass containing heavy metals + Colloidal silica (5 wt%)
- Size: 1–5 μm
- Filler loading: 80–90 wt% or 65–77 vol%.

Properties

Best physical and mechanical properties are observed because of high filler content. These composites are both smoother and durable (Table 6.16).

HYBRID COMPOSITES

These are developed to obtain better surface smoothness than that of small particle composite and maintain other properties, which range

between conventional and small particle composites (Fig. 6.24C).

Composition

The composition described previously in this chapter was same for all varieties of composites except in filler size, type and quantity.
- Type of filler: Colloidal silica + Heavy metal glasses
- Size: < 1 μm (0.6–1 μm)
- Filler loading: Colloidal silica: 10–20 wt%, heavy metal glasses: 75 wt%.

Properties (see Table 6.17)

NANOCOMPOSITES

As the name implies, these include constituents that are mixed on a nanometer-length scale. A nanocomposite has at least part of its grains of size of 1–100 nm.

The nanofiller used includes an aluminosilicate powder having a mean particle size of about 80 nm and a 1:4 ratio of alumina to silica. This nanofiller has a refractive index of 1.508.

Restorative nanocomposites contain a unique combination of individual nanoparticles and nanoclusters. Nanoparticles are discrete particles of 20 nm in size. Nanocluster fillers are loosely bound agglomerates of nanosized particles. The agglomerates act as a single unit enabling high filler loading and strength. These nanoclusters are lightly sintered so that they can break apart during the wear process. So during day to day abrasion of filling due to

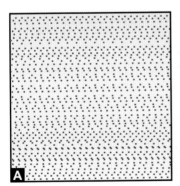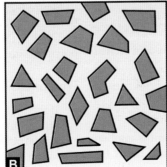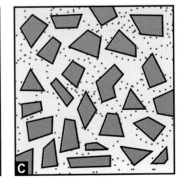

Figs 6.24A to C (A) Microfilled composite (B) Fine-filled composites (C) Hybrid composite

brushing or eating, the optical effect is the loss of a nanometer-sized particle rather than the loss of a micron (e.g. hybrid composite) sized particle.

Since nanocluster filler particles consist of loosely bound agglomerates of nano-sized filler particles, during abrasion, the primary particles (nanosized), not the cluster themselves, can be worn away. This increases the polish retention of the cured composite when compared to traditional hybrid composites. A good quality nanofilled composite resin is formulated using both nanoparticles and nanocluster fillers.

Advantages

- Reduces polymerization shrinkage – as low as 1–1.6%.
- Allows excellent polish.
- More chameleon-like effect with a greater scattering of light.
- No compromise on strength.
- Can be used for posterior and anterior restorations.
- Excellent hardness.
- Excellent flexural strength.
- Superior elastic modulus.

Manipulation

General characters and criteria for selection of selected direct restorative materials were given in Table 6.22.

Cleaning

The tooth is first cleaned with a mild abrasive.

Etching

The enamel at the cavity margins is acid etched with 37% orthophosphoric acid. The acid is rinsed off and the area is dried thoroughly.

Bonding Agent Application

An enamel or dentin-bonding agent is applied and polymerized. The cavity is now ready for the composite.

Technique for Chemically Activated Resins

Dispension

They are supplied in the form of powder and liquid/ 2-paste system/ paste-liquid system.

Mixing

The correct proportions of pastes are dispensed onto a mixing pad and combined by rapid spatulation with a plastic or wooden spatula for 30 seconds. It is important that the material be thoroughly mixed in order to ensure a homogeneous distribution of the curing agent (activator) throughout the mass, yet not so vigorously that air is incorporated.

Insertion

The method of insertion is similar to that of the bulk or pressure technique described for unfilled acrylic resins. When the mixing is completed, the resin should be promptly inserted into the cavity to avoid poor adaptation to the cavity walls and loss plasticity because of the onset of polymerization.

- Working time: 1–1½ minutes
- Setting time: 4–5 minutes.

Care should be taken to avoid incorporating air during mixing and insertion of the resin, because the polymerized mass is oxygen inhibited, such air inclusions can result in soft spots in the restoration.

Contour of the restoration is achieved by the use of a properly placed matrix strip as shown in Figure 6.25, which applies pressure to yield better adaptation to the walls by forcing the material to flow during the plastic stage of the polymerization .

Precautions

- If the materials are furnished in jars, cross-contamination must be avoided, because partial polymerization of the paste may occur in the contaminated container.
- Proportioning should be accurate.

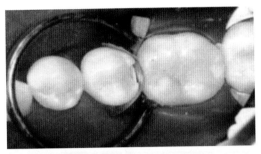

Fig. 6.25 Matrix strip placement

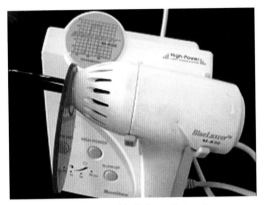

Fig. 6.26 Visible light curing unit

- The mixing should be thorough to ensure homogeneous mixture of the activator and the initiator.
- Avoid using small instruments with sharp edges during insertion, because such instruments often leave imprints that can result in voids when a new portion of composite is added.

Advantages

- The rate of polymerization is uniform throughout the mass.

Technique for Light Activated Composites

Light activated composites are supplied in the form of single paste systems. The polymerization can be initiated when the resin is exposed to light with a suitable wavelength (may be UV light or visible light). Light curing units are available to supply light (Fig. 6.26).

Advantages of light activated resins over chemically activated resins:

- Require no mixing since the material available in the form of single paste system.
- Adequate working time.
- Materials set rapidly once they are exposed to the curing light with a suitable wavelength.

Insertion

The best method to insert the restorative material into the tooth cavity is with a syringe. The depth of cure depends on the material color, quality and location of the light source. Different light

Table 6.18 Different lamps used for curing and their wavelengths

Type of light source	Wavelength
LED lamps (light emitting diodes)	440–480 nm
QTH lamps (Quartz tungsten Halogen bulb)	400–500 nm (Violet blue)
PAC lamp (Plasma arc curing lamps)	400–500 nm (Blue light)
Argon laser lamp	490 nm

sources or lamps (Table 6.18) available that facilitate the operator to choose the lamp with suitable wavelength. If the cavity is so deep the restoration must be built up in increments. Each increment must be cured before the successive increment is added as this procedure can reduce the voids and also polymerization shrinkage can be compensated. The exposure time should not be less than 40 seconds and the resin thickness should be around 2–2.5 mm. Darker shades and microfilled resins require longer exposure times.

Light Sources

There are four types of curing lamps which emit light radiations of different intensities (Table 6.18).

1. *LED Lamps:* LED stands for *Light Emitting Diodes.* These lamps emit radiation only in the blue part of visible spectrum between 440–480 nm.

2. *Quartz-Tungsten Halogen (QTH) Lamps:*
These lamps are having quartz halogen bulbs
with tungsten filament which radiates both
UV and visible light, so filters are required to
remove the unwanted wavelength of light.
These are the most commonly used light
sources as these are inexpensive.
3. *Plasma arc curing lamps:* These lamps use
xenon gas. This gas is ionized and produces
plasma (a high intensity white light). Filters
should be used in these lamps to remove
heat and allow blue light to be emitted.
4. *Argon laser lamps:* These lamps produce high
intensity of light radiation.

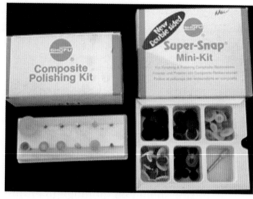

Fig. 6.27 Composite polishing kit

Precautions

• The resin paste should not be dispensed
until it is to be used. Exposure to operatory
lights for any appreciable time can initiate
polymerization of the material.
• Exposure to sunlight should also be avoided.
• Unused composite should never be returned
to the syringe or kept for future use.
• Storage should be in a cool and dry
environment to maintain shelf life for all
composites.
• The high intensity light can cause retinal
damage if one looks at it directly. Protective
eyeglasses should be used.

Disadvantages

• Uniform polymerization is not observed.
• Deep cavities have to be filled incrementally,
which is time consuming.

Finishing and Polishing

Finishing can be initiated upon removal of the
matrix or one minute after removal of the light
in the case of light activated system. However, it
is suggested that when finishing is delayed for 24
hours, better marginal adaptation is achieved.

Carbide finishing burs are commonly used.
Final finishing can be done with abrasive points
slightly coated with silicon grease, a rubber
cup and pumice paste or aluminum oxide and
zirconium silicate strips or disks (Fig. 6.27).

Glazing Agents

These consisting of dilute solutions of bis-GMA
are applied to overcome the roughness in the
finished composite resin restoration surface.
The glazing agent is painted on the surface of
the restoration after final finishing providing a
smooth coating.

ACID-ETCH TECHNIQUE

Bunocore et al in 1955 introduced acid etch
technique to enhance bonding between tooth
surface and restoration which provided scope
for the use of resin bonded metal retainers,
porcelain laminate veneers and orthodontic
brackets as it provides a strong bond between
resin and enamel.

Principle

The process of achieving a bond between
enamel and resin based restorative materials
involves discrete etching of the enamel to
provide selective dissolution of enamel rods with
resultant microporosity.

Etched enamel has high surface energy
allows a resin readily to wet the surface and
penetrate into the microporosity. Then it can be
polymerized to form a mechanical bond to the
enamel. These resin tags may penetrate 10–20
μm into the enamel porosity (Fig. 6.28A).

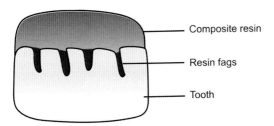

Fig. 6.28A Resin tag formation

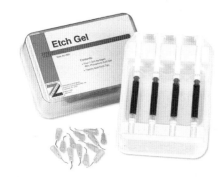

Fig. 6.28B Gel etchant

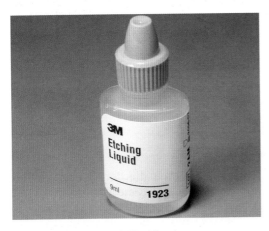

Fig. 6.28C Liquid etchant

Procedure

Acid used: 37% orthophosphoric acid.

If the concentration of phosphoric acid is greater than 50%, it results in the formation of "monocalcium phosphate monohydrate" on the etched surface that inhibits further dissolution.

Types of Etchants

- Liquid etchants (Fig. 6.28C).
- Gel etchants (Fig. 6.28B).

Liquid Etchants

Liquid etchants are used primarily to etch large surface areas of enamel, such as for veneers or sealants. Common types of applicators include small cotton pellets, foam sponges and brushes.

- Gently apply the acid to the appropriate enamel surfaces to be restored, keeping the excess to a maximum of 0.5 mm past the anticipated extent of restoration.
- For preparations involving proximal area a polyester strip is placed before acid etching to prevent the etching of the adjacent tooth.
- The application of acid is repeated every 10–15 seconds to keep the area moist for 30 seconds.
- Shorter etching time is advised as it yields acceptable bond strength in most cases and it also conserves enamel and saves time.
- Care is to be taken not to flood the area with acid or to rub the enamel.
- The acid is rinsed off thoroughly with a stream of water for 10–15 seconds after etching the tooth.
- If cotton roles were used for isolation, it should be replaced at this time, ensuring that the cavity preparation does not become contaminated with saliva.
- Now this tooth surface is dried with clean air for 20 seconds.

Enamel that has been properly air-dried is described as having a ground glass or white frosted appearance.

Gel Etchants

- For application of a gel etchant a brush paper point instrument or syringe are used to place the etchant onto the prepared enamel.
- Leave the surface untouched for 30 seconds after the application etchant.

- Rinse for 20–30 seconds with water.
- Gel etchants are more easily applied with small syringe.
- Dry the tooth surface.

Precautions

- Prevent the formation air bubbles during the acid application.
- Etched surface should not be allowed to contamination, e.g. blood, saliva, etc. such contamination reduces the surface energy, tag formation, and bonding with etched enamel. Contamination should be rinsed off.
- The concentration of phosphoric acid should not be used.

A tooth with high fluoride content derived from a fluoride water supply, i.e. resistant to acid etching doubling or tripling of usual 35 seconds etching time (Fluorapatite resistant to acids).

Bond strength to etched enamel range from 18–25 MPa, depending on the resin and testing method used.

BONDING AGENTS

Bonding agents are the materials similar to unfilled acrylics, which help in bonding between resin and enamel and between resin particles.

Requirements

- It should be nontoxic.
- It should not disintegrate in the oral fluids.
- It should be both hydrophobic to react with the composite resin and hydrophilic to bond with the tooth.
- They should have good bond strength.

ENAMEL BONDING AGENTS

Composites are mainly composed with dimethacrylate resins. As the viscosity of these resins is very high they cannot be able to penetrate into the micro-porosities created by acid etching. So the bonding agents are developed with high flow property and they are mainly unfilled acrylic resins. They provide mechanical bonding between the enamel and the composite resin by resin tag formation within the enamel called as enamel bonding agents (Fig. 6.29A).

DENTIN BONDING AGENTS

Enamel bonding agents fail to provide a strong bonding with the dentin. The reasons for this failure are as follows:

- Dentin is a heterogeneous that consists of 50% inorganic hydroxyapatite, 30% organic material and 20% fluid. Dentin also contains less amount of calcium for chemical bonding.
- Dentinal fluids come onto the surface of the dentin and prevent spreading of bonding agent.
- Presence of smear layer on the exposed dentinal tubules.
- Low surface energy of the dentin.

The agents used for bonding with dentin should contain both hydrophilic and hydrophobic parts. Hydrophobic part provides bonding with dentin by displacing the dentinal fluids and also hydrophobic part will react chemically with resin restorative material. Bonding is better to be polymerized separately to reduce the polymerization shrinkage.

Dispension

Dentin bonding agents are supplied as a kit containing primers/conditioners and the bonding agent.

Primers

Primers condition the dentin surface and improve bonding. They are acidic in nature.

For example, Ethylene–di amine–tetra acetic acid (EDTA), nitric acid, maleic acid, etc.

Functions of Primers

- Removes smear layer and provides subtle opening of dentinal tubules.
- Provides modest etching to the intertubular dentin.
- It exposes collagen to the bonding agent.

Chemistry

Molecules designed for these purposes are represented by formula M–R–X.

Where M is the methacrylate group that reacts with resin matrix.

R is the spacer.

X is the functional group for adhesion to tooth tissue.

Generations of Dentin Bonding Agents

A convenient way of examining the progress in the dentin bonding systems is the categorize dentin adhesives into the so-called "generations". Evolution of bonding agents was briefly discussed in Table 6.19.

First Generation

In 1956, Bunocore et al demonstrated glycerol phosphoric acid dimethacrylate containing resin and cyanoacrylates to bond to acid etched dentin. This bond is believed to be due to production of a bifunctional resin molecule, hydrophilic phosphate group from the glycerol phosphoric acid dimethacrylate resin that increases bonding with Ca ions of the hydroxy apatite. The methacrylate groups were then able to bond to an acrylic restorative resin.

Commercial product: Scotch bond.

Relatively low bond strengths were obtained and decreased with storage in water for these systems.

Nine years later Bowen tried to address this issue using N-phenyl glycerin and glycidyl methacrylate or NPG-GMA. It is a bifunctional molecule; one end of the molecule bonds to dentin while the other bonds to composite resin.

Commercial names: Cervident, Palakav, etc.

Phosphate-based bonding agent

Aminocarboxylate-based bonding agent (NPG-GMA)

The bond strength of these early systems was only 1–3 MPa. The clinical results with these systems were poor.

Second Generation

In the late 1970's, the second-generation systems were introduced. The majority of these are "halo phosphorus esters" of unfilled acrylic resins such as bis–GMA or HEMA.

Mechanism of adhesion: The second-generation systems bonded to dentin by an ionic bonding to Ca by chlorophosphate groups.

Chloro-based bonding agent

The systems were highly soluble in oral fluids and moisture from dentin itself could result in composite resin debonding from the dentin and causing microleakage.

However, these systems resulted in bond strengths to dentin that was weak and unreliable.

Commercial products: Clearfil, Prisma Universal Bond, Johnson and Johnson Dentin-Enamel bonding agent.

Third Generation Systems

As further developments ensured, interaction with the smear layer, the cutting debris smeared over the enamel and dentin and plugging the dentinal tubules was appreciated as having a significant influence on the behavior of adhesive systems. Thus, the third generation of adhesive systems used a dentin conditioning step as well as an intermediate primer in conjunction with a bonding agent. The conditioning agents either modify or remove the smear layer before placement of adhesive resins and attempts have been made to bond chemically with the calcium of dentin.

One of the first of these systems developed by Bowen and employed a 2.5% of nitric acid or ferric oxalate dentin conditioner followed by treatments of NTG–GMA and PMDM (Pyromellitic di anhydrate and 2-hydroxy ethyl methacrylate).

This system was later modified by replacing ferric oxalate with aluminum oxalate.

Commercial names:
- Tenure:
  Conditioner: Phosphoric acid with aluminum oxalate and nitric acid.
- Mirage bond
  Dentin conditioner: HNO_3 and NPG-GMA: 2.5%
  Primer: PMDM.
- **Gluma bonding system**
  Dentin conditioner: EDTA.
  Primers: HEMA + Glutaraldehyde.
- **Scotch bond – II**
  Dentin conditioner: Maleic acid and HEMA.
  Primers: BIS-GMA + HEMA.
- **Prisma universal bond – III:** This is designed to bond both the inorganic and organic parts of dentin.

Significant improvements in bond strengths were obtained with third generation systems.
- Scotch bond – II: 9 Mpa.
- Prisma Universal Bond – III and Tenure: more than 18 Mpa.

Newer Generation Systems

Strategies for dentin adhesion so far have included—
- Bonding via resin tag formation in the tubules of conditioned dentin.
- Formation of precipitate on pretreated dentin surfaces followed by chemical or mechanical bonding of a resin.

- Chemical union to either inorganic or organic components of the dentin.

Modern adhesives rely on a fourth concept, first proposed by Nakabayashi et al; diffusion and impregnation of resins into the substrate of partially decalcified dentin followed by polymerization creating a "hybrid resin reinforced layer".

This hybrid layer is an acid resistant admixture of polymer and tooth structure components creating a resin-dentin composite.

Fourth generation system employing a dentin conditioning step followed by application of a multicomponent resin system and fifth generation system using a dentin conditioning system followed by application of one component system.

Fourth Generation Systems

These generation adhesive systems rely on the hydration of the dentin as a critical parameter for effective bonding. In this generation there was a complete elimination of smear layer has taken place.

Commercial names:
- All bond – II
  Conditioner: Phosphoric acid.
  Primers: Hydrophilic resins such as NTG-GMA + BPDM in acetone.
- **Scotch bond multipurpose** (Fig. 6.29B)
  Conditioner: Maleic acid – 10%.
  Primers: Aqueous solution of HEMA and copolymer.
- **Imperiva bond**
- **Perma quick**
- **Probond**
- **Liner bond–II.**

In addition to dentin and enamel adhesion, bond strength claims are made for cast alloys, amalgam and porcelain. Mean shear bond strengths of these systems are reported to range from 17 Mpa to more than 24 Mpa.

Fifth Generation

To simplify the clinical procedure by reducing the bonding steps and thus the working time, a

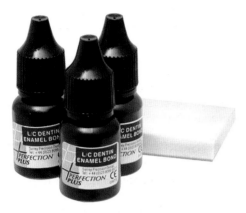

Fig. 6.29A Enamel and dentin bonding agent

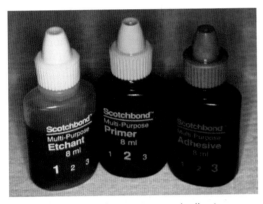

Fig. 6.29B Etchant, primer and adhesive

better system was needed and also to prevent the collagen collapse of demineralized dentin. The fifth generation bonding systems were developed to make use of adhesive materials more reliable for practitioners.

The distinguishing characteristic of the fifth generation system is the combination of the priming and bond resin application steps to achieve bonding with a one component resin formula. These systems are marketed as faster and easier to use. These systems required the following procedures:

- Acid conditioning for maximal adhesion to enamel to enamel and dentin.
- These materials rely on the hybridization of dentin for achieving adhesion as in fourth generation systems.

- These materials also generally rely on residual moisture in the dentin and hydrophilic water-chasing compositions to effect resin penetration into the dentin.

The fifth generation system consists of single bottle system.

One bottle system: To facilitate clinical use one-bottle systems combined the primer and adhesives into one solution to be applied after etching enamel and dentin simultaneously.

Commercial names: One-bond, prime and bond, optibond solo, scotch bond multipurpose, etc.

Sixth Generation

These generation systems consist of two different types:

Self-etching primer: Self-etching primer is an aqueous solution of 20% of phenyl – P in 30% HEMA for bonding to enamel and dentin simultaneously.

The combination of etching and priming steps reduce the working time, eliminate washing out of the acid gel and also eliminate the risk of collagen collapse.

Disadvantages
- Less shelf-life.
- A residual smear layer remained in between adhesive material and resin.
- Less effectiveness and etching.

Self-etching adhesives: These are all-in-one adhesives contain acidic unreacted monomer that contacts the composite restorative material directly. The etching, priming, and bonding together in a single solution are now available. All-in-one provides similar enamel bond strengths but the dentin bond strengths are significantly lower than those obtained with total-etch adhesives.

Commercial products: Adper Prompt L-Pop (3M ESPE), One-Up Bond F (Tokuyama Dental), Xeno III (Dentsply).

Seventh Generation

The latest category, seventh-generation bonding systems, is the "all in one" adhesives that combine etch, prime, and bond in a single solution. Laboratory studies show bond strengths and margin sealing to be equal to sixth-generation systems. The all-in-one adhesives are user-friendly, and most offer both a bottle and a unit-dose version. See Table 6.19 for the comparison of different dental adhesive systems.

Table 6.19 Evolution of bonding agents

First and second degeneration (1960s and 1970s)
Did not recommend dentin etching.
Relied on adhesion to smear layer.
Weak bond strengths

Third generation (1980s)
Acid-etching of dentin
Separate primer
Increased bond strength
Margin staining caused clinical failure over time

Fourth generation (early 1990s)
Hybrid layer of dentin and collagen
Dentin seal
Concept of "wet bonding" introduced
Technique sensitive

Fifth generation (mid 1990s)
Combined primer and adhesive in one bottle
Maintained high bond strength
Unit-dose packaging introduced

Sixth generation (late 1990s, early 2000s)
"Self-etching" primers
Reduced incidence of post-creatinine sensitivity
Bond strengths lower than fourth and fifth generations

Seventh generation (late 2002)
All-in-one combines etching, printing and bonding
Single solution
Good bond strength and margin sealing

Commercial products: *iBond™ (Heraeus), Xeno® IV (Dentsply), G-Bond™ (GC), Complete (Cosmedent), and OptiBond® All-In-One (Kerr).*

Both OptiBond All-in-One and Xeno IV are fluoride releasing, while iBond and G-Bond are non-fluoride containing.

Xeno IV self-etch seventh generation adhesive is available in a bottle or unit dose delivery and does not require mixing. Xeno IV is pH balanced to reduce gingival irritation and sensitivity.

Clearfil S3 Bond, G-Bond and iBond are available in a bottle. Clearfil S3 Bond contains water to alleviate the need for a surface with a specific degree of wetness and to resist hydrolysis, providing for a lasting and reliable adhesion. It resists hydrolysis which provides for reliable and durable adhesion. G-Bond offers versatility in the degree of wetness on the tooth surface at the time of adhesive application.

Comparison of dental adhesives were given in the Tables 6.20 and 6.21.

RECENT ADVANCES IN COMPOSITES

Condensable Composites

These are also called as packable composites or polymeric rigid inorganic matrix material (PRIMM), was developed by Dr Lars Ehrnford of Sweden in 1995. This system is composed of a resin matrix, and an inorganic ceramic component. In this system, the resin is incorporated into the fibrous ceramic filler network rather than incorporating the filler particles into the composite resin matrix. The filler mainly consists of aluminum oxide and silicone dioxide glass particles or barium aluminum silicate or strontium glasses. Colloidal silica ultrafine particles are also incorporated to control the handling characteristics such as viscosity, resistance to flow, condensability and reduced stickiness.

The glass particles are liquefied to form molten glass which is forced through a die to form thin strands of glass fibers with a diameter of approximately 2–3 µm. These glass fibers are crushed into small fragments and then reheated to a sufficient temperature to cause superficial

Table 6.20 Comparison of 4th, 5th, 6th and 7th Generation dental adhesive systems

Generations	Etching of enamel and dentin	Steps Priming of dentin	Sealing of enamel and dentin
4th Generation	Etchant	Primer	Resin/sealer
5th Generation	Etchant	Self-priming resin/sealer	Self-priming resin/sealer
6th Generation	Self-etching primer	Self-etching primer	Resin/sealer
6th Generation (Mixing Required)	Self-etching, Self-priming resin/Sealer	Self-etching, Self-priming resin/Sealer	Self-etching, Self-priming resin/Sealer
6th Generation (No Mixing required)	Self-etching, Self-priming resin/ Sealer desensitizer disinfectant	Self-etching, Self-priming resin/ Sealer desensitizer disinfectant	Self-etching, Self-priming resin/ Sealer desensitizer disinfectant

Table 6.21 Comparison of the number of system components, number of steps required and shear bond strength of dental adhesive systems

Generation	Number of components	Description	Number of steps required	Shear band strength (MPa)
1st	2	Etch enamel, apply adhesive	2	2
2nd	2	Etch enamel, apply adhesive	2	5
3rd	2–3	Etch enamel, apply primer	3	12
4th	3–5	Total etch, apply primer	3	24
5th	2	Etch enamel, apply adhesive	2	25
6th	2	Apply self-etch adhesive	1	20
7th	1	Apply self-etch adhesive	1	25

fusion of glass fibers at selected sites (silanation). This forms a continuous network of small chambers or cavities with 2 μm dimensions. Resin is infiltrated into these spaces or chambers. This concept provides a basis for fabricating packable or condensable posterior composite resin.

Advantages

- Greater ease in achieving a good contact point.
- Better reproduction of occlusal anatomy.
- Physical and mechanical behavior is similar to that of silver amalgam.
- Clinical behavior is similar to that of hybrid composites.

Disadvantages

- Difficulties in adaptation between one composite layer and another.
- Difficult handling.
- Poor esthetics in anterior teeth.

Indications

- Class II cavity restoration in order to achieve a better contact point.

Indirect Composite Resins

Because of major clinical problems with direct posterior composite resins, the indirect composite inlay/onlay system was introduced. Since the restoration is generated on a die rather than directly in the cavity preparation, superior marginal adaptation, contour and proximal contact can be achieved. Most clinical studies have demonstrated a dramatic improvement in general clinical performance.

Advantages

- Has superior adaptation.
- Contour and proximal contact.
- Wear resistance.
- Good esthetics.
- Control over polymerization shrinkage.

ORMOCER

ORMOCER is an Organically Modified Ceramic that contains inorganic-organic copolymers in addition to the inorganic silanated filler particles such as *urethane and thioether (meth)acrylate alkoxysilanes*. ORMOCER is synthesized through a *sol-gel* process. ORMOCERs are described as 3-dimensionally cross-linked copolymers.

Indications

- For cavities classes I to V.
- Reconstruction of traumatically affected anteriors.
- Veneering of discolored anteriors.
- Correction of shape and shade for better esthetics.
- Repair of veneers.
- Core build-up.
- Protective sealant for child teeth.
- Orthodontic bonding adhesive.
- Indirect inlays.

Advantages

- Reduced polymerization shrinkage.
- Improved marginal adaptation.
- Best biocompatibility as no diluent monomer is required.
- High abrasion resistance.
- Protection against caries.
- Does not liberate any residual monomer after polymerization.

Fiber Reinforced Composites (FRC)

Fiber reinforcement has further increased the potential uses of composites within restorative dentistry. Glass fibers, carbon fibers, polyethylene fibers, aramid fibers, etc are the most commonly used fibers in dental composites. These fibers can be oriented in different directions; unidirectional, weave type, mesh type, etc, in the resin matrix to improve the physical and mechanical properties of composites. The durability of the fiber-reinforced composites mainly depends on the following factors:

- The individual properties of the fibers and resin matrix.
- Fiber loading within the resin.
- Adhesion of fibers to matrix.
- Volume of fibers in the composite matrix.
- The orientation of the fibers.
- Location of fibers in the prosthesis construction.

Silane coupling agents are commonly used to provide bonding between resin matrix and fibers.

Clinical Applications

- Reinforced direct composite restoration.
- Single indirect restoration (inlay, onlay, partial/full veneer crowns).
- Periodontal splinting/post-trauma splints.
- Immediate replacement transitional and long-term provisional bridges.
- Fixed bridge work—anterior and posterior such as simple cantilever, fixed-fixed, implant supported.
- Reinforcing or repairing dentures.
- Fixed orthodontic retainers.

PIT AND FISSURE SEALANTS

Pits and fissures on the occlusal surfaces of the posterior teeth are very susceptible to decay especially in the child patient. Deep pits and fissures provide shelter for carcinogenic factors and obstruct oral hygiene procedures.

Table 6.22 Comparison of direct restorative dental materials

Factors	Amalgam	Resin-based composite (Direct and Indirect)	Glass ionomer	Resin-modified glass ionomer
General description	A mixture of mercury and silver alloy powder that forms a hard solid metal filling. Self-hardening at mouth temperature.	A mixture of submicron glass filler and acrylic that forms a solid tooth-colored restoration. Self- or light-hardening at mouth temperature.	Self-hardening mixture of fluoride containing glass powder and organic acid that forms a solid tooth colored restoration able to release fluoride.	Self- or light-hardening mixture of sub-micron glass filler with fluoride-containing glass powder and acrylic resin that forms a solid tooth-colored restoration able to release fluoride.
Principal uses	Dental fillings and heavily loaded back tooth restorations.	Esthetic dental fillings and veneers.	Small non-load-bearing fillings, cavity liners and cements for crowns and bridges.	
Leakage and recurrent decay	Leakage is moderate, but recurrent decay is no more prevalent than other materials.	Leakage low when properly bonded to underlying tooth; recurrent decay depends on maintenance of the tooth-material bond.	Leakage is generally low, recurrent decay is comparable to other direct materials, fluoride release may be beneficial for patients at high risk for decay.	Leakage is low when properly bonded to the underlying tooth; recurrent decay is comparable to other direct materials; fluoride release may be beneficial for patients at high risk for decay.
Overall durability	Good to excellent in large load-bearing restorations.	Good in small-to-moderate size restorations.	Moderate to good in non-load-bearing restorations; poor in load-bearing.	
Cavity preparation considerations	Requires removal of tooth structure for adequate retention and thickness of the filling.	Adhesive bonding permits removing less tooth structure.		
Clinical considerations	Tolerant to a wide range of clinical placement conditions, moderately tolerant to the presence of moisture during placement.	Must be placed in a well-controlled field of operation; very little tolerance to presence of moisture during placement.		
Resistance to wear	Highly resistant to wear.	Moderately resistant, but less so than amalgam.	High wear when placed on chewing surfaces.	
Resistance to fracture	Brittle, subject to chipping on filling edges, but good bulk strength in larger high-load restorations.	Moderate resistance to fracture in high-load restorations.	Low resistance to fracture.	Low to moderate resistance to fracture.

Contd...

Contd...

Factors	Amalgam	Resin-based composite (Direct and Indirect)	Glass ionomer	Resin-modified glass ionomer
Biocompatibility	Well-tolerated with rare occurrences of allergenic response.			
Post-placement sensitivity	Early-sensitivity to hot and cold possible.	Occurrence of sensitivity highly dependent on ability to adequately bond the restoration to the underlying tooth.	Low	Occurrence of sensitivity highly dependent on ability to adequately bond the restoration to the underlying tooth.
Esthetics	Silver or gray metallic color does not mimic tooth color.	Mimics natural tooth color and translucency, but can be subject to staining and discoloration over time.	Mimics natural tooth color, but lacks natural translucency of enamel.	
Relative cost to patient	Generally lower; actual cost of fillings depends on their size.	Moderate; actual cost of fillings depends on their size and technique.		
Average number of visits to complete	One	One for direct fillings; 2+ for indirect inlays, veneers and crowns.	One	One

Cross-sectional views of typical fissure morphology, varies from a wide "V" shape to a bottleneck shape (Fig. 6.30B). Fluorides are least effective in preventing caries in these areas.

The objective of sealant (Fig. 6.30A) use is for the resin to penetrate into pit and fissures and to polymerize and seal these areas against oral bacteria and debris preventing occlusal caries (Figs 6.30C). Success of sealant technique is dependent on obtaining and maintaining an intimate adaptation of sealant to tooth surface.

Requirements

- They should be biocompatible.
- They must have low viscosity so that they will flow readily.
- Should possess anticariogenic property.
- Good esthetic quality.
- Good mechanical properties.
- They should maintain surface integrity and tooth structure.

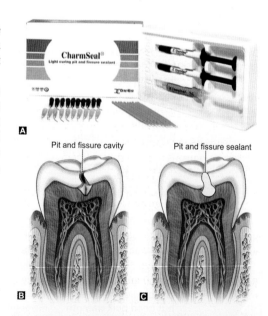

Figs 6.30A to C (A) Light curing pit and fissure sealant; (B) Pit and fissure cavity with caries; (C) Sealant filled in pit and fissure cavity

Materials

Both filled and unfilled resins are employed as pit and fissure sealants.

- Unfilled resins: Colorless or tinted transparent materials.
- Filled resins: Opaque and available either as tooth colored or white material.

The resin systems include cyanoacrylates, polyurethanes and UEDMA. Glass ionomer cements also can be used as pit and fissure sealants.

The properties of the sealants are similar to those of the resin matrix component of composite materials. The composites because of high viscosity does not penetrate narrow pit and fissures hence are not good sealants.

Sealant should be examined every six months. If the sealant is missing, it should be reapplied.

DIRECT FILLING GOLD

Very few materials are used in dentistry in the pure state for restorative purposes, for example, gold and titanium.

CHARACTERISTICS OF PURE GOLD

- Pure gold is the noblest of all metals.
- Chemically inactive.
- It is one of the most malleable of dental alloys, thus gold restorations can be easily inserted and adapted to the cavity wall. They can be hammered to a thin sheet of 0.13 mm thickness (0.00013 mm).
- It is ductile, i.e. it can be drawn over the margins of the prepared cavity. It exhibits excellent marginal seal. (12.8% elongation).
- Pure gold is extremely soft (25 BHN) but it can be work hardened to approximately the hardness of type-II casting gold, which ranges between 70 and 100 BHN.

Pure gold is an almost ideal dental restorative material for permanently pressing the tooth structure in nonesthetic, low stress bearing areas.

DISADVANTAGES

1. It has a rich yellow color with a strong metallic luster.
2. It has high thermal conductivity.
3. It is lower in strength.
4. Technical difficulties in forming a dense restoration.
5. It has one of the highest densities of all elements 19.3 g/cc. Thus, requires more material to restore the cavity.

FORMS OF DIRECT FILLING GOLD

I. According to the microstructure of the piece
   1. Gold foil or fibrous gold
      a. Sheet
         i. Cohesive
         ii. Noncohesive
      b. Ropes
      c. Cylinders
      d. Laminated foil
      e. Platinized foil
   2. Electrolytic precipitate
      a. Mat gold
      b. Mat foil (gold foil + mat gold)
      c. Gold-calcium alloy
   3. Powdered gold or encapsulated gold powder
II. According to the surface condition of the piece
      a. Cohesive (clean)
      b. Noncohesive (containing adsorbed gases)
III. According to the geometric form in which it is supplied
      a. Sheets
      b. Ropes
      c. Strips
      d. Pellets.

COMPOSITION

All the types of direct filling gold is essentially 100% pure gold with exceptions of platinized foil and gold calcium alloy (alloyed electrolytic precipitate).

GOLD FOIL

A process known as gold beating forms gold foil. Gold is first passed through a series of rolls (rolling). For dental use 25 μm is starting thickness for beating operation and that reduces it to a ribbon form of about 0.0025 mm thick (tissue paper thickness).

The gold is cut into small pieces of 3.5 × 3.5 cm and each piece is placed in between two sheets of parchment paper to form a 'cutch', which are placed one over other to form a packet.

A hammer of 16 pounds then beats the packet, which may contain 200–250 pieces of small gold ribbons, for 1–½ hours. The final thickness of the gold (0.00064 μm) can be determined only by its weight.

Pure gold work hardens readily. Consequently, it must be heat treated (stress relieving anneal) to increase its ductility and malleability.

Gold foil is supplied in flat square sheets of varying thickness. For example, Standard number gold foil is supplied in 4″ × 4″ sheets (100 mm × 100 mm) that weigh four grains (0.259 grams) and are about 0.51 μm thick. Similarly, number 3 gold foil weighs (0.194 grams) and is about 0.38 μm.

Although foil may be obtained in thin sheets, it is normally purchased in pellet/cylinder form. Sheets may be cut into 1/8, 1/16, 1/32, 1/64, etc. and then compressed into pellet/cylinder. This particular shape is developed by loosely rolling each of the sheets into cylinders of desired thickness. Because of its softness and lack of mass, gold foil takes longer time to build up and for this reason it is used only in small lesions. However, it can be used throughout the cavity and is suitable as a surface material.

Advantages

• Ease of manipulation and workability.

Disadvantages

• Requires considerable time to build up the restoration.

Gold Foil Cylinders

This form is produced by rolling cut segments of number 4 foils into a desired width usually 3.2 × 4.8 × 6.4 mm.

Laminated Gold Foil

Laminated foils are made by placing a number of sheets on top of each other and cutting the laminate into pieces of a desired size.

Preformed or Corrugated or Carbonized Gold Foil

This is produced by placing sheets of gold between papers and enclosing both in iron box. The contents are then smoldered (fired without flame). Then the paper is carbonized. When carbon is blown off each sheet, the corrugated (small folded) gold remains.

This form of gold foil is of historical interest because it was an outcome of the great Chicago fire in 1871. During this the foil was unharmed.

Platinized Gold Foil

It is produced by placing a layer of pure platinum foil between two sheets pure gold foil (sandwiched) and hammered until the thickness of no:4 sheet is obtained.

Platinized gold foil increases the hardness and wear resistance.

ELECTROLYTIC PRECIPITATE OR CRYSTALLINE GOLD

Crystalline gold powder formed by electrolytic precipitation. It cannot be described as foil because it is not formed by a thickness reduction process.

Mat Gold

Sometimes referred to as 'sponge gold'.

Manufacture

• A gold bar anode and a thin gold cathode are used in an electrolytic bath. Here the voltage is so increased such that the gold atoms are attracted so rapidly to the cathode that they do not orient themselves into a dense solid metal. Instead, they form crystals in a helter-skelter pattern over the surface with large voids between them, creating the characteristic porosity of uncondensed mat gold (Fig. 6.31).

- The gold is removed, washed and dried.
- The gold is sized through sonic (vibrating) sifter. The average size of the particle is 10–20 μm.
- Then the gold is shaped which involves making the particles 3–6 mm wide and sintered to make the cohesive crystals and grow together.

Mat Foil

This is the combination of mat gold and gold foil. Mat foil is a sandwich of electrolyte precipitated gold powder between sheets of number 3 gold foil. The sandwich is sintered and cut into strips of different widths.

It has rapid filling properties and is especially suited for use as an internal filling material in a preparation. In addition, it combines the adaptability of mat gold with the surface density of the gold foil, making it effective throughout the restoration. It facilitates in eliminating the need to veneer the restoration with a foil.

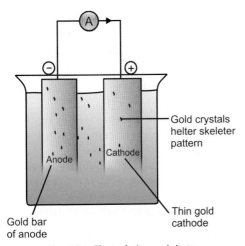

Fig. 6.31 Electrolytic precipitate

Alloyed Electrolytic Precipitate or Alloyed Gold or Gold-Calcium Alloy

Alloyed gold is a mat foil-calcium alloy marketed as Electralloy RV. It involves alloying of pure gold powder with a small amount of calcium. The calcium content in a finished product is about 0.1% and is added to produce stronger restoration by dispersion strengthening.

POWDERED GOLD

Powdered gold is a blend of atomized and chemically precipitated gold powders in pellet with maximum particle size is about 74 mm and the average is about 15 mm.

The atomized and chemically precipitated powders are first mixed with a soft wax to made pellets, then wrapped with foil.

Cohesive and Noncohesive Gold

The surfaces of the gold foil sheets must be clean without any impurities to provide proper cohesion and compaction between the gold foil sheets during cold working in the tooth cavity. But pure gold foils have the tendency to adsorb gases like O_2, N_2, H_2, etc. These gases prevent the cohesion between the two gold foil sheets. These kinds of gold foils with adsorbed gases are called as non-cohesive foils.

Manufacturers usually supply gold foils in non-cohesive state to prevent cohesion between them during storage and transport.

Before condensing the gold foil sheets into prepared tooth cavity non-cohesive gold foils must be heated to remove the adsorbed gases. Once the adsorbed gases are removed they can be bonded very well on cold working. The gold foils without contamination of gases are called as cohesive gold foils.

Manipulation

Removal of Surface Impurities

In order to achieve good welding between the pieces of gold, the surface of the gold should be clean. With the exception of noncohesive gold, direct filling golds are received by the dentist in a cohesive condition. However, during packaging and storage, they may be contaminated. Therefore, it is necessary to heat the direct filling gold to relatively high temperature immediately before it is carried into the prepared cavity. This step is commonly called as annealing heat treatment or degassing.

Objective

The main objective of heating is to remove the adsorbed impurities and they are by producing an atomically clean surface to achieve cold welding during condensation procedure. Consequently, a more appropriate term would be desorption.

Desorption is essential to remove possible surface contaminants such as oxygen, nitrogen, water vapor, sulfur dioxide and ammonia (intentional contamination).

During desorption, it is possible that some amount of recrystallization or stress relief may occur but these are unintentional. Both over and under heating should be avoided to achieve good cohesion.

Methods

Tray Method

In tray method, numerous pellets heated simultaneously on a mica tray (Fig. 6.32A) over an alcohol flame or an electric hot plate for 10 minutes at 454°C. The time required varies from 5 to 20 minutes depending on the temperature and quantity of gold on the tray. Problems that may cause incomplete tray desorption include:

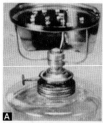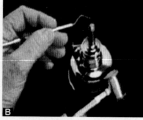

Figs 6.32A and B (A) Mica tray (B) Alcohol flame method

- Adhesion of pellets.
- Air currents that are effecting heating uniformly.
- Use of an excessive amount of gold to heat.
- Over sintering.
- Greater exposure to contamination.

Precautions

- Excessive amount of gold overheating or repeated heating should be avoided.
- Care should be taken to handle the pieces with stainless steel wire points that will not contaminate the gold.

Alcohol Flame Method

In this, individual pellets are heated in a methyl or ethyl alcohol flame at 593 to 694°C. The pellet is held by a pointed nichrome wire and passed through the tip of the inner blue cone of flame with a slow continuous motion to allow the gold to acquire a dull red glow (Fig. 6.32B).

Overheating to a bright red color makes the gold difficult to condense. Insufficient heating leaves impurities on the surface of the gold and prevents complete welding.

In mechanical condensing, a pneumatic condenser or an electromallet condenser may be used. Placing a condenser in contact with the foil and striking the other end of the condenser with mallet can accomplish compaction. Subsequently additional foil is welded to these pieces in the same manner (cold welding). Condensers used are:

1. Hand condenser with mallet.
2. Mechanical condenser or pneumatic vibratory condenser (Fig. 6.33A).
3. Electrical condenser (Fig. 6.33B).

Each increment must be carefully condensed by applying adequate compaction force to produce a void free restoration.

There are several controlling factors in the condensation process.

- Force of the condensing blow.
- Character of supporting bone and periodontal membrane resistance.
- Size of the condensing point.
- Proper stepping.

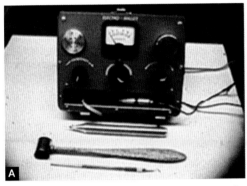 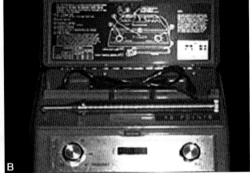

Figs 6.33A and B (A) Pneumatic vibratory condenser (B) Electrical condenser

During condensation, the strength is increased by work hardening. Once the preparation has been restored, the entire surface is subjected to additional condensation for the purpose of increasing surface hardness – Burnishing. Finishing follows this procedure.

SUITABILITY OF DIRECT FILLING GOLD AS A RESTORATIVE MATERIAL

Advantages

1. Direct filling gold is insoluble in oral fluids and will not readily tarnish or corrode, maintaining a high polish.
2. Due to its high ductility, it is capable of perfectly adapting to cavity walls.
3. It may be welded in a cold state and has a thermal expansion almost similar to that of the dentin (16.2 ppm/°C).
4. Oral tissues accept readily the polished surface of direct gold restorations.
5. Although the initial cost may seem high, the long-term cost of a direct gold restoration is relating low compared with other restorative materials.
6. Although there is a yellow hue in gold, this is harmonious with color of tooth structure and in contrast to silver alloy filling materials, direct gold cause no tooth discoloration.

Disadvantages

1. Direct filling gold is difficult to manipulate, requiring patience and skill of clinician.

2. Due to its low surface hardness, it is unacceptable in areas of high shear stress.
3. With some patients the initial high cost of direct filling gold restoration may prohibit its use.
4. Not adhesive to tooth structure.
5. Nonesthetic.
6. High thermal conductivity.

Uses

1. They are used primarily for pits and small class I restorations.
2. For repairing of casting margins.
3. For class III and V restorations.

SUGGESTED READING

1. Abby F Fleisch, Perry E Sheffield, Courtney Chinn, Burton L Edelstein, Philip J Landrigan, Bisphenol A. Related compounds in dental materials. Pediatrics; 2010. pp. 760-8. Published online Sep 6, 2010; DOI: 10.1542/peds.2009-2693.
2. Adela Hervás García, Miguel Angel Martínez Lozano, Jose Cabanes Vila, Amaya Barjau Escribano, Pablo Fos Galve. Composite resins. A review of the materials and clinical indications. Med Oral Patol Oral Cir Bucal. 2006;11:E215-20.
3. Andresa CO, Mário Alexandre Coelho S, Lourenço C-S, Mário Fernando de GÓES, Simonides C. Evaluation of Mechanical Properties of Z250 Composite Resin Light-Cured by Different Methods. J Appl Oral Sci. 2005;13(4):393-8.
4. Arrondo JLR, Collado MI, Soler I, Triana R, Ellacuria J. Setting reaction of polyacid modified

composite resins or compomers. The Open Dent J. 2009;3:197-201.

5. Asli Topaloglu Ak, A Riza Alpoz, Oguz Bayraktar, Fahinur Ertugrul. Monomer release from resin based dental materials cured with LED halogen lights. Eur J Dent. 2010;4:34-40.

6. Athina B, Triantafillos P, Pavlos G. Molecular toxicology of substances released from resin-based dental restorative materials. Int J Mol Sci. 2009;10:3861-99; doi:10.3390/ijms10093861.

7. Atkinson JC, Diamond F, Eichmiller F, Selwitz R, Jones G. Stability of bisphenol A, triethylene-glycol dimethyacrylate, and bisphenol A dimethyacrylate in whole saliva. Dent Mater. 2002; 18:128-35.

8. Azarsina M, Kasraei SH, Masoum T, Khamverdi Z. Effect of surface polishing on mercury release from dental amalgam after treatment 16% carbamide peroxide gel. J Dent. 2011;8(1):33-8.

9. Bauer JG, Henson JL. Microleakage: a measure of the performance of direct filling materials. Oper Dent. 1984;9(1):2-9.

10. Bennetts AJ, Wilde CG, Wilson AD. Adhesive cement. UK Patent 2386121; 2003.

11. Bitter K, Paris S, Pfuertner C, Neumann K, Kielbassa AM. Morphological and bond strength evaluation of different resin cements to root dentin. Eur J Oral Sci. 2009;117:326-33.

12. Bumgardner JD, Johansson BI. Galvanic corrosion and cytotoxic effects of amalgam and gallium alloys coupled to titanium. Eur J Oral Sci. 1996;104(3):300-8.

13. Burgess JO, DeGoes M, Walker R, Ripps AH. An evaluation of four light-curing units comparing soft and hard curing. Pract Periodontics Aesthet Dent. 1999;11(1):125-32.

14. Camile S Farah, Vergil G Orton, Stephen M Collard. Shear bond strength of chemical and light-cured glass ionomer cements bonded to resin composites. Aust Dent J. 1998;43:(2):81-6.

15. Cenci MS, Piva E, Potrich F, Formolo E, Demarco FF, Powers JM. Microleakage in bonded amalgam restorations using different adhesive materials. Braz Dent J. 2004;15(1):13-8.

16. Christensen GJ. Compomers vs. resin-reinforced glass ionomers. J Am Dent Assoc. 1997;128:479-80.

17. Dana G Colson. A safe protocol for amalgam removal. J of Environmen and Pub Health, Vol 2012; Article ID:517391, doi:10.1155/2012/517391.

18. Deborah S Cobb, Katherine M Macgregor, Marcos A Vargas, Gerald E Denehy. The physical properties of packable and conventional

19. de Souza Costa C, Hebling J, Hanks C. Current status of pulp capping with dentin adhesive systems: a review. Dent Mater. 2000;16:188-97.

20. Dunne SM, Gainsford ID, Wilson NH. Current materials and techniques for direct restorations in posterior teeth. Part 1: Silver amalgam. Int Dent J. 1997;47(3):123-36.

21. Ferracane JL, Antonio RC, Matsumoto H. Variables affecting the fracture toughness of dental composites. J Dent Res. 1987;66: 1140-5.

22. Finer Y, Santerre JP. The influence of resin chemistry on a dental composite's biode-gradation. J Biomed Mater Res. 2004;69A:233-46.

23. Gemalmaz D, Pameijer CH, Latta M, Kuybulu F, Alcan T. In vivo disintegration of four different luting agents. Int J Dent. 2012;2012:831508. Epub 2011 Oct 5.

24. GO Mec Y, Dorter C, Dabanoglu A, Koray F. Effect of resin-based material combination on the compressive and the flexural strength. J of Oral Rehabili. 2005;32:122-7.

25. Gladys S, Van Meerbeek B, Lambrechts P, Vanherle G. Evaluation of esthetic parameters of resin modified glass-ionomer materials and a poly-acid modified resin composite in Class V cervical lesions. Quint Inter. 1999;30(9):607-14.

26. Guertsen W. Substances released from dental resin composites and glass ionomer cements. Eur J of Oral Sci. 1998;106:687-95.

27. Habu H, Ohta K, Tanabe N, Hiraguchi H. Amalgam corrosion determined by dissolution of component elements and microstructural changes. Dent Mater J. 1986;5(1):26-36.

28. Harini K, Neil B Cramer, Lauren H Schneidewind, Parag Shah, Jeffrey W Stansbury, Christopher N Bowman. Evaluation of highly reactive mono-(meth)acrylates as reactive diluents for Bis-GMA-based dental composites. Dent Mater. 2009;25(1): 33-8. doi:10.1016/j.dental.2008.05.003.

29. Harold R Stanley. Local and systemic responses to dental composites and glass ionomers. Adv Dent Res. 1992;6:55-64.

30. Herod EL. Use of cyanoacrylate adhesive in dentistr. J Can Dent Assoc. 1990;56(4):331-4.

31. Hersek N, Canay S, Akça K, Ciftçi Y. Comparison of microleakage properties of three different filling materials. An autoradiographic study. J Oral Rehabil. 2002;29(12):1212-7.

32. Hilton TJ. Keys to clinical success with pulp capping: a review of the literature. Oper Dent. 2009;34(5):615-25.

33. Hiroyuki A, Hideo T, Takahito K, Seiji BAN. Effect of various visible light photoinitiators on the polymerization and color of light-activated resins. Dent Mater J. 2009;28(4):454-60.

34. Isil Cekic-Nagasa, Ferhan Egilmezb, Gulfem Ergun. The effect of irradiation distance on microhardness of resin composites cured with different light curing units. Eur J Dent. 2010;4:440-6.

35. James L. Drummond, degradation, fatigue and failure of resin dental composite materials. J Dent Res. 2008;87(8):710-9.

36. Jens F, Svenja R, Bogna S, Christoph H, Hämmerle F. Investigations in the correlation between Martens hardness and flexural strength of composite resin restorative materials. Dent Mater J. 2010;29(2):188-92.

37. Jing LI, Yoshihito N, Jian-Rong C, Takaharu G, Yuichi I, Takanori K, et al. New glass polyalkenoate temporary cement for cement-retained implant restoration: Evaluation of elevation and retentive strength. Dent Mater J. 2010;29(5):589-95.

38. Juan P, Loyola-Rodriguez, Franklin Garcia-Godoy, Renicko Lindquist. Growth inhibition of glass ionomer cements on mutans streptococci. Pediatric Dentistry. 1994;16(5):346-9.

39. Juergen M, Hong Y Chen, Reinhard Hickel. The suitability of packable resin-based composites for posterior restorations. J Am Dent Assoc. 2001;132;639-45.

40. Justin NR, O'Donnell, Gary E Schumacher, Joseph M Antonucci, Drago Skrtic. Structure-composition-property relationships in polymeric amorphous calcium phosphate-based dental composites. Materials. 2009;2:1929-54; doi:10.3390/ma2041929.

41. Kunio I, Takeshi E. A review of the development of radical photopolymerization initiators used for designing light-curing dental adhesives and resin composites. Dent Mater J. 2010;29(5): 481-501.

42. Leinfelder KF. New developments in resin restorative systems. J Am Dent Assoc. 1997; 128:573-81.

43. Lia W, Swain MW, Lic Q, Ironside J, Steven GP. Fibre reinforced composite dental bridge. Part II: numerical investigation. Biomaterials 2004;25:4995-5001.

44. Libonati A, Marzo G, Klinger FG, Farini D, Gallusi G, Tecco S, et al. Embryotoxicity assays for leached components from dental restorative materials. Reproductive Biology and Endocrinology. 2011;9:136.

45. Lim SD, Takada Y, Kim KH, Okuno O. Ions released from dental amalgams in contact with titanium. Dent Mater J. 2003;22(1): 96-110.

46. Lihua E, Masao I, Noriyuki N, Takashi Y, Kazuomi S. Mechanical properties of a resin-modified glass ionomer cement for luting: effect of adding spherical silica filler. Dent Mater J. 2010;29(3): 253-61.

47. Ling L, Xu X, Choi GY, Billodeaux D, Guo G, Diwan RM. Novel F-releasing composite with improved mechanical properties. J Dent Res. 2009;88(1):83-8. doi:10.1177/0022034508328254.

48. Lippo VJ Lassila, Sufyan Garoushi, Johanna Tanner, Vallittu PK, Söderling E. Adherence of Streptococcus mutans to fiber-reinforced filling composite and conventional restorative materials. The Open Dent J. 2009;3:227-32.

49. Lombard R, du Preez IC, Oberholzer TG, Microleakage of different amalgams bonded with dual cure resin cements. SADJ. 2007;62(2):056, 058-61.

50. Lutfi AN, Kannan TP, Fazliah MN, Jamaruddin MA, Saidi J. Proliferative activity of cells from remaining dental pulp in response to treatment with dental materials. Aust Dent J. 2010; 55:79-85.

51. Marc A Gauthier, Zhao Zhang, Zhu XX. New dental composites containing multimethacrylate derivatives of bile acids: a comparative study with commercial monomers. Applied Materials and Interfaces. 2009;1(4):824-32.

52. Maryam Khoroushi, Atieh Feiz, Maysam Ebadi. Influence of intermediary filling material on microleakage of intracoronally bleached and restored teeth. Dent Res J. 2009;6(1):17-22.

53. Maryam T, Fatemeh M, Ali Reza Sarraf, Sina Sanaie Zaker. Clinical study of a polyacid-modified resin composite-based fissure sealant in young permanent molars. Dent Res J. 2008; 5(1):31-5.

54. Mayanagi G, Igarashi K, Washio J, Nakajo K, Domon-Tawaraya H, Takahashi N. Evaluation of pH at the bacteria-dental cement interface. J Dent Res. 2011;90(12):1446-50.

55. McKenna JE, Ray NJ, McKenna G, Burke FM. The effect of variability in the powder/liquid ratio on the strength of zinc phosphate cement. Int J Dent. 2011;2011:679315. Epub 2011 Dec 8.

56. McKinney JE, Wu W. Chemical softening and wear of dental composites. J Dent Res. 1985;64:1326-31.

57. Miller BH, Woldu M, Nakajima H, Okabe T. Strength and microstructure of gallium alloys. Dent Mater J. 1999;18(1): 96-107.

58. Ming Tian, Yi Gao, Yi Liu, Yiliang Liao, Nyle E.Hedin, Hao Fong. Fabrication and evaluation of Bis-GMA/TEGDMA dental resins/composites containing nano fibrillar silicate. Dent Mater. 2008;24(2):235-43.

59. Mirmohammadi H, Aboushelib MN, Salameh Z, Feilzer AJ, Kleverlaan CJ. Innovations in bonding to zirconia based ceramics: Part III. Phosphate monomer resin cements. Dent Mater. 2010; 26:786-92.

60. Mount GJ. Buonocore memorial lecture. Glass ionomer cements: past, present and future. Oper Dent. 1994;19:82-90.

61. Nagaraja Upadhya P, Kishore G. Glass ionomer cement—The different generations, trends biomater. Artif Organs. 2005; 18(2):158-62.

62. Nakai H, Suzuki K, Hashimoto H. Effect of mercury to alloy ratio on the hardness of low and high copper amalgams: a comparison with central and marginal regions. Dent Mater J. 1985;4(2): 125-33.

63. Nakai H, Suzuki K, Irie M, Nagayama K, Hashimoto H. Characterization of low and high copper amalgam alloys and the effect of mixing time on their physical properties. Dent Mater J. 1984;3(2):170-92.

64. Nomoto R, Uchida K, Hirasawa T. Effect of light intensity on polymerization of light cured composite resins. Dent Mater J. 1994;13(2):198-205.

65. Okabe T, Mitchell RJ. Setting reactions in dental amalgam. Part 2. The kinetics of amalgamation. Crit Rev Oral Biol Med. 1996; 7(1):23-35.

66. Olea N, Pulgar R, Perez P, Olean-Serrano F, Rivas A, Novillo-Fertell A, et al. Sonnenschein, estrogenicity of resin-based composites and sealants used in dentistry. Environmental Health Perspectives. 1996;104:298-305.

67. Pascal Magne. Composite resins and bonded porcelain: The postamalgam era?, cda journal. 2006;34(2):135-47.

68. Payot P, Cattani-Lorente M, Godin CH, Bouillaguet S, Forchelet J, Meyer JM. Efficiency of curing devices for dental composites. Eur Cells Mater. 3(1):30-1.

69. Philips RW, Swartz ML, Lund MS, Moore BK, Vickery J. In vivo disintegration of luting cements. J Am Dent Assoc. 1987;114: 489-92.

70. Quan Wan, Joel Sheffield, John McCool, George Baran. Light curable dental composites designed with colloidal crystal reinforcement. Dent Mater. 2008;24(12):1694–1701. doi:10.1016/j. dental.2008.04.003.

71. Rafael L Bowen, William A Marjenhoff. Dental Composites/Glass Ionomers: the Materials. Adv Dent Res. 1992;6:44-9.

72. Richard S, Walker A, Gardiner Wade, Gelsomina Iazzetti, Nikhil K Sarkar. Galvanic interaction between gold and amalgam: Effect of zinc, time and surface treatments. J Am Dent Assoc. 2003; 134(11):1463-7.

73. Ripa LW. Sealants revisited: an update of the effectiveness of pit-and-fissue sealants. Caries Res. 1993;27.

74. Riza Alpöz A, Fahinur Ertuðrul, Dilsah Cogulu, Asli Topaloðlu Ak, Metin Tanoðlu, Elçin Kaya. Effects of light curing method and exposure time on mechanical properties of resin based dental materials. Eur J Dent. 2008;2:37-42.

75. Robin A Bernhoft. Mercury toxicity and treatment: a review of the literature, journal of environmental and public health volume 2012, Article ID 460508, doi:10.1155/2012/460508.

76. Rochelle G Lindemeyer. The use of glass ionomer sealants on newly erupting permanent molars. J Can Dent Assoc. 2007;73(2): 131-4.

77. Rosenstiel SF, Land MF, Crispin BJ. Dental luting agents: a review of the current litterature. J Prosthet Dent. 1998;80: 280-301.

78. Ruya Yazici A, Cigdem Celik, Berrin Dayangac, Gul Ozgunaltay. Effects of different light curing units/modes on the microleakage of flowable composite resins. Eur J Dent. 2008;2:240-6.

79. Safaa KH Khalil, Mousa A Allam, Wael A Tawfik. Use of FT-Raman spectroscopy to determine the degree of polymerization of dental composite resin cured with a new light source. Eur J Dent. 2007;1:72-9.

80. Santerre JP, Shajii L, Leung BW. Relation of dental composite formulations to their degradation and the release of Hydrolyzed Polymeric-Resin-Derived Products. CROBM. 2001;12:136.

81. Saraf KK, Kumar A, Mishra SK. Bonding systems for the new millennium. J Ind Dent Assoc. 2002;73(10):163-70.

82. Sayed Mostafa Mousavinasab, Ian Meyers. Fluoride release by glass ionomer cements, compomer and giomer. Dent Res J. 2009; 6(2):78-84.

83. Seitaro S, Hirotomo K, Rogelio J, Scougall-Vilchis, Shizue O, Masato H, et al. Antibacterial activity of composite resin with glass-ionomer filler particles. Dent Maters J. 2010;29(2):193-8.

84. Seyed MM, Kazem K, Nasrin T. Microleakage assessment of class V composite restorations rebonded with three different methods. Dent Res J. 2008;5(1):21-6.

85. Sidhu SK, Sherriff M, Watson TF. The effects of maturity and dehydration shrinkage on resin-modified glass-ionomer restorations. J Dent Res. 1997;76.

86. Skrticl D, Antonucci JM. Dental composites based on amorphous calcium phosphate – resin composition/physicochemical properties study. J Biomater Appl. 2007;21(4):375-93.

87. Soderholm K, Mariotti A. Bis-GMA based resins in dentistry: are they safe? J Am Dent Assoc. 1999;130:201-9.

88. Sridhar V, Sowmya NK, Deivanayagam K, Nagendrababu V. Fourier transform infrared spectroscopic evaluation - degree of conversion of a packable, hybrid and flowable composite resin cured using a light transmitting post. J Conservative Dent. 2007;10(1):38-42.

89. Tae-Sung J, Ho-Seung K, Sung-Ki KIM, Shin KIM, Hyung-Il KIM, Yong Hoon K. The effect of resin shades on microhardness, polymerization shrinkage, and color change of dental composite resins. Dent Mater J. 2009;28(4):438-45.

90. Taira M, Hiroyuki O. Dimensional change measurements of conventional and flowable composite resins using a laser displacement sensor. Dent Mater J. 2009;28(5):544-51.

91. Takeshi M, Yoshitaka Y, Masahiro I, Naohisa K, Itaru M. Force and amount of resin composite paste used in direct and indirect bonding. Angle Orthod. 2010;80:1089-94.

92. Theodore P Croll, DDS John W Nicholson. Glass ionomer cements in pediatric dentistry: review of the literature. Pediatr Dent. 2002;24:423-9.

93. Thiago A Pegoraro, Nelson RFA, da Silva, Ricardo M Carvalho. Cements for use in esthetic dentistry. Dent Clin N Am. 2007;51:453-71.

94. Tinca B, Violeta M, Florentina J, Emil CB. Evaluation of some multifunctional monomers for use in dental purposes. Revue Roumaine de Chimie. 2009;54(11-12):1001-5.

95. Toman M, Toksavul S, Akin A. Bond strength of all-ceramics to tooth structure using new luting systems. J Adhes Dent. 2008;5: 373-8.

96. Toksoy F, Sahinkesen TG, Yaman el K, Oktaya UEEA, Ersahan S. Influence of different drinks on the color stability of dental resin composites. Eur J Dent. 2009;3:50-6.

97. Ulrich Lohbauer. Dental glass ionomer cements as permanent filling materials? Properties, limitations and future trends. Materials. 2010;3:76-96.

98. Unterbrink GL, Muessner R. Influence of light intensity on two restorative systems. J Dent. 1995;23(3):183-9.

99. Vincenzo Fano, Mohamed Shatel, Maria Luisa Tanzi. Release phenomena and toxicity in polymer-based dental restorative materials. ACTA Biomed. 2007;78:190-7.

100. William J Dunn, Anneke C Bush. A comparison of polymerization by light-emitting diode and halogen-based light-curing units. J Am Dent Assoc. 2002;133:335-41.

101. Yong-Keun LEE, Bin YU, Guang-Feng ZHAO, Jin Ik LIM. Effects of aging and HEMA content on the translucency, fluorescence, and opalescence properties of experimental HEMA-added glass-ionomers. Dent Mater J. 2010;29(1):9-14.

102. Yoshiko K, Tomohiro T, Makoto O, Masaomi I, Yoshinori K, Junichi Y, et al. Effect of PMMA filler particles addition on the physical properties of resin composite. Dent Mater J. 2010;29(5): 596-601.

103. Yurdanur Ucar, William A Brantley. Biocompatibility of dental amalgams. Int Jl of Dent Volume 2011, Article ID 981595, doi:10.1155/2011/981595.

104. Zhang C, Degrange M. Shear bond strengths of self-adhesive luting resins fixing dentine to different restorative materials. J Biomater Sci Polym Ed. 2010;21:593-608.

Impression Materials

7

Impression

An impression is an exact negative replica of the oral structure with an accurate reproduction of all the finer details maintaining the correct spatial dimensions.

Impression materials are generally transferred to the patient's mouth in an impression tray. The tray is required because these materials are initially quite fluid and require support. Once positioned in the patient's mouth, the material undergoes setting either by physical or chemical process. After setting, the impression is removed from the patient's mouth. This negative replica is converted into a positive replica by pouring it with cast or die materials.

Cast

Cast is the dimensionally accurate positive reproduction of a portion of the oral cavity and extra oral facial structures, produced in a durable hard material and is used as a base for the construction of orthodontic and prosthodontic appliances.

Model

Model is a positive replica of the dentition and surrounding or adjoining structures and is used as a diagnostic aid for example to observe the progress of treatment in orthodontics.

Die

The term die is normally used when referring to a positive replica of single tooth or reproductions of multiple teeth with prepared cavities used in constructing restorations such as crowns, bridges inlays and onlays.

Purpose of Making Impression

Many dental appliances are constructed outside the patient's mouth on a cast of hard and / or soft tissues. As the fabrication required many laboratory procedures and the patient cannot be asked to sit in dental office during this considerable period of fabrication. Therefore, they are constructed on the cast in the absence of patient. The accuracy of fit and the functional efficiency of the appliance depend upon how well the cast replicates the natural oral tissues. The accuracy of the cast depends on the accuracy of the impression in which it was cast.

Impression Trays

Impression trays are used as rigid containers for carrying the impression material into the patient's mouth, for maintaining it in position during setting or hardening and supporting it during removal from the mouth and when casting the model.

Classification of Impression Trays

Impression trays may be classified as Stock trays and special trays (Table 7.1).

Selection of Trays

Impression trays are selected based on:
i. Relative need for retention
   For example, perforated trays for hydro-colloids – Perforations will produce

Table 7.1 Differences between stock trays and special trays

Stock trays	Custom or Special or Individual trays
Available in standard size.	Fabricated from a cast of patient's mouth and all are disposable
a. Reusable: These are supplied either with or without perforations	These are made up of: a. Shellac or similar thermoplastic material
b. Disposable: Usually perforated made up of a polymer such as nylon or polystyrene.	b. Acrylic resins
Advantages	*Advantages*
a. Eliminates time and expense of fabricating special trays	a. Moderate impression material is required
b. Metal stock trays are rigid	b. Sterilization not needed since it cannot be used for other patient
c. Nonsusceptible to corrosion	
Disadvantages	*Disadvantages*
a. Must be sterilized before using for other patient	a. Trays are fabricated in laboratory so time consuming process
b. Require more bulk of material	

mechanical interlocking as the material flows through holes.

ii. Special trays for free flowing impression materials.
For example, ZOE impression paste, and elastomers, for elastomers retention is achieved by the application of tray adhesive prior to the insertion of impression material.

iii. Based on the type of impression materials used
For example, perforated – Hydrocolloids
Nonperforated – Impression compound
Special trays – ZOE impression paste and elastomers.

iv. Based on the patient's arch shape and size.
$U_1, U_2, U_3, U_4 / L_1, L_2, L_3, L_4$

REQUIREMENTS AND CLASSIFICATIONS

Impression Materials

Impression materials are used to register or reproduce the form and relationship of teeth and oral tissues or used to accurately record the dimensions of oral tissues and their spatial dimensions.

The various types of impression materials used are as follows:

Inelastic materials/ Rigid materials	Elastic materials
Impression compound	Hydrocolloids
	i. Reversible: Agar–Agar
Impression waxes	ii. Irreversible: Alginate
Impression plaster	Elastomers
	a. Poly sulfides
ZOE impression paste	b. Poly silicones
	i. Condensation silicone
	ii. Addition silicone
	c. Poly ether
	i. Chemically activated poly ether
	II. Light activated poly ether

Ideal Requirements

Many materials have been used for taking impressions. But none of them is perfect. Each material is superior to other in some respects. So in order to have some means of comparison it is useful to enumerate the properties, which should be possessed by an ideal impression material.

Biological Requirements

Biocompatibility: An ideal impression material should be non-toxic and nonirritant.

An exception is ZOE impression paste. Reactor paste contains eugenol, which may cause irritation, allergy, burning sensation or chronic gastric disturbance in some patients.

Disinfection: It should be possible to decontaminate an impression to render it safe for further handling without affecting the accuracy or fine details. They can be decontaminated by soaking in aqueous solution of glutaraldehyde (widely used) or formaldehyde or hypochlorite.

Chemical Requirements

Inertness: An ideal impression material should be:
  i. Chemically inert in the mouth.
  ii. Not dissolve or disintegrate in oral conditions.

Moisture compatibility: An ideal impression material should be hydrophilic for better reproduction of details.

Some are hydrophobic (e.g. addition polysilicones) they require dryfield of operation, otherwise they may be repelled by moisture in a critical area of the impression. This normally results in the formation of 'blow hole' in the impression. For hydrophilic materials no special precautions are necessary.

Compatible with cast or die materials: Impression material should be compatible with model and die materials.

Rheological Requirements

Rheology is the science that explains the fluid or flow characteristics of materials.

Fluidity and viscosity: Viscosity is the resistance offered by a fluid to flow. Impression material should have good flow property (less viscosity)

before setting so that all finer details can be recorded and less flow property (high viscosity) after setting so that impression can be withdrawn from the mouth without any distortion. Based on viscosity, impression materials can be classified into mucostatic and mucocompressive materials.
  i. *Mucostatic:* These are initially fluid and compress soft tissues to a lesser extent. They are more fluid so all the finer details can be recorded and are used for taking secondary or corrective wash impressions, e.g. light body elastomers, ZOE impression paste, impression plaster, Agar-Agar, and alginate.
  ii. *Mucocompressive:* Initially more viscous, exert more pressure and displaces soft tissues to a greater extent. They are used to record primary or preliminary impression, e.g. impression compound and Putty body elastomers.

Pseudoplasticity: Certain materials those appear fairly viscous while under low stress conditions may become fluid during recording of the impression, when the material is placed under high stress. When a substance behaves in this way, it is said to be pseudoplastic, e.g. addition polysilicone is supplied in only one consistency (monophase material).

Mixing time, working time, and setting time
  i. *Mixing time:* Mixing time is the time from the start of mixing until a proper smooth creamy homogeneous mix is obtained.
  ii. *Working time:* Working time is the time from the start of mixing until the material is no longer suitable for recording an impression. It is normally characterized by the time taken for the viscosity to increase by a given amount above that of freshly mixed material (Fig. 7.1).
  iii. *Setting time:* The setting time of an impression material may be defined in terms of the required time to complete the setting reaction or it is the time required to reach a certain degree of rigidity hardness or elasticity.

Ideally, an impression material should have longer working time and shorter setting time.

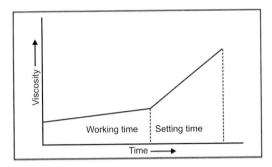

Fig. 7.1 Relationship between viscosity and time, that defines working and setting time

Mechanical Requirements

Accuracy: Must be capable of reproducing all the finer details with greatest accuracy. For greatest accuracy the dimensional change should be minimum ($\pm$ 20 μm).

Material that expands during setting, results in under sized die or cast and vice-versa (Fig. 7.2).

Elasticity: Impression materials should be sufficiently elastic (after setting) on removing from the mouth so that under cuts can be recorded without distortion or it should have large recovery and less permanent deformation. Tooth shape and curvature provide undercuts.

Tear strength: On removing the elastic impression material from undercut areas they are often put under a considerable tensile stress. So the material should have sufficient tear strength to withstand such stresses without tearing.

The thickest parts of the impression are compressed against the tray when they pass the widest part of the tooth (Figs 7.3 and 7.4).

Flexibility or strain in compression: Should be sufficiently flexible to permit easy removal over undercuts.

Adhesion or retention: Should be adhesive or remain attached to the tray during recording the impression. Partial detachment may cause distortion of the impression and will lead to ill-fitting of restorations.

Retention can be achieved by using tray adhesive (for elastomers) or by using a perforated tray (for hydrocolloids).

Dimensional stability: Should have no dimensional changes in or out of the mouth at all temperatures and humidity or should have perfect dimensional stability such that impression would retain its original accuracy indefinitely, e.g. Hydrocolloids are not dimensionally stable due to syneresis and imbibition.

Majority of material accuracy is best maintained by pouring gypsum cast soon after recording the impression.

Thermal Requirements

Coefficient of thermal expansion (α) Must be zero or minimum to minimize dimensional change on cooling or heating.

On being withdrawing from the mouth at 37°C to room temperature of 27°C, the impression undergoes approximately 10°C cooling. This results in thermal contraction, the magnitude of which depends on the value of COTE of the impression material and impression tray, thermal contraction can be minimized if the values of COTE of the impression material and tray are same.

Thermal conductivity: Should be a good conductor of heat so that it can soften or harden uniformly which minimizes distortion. But practically, all impression materials are poor conductors of heat. Hence they do not set simultaneously.

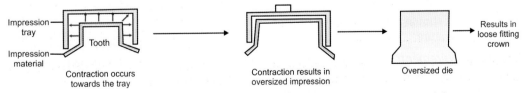

Fig. 7.2 When impression material undergoes contraction, results in oversized die

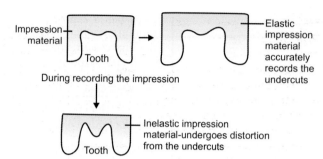

Fig. 7.3 Comparison of elastic and inelastic impression materials while they are removing from undercuts

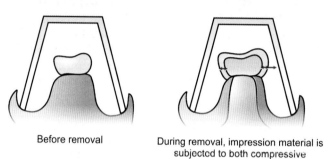

Before removal

During removal, impression material is subjected to both compressive and tensile stresses

Fig. 7.4 On removing impression material which will be subjected to both compressive and tensile stresses

For example,

1. Agar-Agar
   Impression — cooling/physical
   Impression compound → change setting
   Impression wax — starts from cooler tray side to warmer tissue side.

2. Alginate
   ZOE impression paste — Chemical change →
   Elastomers, and — starts from warmer
   Impression plaster — tissue setting side to cooler tray side.

Softening temperature: In case of thermoplastic material, the range of softening temperature should not be greater than 50–55°C. Otherwise on placing it in patient's mouth it may burn the oral tissues. It should set or harden at or near mouth temperature.

Esthetic Requirements

Color contrast: Suitable colors are used to distinguish materials of different viscosities. Two paste materials must be supplied in contrasting colors so that it is easy to see when mixing has been completed satisfactorily, there are no streaks of individual color left in the mix.

Minor Requirements

Acceptable taste and odor: Materials should have good taste and odor.
　　Exceptions – Impression plaster – bad taste.
　　Polysulfide – Bad odor.

Shelf-life: Materials should have longer shelf-life so that the unused material can be stored.

Economic: Be relatively inexpensive, simple, and easy to use.

Availability: Be easily available.

Ease of manipulation: Should be easy to proportionate, mix and clean. Should not require any elaborate equipment for manipulation.

Sterilization: Should be easy to sterilize if used for more than once.

Reusability: To be used again and again without any loss of useful properties of material.

Should permit multiple die pours.

Be capable of having additions made and insertion in the mouth without distortion. This will allow minor corrections to be made without having to take an entirely new impression. None of the available materials satisfies all the above requirements hence suitable material could be selected according to the clinical condition of patient's mouth.

Classification of Impression Materials

I. According to their chemical name–
  a. Impression compound
  b. Impression waxes
  c. Impression plaster
  d. ZOE impression paste
  e. Hydrocolloids
      i. Reversible – Agar-Agar
      ii. Irreversible – Alginate
  f. Elastomers
      i. Polysulfides
      ii. Polysilicones (Addition and Condensation silicones)
      iii. Polyether (Chemically activated and light activated)

II. According to their mechanical properties–
  a. Elastic
      i. Hydrocolloids
          Reversible – Agar-Agar
          Irreversible – Alginate
      ii. Elastomers
          Polysulfides
          Polysilicones (Addition and condensation silicones)
          Polyether (Chemically activated and light activated)
  b. Nonelastic or rigid
      i. Impression compound
      ii. Impression waxes
      iii. Impression plaster
      iv. ZOE impression paste

III. According to the force exerted on the soft tissues–
  a. Mucostatic
      i. Impression plaster
      ii. Agar-Agar
      iii. Alginate
      iv. Light body elastomer
      v. Impression waxes
      vi. ZOE impression paste.
  b. Mucocompressive
      i. Impression compound
      ii. Putty elastomer

IV. According to the nature of hardening or setting–
  a. By a physical change
      i. Impression compound
      ii. Impression waxes
      iii. Agar-Agar
  b. By a chemical change
      i. ZOE impression paste
      ii. Alginate
      iii. Impression plaster
      iv. Elastomers

V. According to their viscosity–
  a. High viscosity—Impression compound and putty body elastomer
  b. Medium viscosity—Regular body elastomers
  c. Low viscosity—Impression plaster
      ZOE impression paste
      Hydrocolloids
      Light body elastomers

VI. According to their dispensing system–
  a. Cakes, cylinders, sticks, and cones – Impression compound and impression wax
  b. Powder – Impression plaster and alginate
  c. Two-paste system – ZOE impression paste, poly- sulfide, and polysilicone.
  d. Three-paste system – Chemically activated polyether.
  e. Single paste system – Light activated polyether.

VII. According to their clinical applications–
  a. Preliminary impression of edentulous arches—impression compound
  b. Secondary or corrective wash impression
      i. ZOE impression paste
      ii. Impression plaster
      iii. Alginate
      iv. Light body elastomer.
  c. Cavity preparations of inlays and onlays – Elastomers.

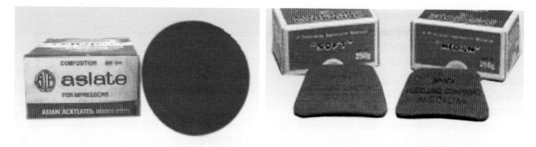

Fig. 7.5 Impression compound—cake form

d. Partial denture impressions – Hydro-colloids, and elastomers.
e. Special uses
   i. Syringe material, e.g. Light body elastomer.
   ii. Tray material, e.g. Tray compound, heavy body and putty body elastomers.
VIII. According to the mouth condition-
   a. Edentulous arches—All impression materials can be used.
   b. Dentulous arches—Hydrocolloids and elastomers.

IMPRESSION COMPOUND

Impression compound is one of the oldest impression materials. It is classified as nonelastic (rigid), mucocompressive and reversible (thermoplastic) impression material, which sets by physical change.

Alternative Names

- Dental compound
- Model compound
- Model plastic
- Impression composition.

ADA Specification Number 3

Types

According to ADA specification number 3, which is classified into two types. They are:
   Type I – Low fusing material, e.g.

a. Impression compound
   - It is supplied in the form of sheets about 4 – 5 mm thick (Fig. 7.5).
   - It is used for making preliminary impression of edentulous arches.
b. Green stick compound
   - Supplied in stick form and available in different colors (Fig. 7.8).
   - Used for copper band impressions of inlays, crowns and border extension of special trays.
   Type II – High fusing material, e.g. Tray compound
   - Used for constructing impression tray into which another impression material is carried to make a corrective wash impression.

Dispensing

Impression compound is dispensed in the form of cakes, sticks, and cones (Fig. 7.5).

Composition: (See Table 7.2)

Setting Reaction

Impression compound is a thermoplastic material, i.e. they soften when heated and harden when cooled, without occurrence of a chemical reaction.

$$\text{Hard} \xleftarrow{\text{Heating}}_{\text{Cooling}} \text{Soft}$$

Desirable Properties

The impression compound should–
   1. Be free of toxic or irritating ingredients.

Table 7.2 Composition of impression compound

Component	Wt%	Functions
Natural or synthetic resin Copal resin – 20% flow and cohesion. rosin – 20%	40	• Provides thermoplasticity. • Gives the qualities of flow and cohesion.
Waxes (Bee's wax, carnauba wax, paraffin wax)	7	• Provides thermoplasticity. • Characterizes the softening temperature and produces smooth surface.
Stearic acid, shellac, and gutta-percha	3	Acts as a plasticizer, which improves plasticity and workability.
Diatomaceous earth, French chalk, or talc	50	Acts as filler. • Increases strength. • Reduces flow at mouth temperature. • Reduces COTE.
Coloring agent	Trace	Gives characteristic color

2. Be well tolerable by the patients, i.e. soften at a temperature, which will cause no discomfort to the patient.
3. Be hardened at or slightly above the mouth temperature without warpage or distortion of any salt.
4. Have sufficient flow at setting temperature, so that all the fine details of oral structures are recorded.
5. Have less flow at hardening temperature to prevent distortion of impression during removal.
6. Exhibit a smooth glossy appearance after it has been passed through a flame.
7. Be capable of being carved or trimmed without chipping or fracturing.
8. Be a good conductor of heat for uniform softening and hardening.
9. Be capable of being sterilized without loss of properties.
10. Be adhesive to the trays and not to the tissues.

Properties

Biological Properties

Impression compound is nontoxic and non-irritant.

Rheological Properties

It is highly viscous (4000 centipoise). The very high viscosity is significant in two ways:
    i. Limits the degree of fine detail, which can be recorded.
    ii. Characterizes compound as a muco-compressive material.

When recording the impressions of some edentulous patients, it is necessary to record the full depth of the sulcus so that a denture with adequate retention can be designed. Only a viscous material such as impression compound is able to displace the labial and buccal soft tissues sufficiently.

Impression compound is mainly used for preliminary impression of edentulous arches. This gives a model (intermediate cast) on which a special tray can be constructed. A secondary impression is recorded in the special tray using a less viscous material such as ZOE impression paste. Pouring this with gypsum product will give a master cast over which the denture is fabricated.

Flow: Flow is the ability of a material to undergo plastic deformation under the influence of external forces or by its own weight.

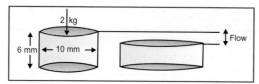

Fig. 7.6 Measurement of flow of impression compound

The flow of the impression compound can be beneficial or a source of error.

- The impression compound should soften at a point just above the mouth temperature and should exhibit high flow to conform to the tissues and register surface detail.
- The impression compound should harden at mouth temperature and exhibit a minimum flow so that it can be withdrawn with out any distortion.
  i. *Measurement:* As shown in Figure 7.6, a cylindrical specimen with 10 mm in diameter and 6 mm in height, is loaded at a definite temperature (37° and 45° C) with a weight of 2 kg for 10 minutes. The flow is designated as the shortening in length of such specimen during the test. Flows of type I and II compounds at different temperatures are given in Table 7.3.

$$\text{Percentage of deformation} = \frac{\text{Change in length}}{\text{Original length}} \times 100$$

  ii. *Factors affecting flow*
  - Flow of the impression compound is increased with the temperature, time and amount of load.
  - Wet kneading should be avoided as it increases the flow of the hardened compound, which may lead to distortion on removal from the mouth.

Wet kneading increases the flow of both the softened compound and hardened impression. This effect on flow is believed to be caused by the incorporation of water in the compound that acts as a plasticizer. Excessive wet kneading can increase the flow qualities of the hardened material at mouth temperature that exceeds the 6% permissible in the specification at which distortion may occur on removal. So it should be avoided.

Table 7.3 Flow of impression compounds at 37 and 45°C

Material	Flow	
	At 37° C	At 45° C
Type I Impression compound	<6%	>85%
Type II Tray compound	<2%	

Thermal Properties

Fusion temperature: Fusion temperature is probably the temperature at which the crystalline fatty acids solidify. The noncrystalline components solidify more slowly and at a lower temperature.

The practical significance of fusion temperature is that indicates a definite reduction in plasticity during cooling. Above this temperature, the fatty acids are liquid and probably plasticize or lubricate the softened material to form a smooth plastic mass while the impression is being obtained. Thus, every detail of the mouth tissues is more likely to be produced. Below this temperature an accurate impression cannot be expected.

Thermal conductivity: Thermal conductivity of impression compound is low. Due to lack of conductivity setting is not uniform (starts from cooler tray side to warmer tissue side). So the impression must be given adequate time to soften or harden uniformly.

When immersed in the water bath or heated over a flame, they soften on outside rapidly whereas the inner region remains hard. It is important that the material be uniformly soft at the time it is placed in the tray and thoroughly cooled in the tray before the impression is withdrawn from the mouth.

Coefficient of thermal expansion (COTE) Impression compound has a high COTE (200–500 ppm) and undergoes considerable shrinkage on removal from the mouth. The average linear contraction of compound on cooling from mouth temperature (37°C) to room temperature (25°C) varies between 0.3 to 0.4%. This can result in inaccuracy. One way to reduce the error due to thermal contraction is first to obtain an impression as usual. Then pass the impression through a flame until the surface is softened and retake the impression. During second impression the shrinkage is relatively less since only the surface layer has been softened.

Another modification of this technique is to spray cold water on the metal tray just before it is inserted in the mouth. Thus the portion adjacent to the tray will be hardened while the surface layer is still soft and records all the finer details.

Mechanical Properties

Dimensional stability: Dimensional changes or distortion can occur on standing the impression due to the relaxation of stresses. Stresses are incorporated due to the following reasons:
- High value of COTE.
- Poor thermal conductivity, and
- Relatively large temperature drop from mouth to room temperature.

To minimize distortion, the safest procedure is to allow thorough cooling of the impression before removal and to construct the cast immediately after removal from the mouth (at least within the first hour).

Manipulation

Softening: Impression compound can be softened by using a thermostatically controlled water bath (Fig. 7.7) or open flame, but they

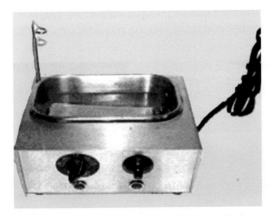

Fig. 7.7 Thermostatically controlled water bath

are normally softened by using a water bath at 55°C–60°C.

The compound is softened by immersing in the water bath at 55°C–60°C. Since the material has low thermal conductivity it must be immersed in the water bath for sufficient time to ensure complete softening.

Kneading: The compound is removed from the water bath and kneaded with the fingers in order to obtain uniform plasticity throughout the mass.

Loading: The compound is kneaded to suitable shape and placed in an impression tray (nonperforated stock tray).

Tempering: The outer surface (tissue side) of the compound can be waved over the flame or spray cold water on metal tray just before it is inserted into the mouth.

Making impression: The compound along with tray is then inserted into the mouth. The impression is retained until it cools to mouth temperature at that might take several minutes due to its lack of conductivity.

Removal: After it has completely hardened the impression is removed from the mouth and washed, dried and trimmed.

Casting: A mix of stone/plaster and water poured into the impression and allow it to set. The safest method for removal of the impression is to immerse it in warm water until the compound softens sufficiently to allow it to be separated easily from the cast.

Precautions

- When direct flame is used, the compound should not be allowed to boil or ignite so that important constituents are volatilized.
- Prolonged immersion or over-heating in water bath is not indicated. The compound may become brittle and grainy because some of the low molecular weight ingredients may be leached out.
- Undue kneading should be avoided as it increases the flow of hardened compound.
- The temperature of the water bath should not be too low. If it is too low, the material does not soften properly.

- The temperature of the water bath should not be more than 60°C. Otherwise the material becomes sticky and unmanageable due to leaching of some of the components (Stearic acid) into the water bath can also burn the patient's mouth.
- The water bath should be lined with napkin, otherwise the material will adhere to the bath.
- Impression must be given adequate time to soften or harden uniformly.
- Premature removal of the impression from the mouth should be avoided as it may result in distortion of impression.
- Cast should be constructed as soon as possible after the removal (at least within the first hour). If longer period elapses, warpage may occur due to relaxation of internal stresses.
- During the separation of the cast from the impression, compound should not be overheated. Otherwise, it may adhere to the cast and causes discoloration of the stone.

Advantages

- Can be used for compressing soft tissues.
- Can be used for any technique requiring a close peripheral seal.
- Can be used in combination with other materials.
- Can be added and readopted.
- Relatively cheap.

Disadvantages

- Distorts easily and should not be used when undercuts exist.

- Does not reproduce fine surface detail.
- Can only give an accurate impression with a long and difficult technique.
- As it can be resoftened and reused it tends to become unhygienic since it cannot be sterilized without affecting its properties.
- Its thermal properties are not ideal – large COTE and low thermal conductivity.

Uses

- Used for recording preliminary impressions of edentulous arches for the construction of special trays.

Green Stick Compound

It is a low fusing compound (type-I), introduced by Green brothers, supplied in cylindrical rods or sticks of about 10 cm length and 6 mm diameter and is available in variety of colors such as green, black, gray, brown and white (Fig. 7.8). The composition of green stick compound is almost similar to that of impression compound with more plasticizers. It is softened by waving over a gas flame and kneaded (dry kneading).

Copper Ring Technique or Tube Impression Technique

Occasionally, green stick compound is used in operative dentistry to obtain an impression of a single tooth preparation (crowns, inlays and onlays). In this technique, green stick compound is softened and placed in a cylindrical copper band. The filled band is then passed over the tooth and compound flows into the prepared cavity. After

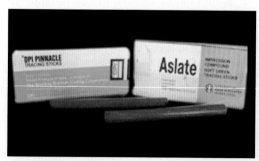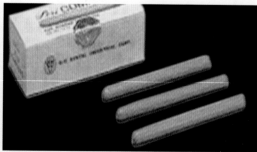

Fig. 7.8 Impression compound—stick form

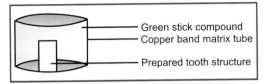

Fig. 7.9 Copper band matrix impression

the compound has been cooled the impression is withdrawn from the mouth (Fig. 7.9).

The contour of the entire tooth may not be reproduced accurately because of flow or fracture of compound on removal. Secondary or corrective wash impression is taken with light body elastomer.

The function of green stick compound is to strengthen the copper tube otherwise the impression will be squeezed with fingers when it is removed from the tooth and distortion will occur.

Uses

- It is used for border extensions of special trays (border molding technique).
- To obtain an impression of single tooth preparations using copper band.
- Peripheral seal material.

Tray Compound

The tray compound is high fusing compound and somewhat more viscous when it is softened and more rigid when it is hardened. They are similar in composition and working qualities to the impression compound except that the temperature at which they soften, i.e. higher (70° C) and the property of flow at mouth temperature is minimal (less than 2%).

They are usually supplied in the shape of tray, which may be black or white in color.

They are used to prepare custom made preliminary impression (special tray) that will later hold a second impression material, which will record final impression (secondary impression). Tray compounds lack strength and dimensional stability; hence they have been replaced to a large extent by trays made from self-cure acrylic resins.

ZINC OXIDE EUGENOL IMPRESSION PASTE

It is classified as rigid or inelastic and mucostatic impression material that sets by a chemical reaction. These materials are normally used to make secondary or corrective wash impressions of edentulous arches. It is abbreviated as ZOE impression paste or metallic oxide paste (Fig. 7.10).

ADA Specification Number: 16

Types

Type I – Hard
Type II – Soft

The difference between two types related to their hardness after setting. Krebs's penetrometer is used to find out the hardness of the set material.

Dispensing

Usually supplied as two pastes in collapsible metal tubes (Fig. 7.10). Tube-1 is base (white in color) and tube-2 is reactor (red in color). They are also available in powder (ZnO) and liquid (Eugenol) system.

Composition

Compositions of base and catalyst paste are given in Table 7.4.

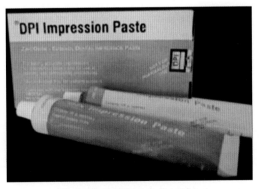

Fig. 7.10 ZOE impression paste

Table 7.4 Composition of zinc oxide eugenol impression paste

Base paste		
Ingredient	*Wt%*	*Functions*
Zinc oxide (French processed or USP)	87	• Reactive ingredient, which takes part in setting reaction. • It should be finely divided and should contain less amount of water.
Fixed vegetable oil or mineral oil (Olive or linseed oil)	13	• Paste former. • Plasticizer – provides smoother and more fluid mix. • Retarder—retards the rate of reaction and increases the setting time. • Aids in masking the action of eugenol as an irritant.
Reactor paste		
Ingredient	*Wt%*	*Functions*
Oil of cloves or eugenol	12	• Reactive ingredient, which takes part in setting reaction. • Oil of cloves contain 70–80% of eugenol it reduces the burning sensation in the soft tissues of the mouth when the mixed paste is first placed in contact with them.
Gum or polymerized rosin	50	• Facilitates the speed of reaction and produces a smoother homogeneous mix. • Gives body and coherence to the mixed material. • Imparts thermoplastic property to the set impression so that it can be softened in hot water for removal from the cast.
Filler (silica type) Kaolin, talc, etc.	20	• Used to form a paste with eugenol. • Increases strength of the mixed paste.
Lanolin	3	Plasticizer.
Resinous balsam (Canada or Peru balsam)	10	To increase flow and improve mixing qualities.
Accelerator solution ($CaCl_2$, or $MgCl_2$)	5	Accelerates the setting reaction.
Color pigments	Trace	• To distinguish from other paste. • Enables thorough mixing to be achieved as indicated by a homogeneous color, free of streaks in the mixed material.

Setting Reaction

On mixing the two pastes, a reaction between zinc and eugenol begins. The basis of the reaction is that the phenolic – OH groups of eugenol acts as a weak acid and undergoes an acid-base reaction with ZnO to form a salt, "zinc eugenolate".

The reaction consists of ZnO hydrolysis and a subsequent reaction between Zn hydroxide and eugenol to form a chelate, i.e. zinc eugenolate.

It can be seen that ionic salt bonds are formed between zinc and phenolic oxygen of each molecule of eugenol. Two further coordination bonds formed by donation of a pair of electrons form methoxyoxygen to zinc.

Water is needed to initiate the reaction and it is also a byproduct of the reaction. This type of reaction is often called "autocatalyzation".

Some manufacturers do not incorporate water into the paste and for these materials setting is delayed until the mixed material

Setting reaction of zinc oxide eugenol impression paste

contacts moisture in the patient's mouth. Water is then absorbed and setting is accelerated.

Water that is formed aids in binding the individual chelate units together in a chain or octahedral structure. The stoichiometric ratio of ZnO to eugenol is approximately 0.25 g/ml. The set impression consists of an amorphous zinc eugenolate matrix, which binds unreacted zinc oxide particles together.

Properties

These materials are nontoxic but those containing eugenol can be irritant giving stinging or burning sensation to the patient and leaving a persistent taste, which some patients may regard as unpleasant.

Relatively low viscosity (mucostatic) coupled with its pseudoplastic nature allows all the finer details to be recorded in the impression.

Setting Time

Setting time should not be too long as it causes inconvenience to the patient and should not be too short so that the material cannot be manipulated.

Factors affecting setting time are discussed in Table 7.5.

Initial Setting Time

It is the time from beginning of mixing until the material ceases to pull away or string out when its surface is touched with a metal rod of specified

Table 7.5 Factors affecting setting time of zinc oxide eugenol/eugenol impression paste

Factors affecting setting time		
Factors	To decrease setting time	To increase setting time
Temperature	Increase (Glass slab and spatula can be heated)	Decrease (Glass slab and spatula can be cooled but not below the dew point)
Humidity	Increase	Decrease
Altering the ZnO paste to eugenol	More eugenol paste (reactor)	More ZnO paste (Base)
Mixing time (within limits)	Faster and longer	Slower and shorter
Chemical modifiers	Add accelerators ($CaCl_2$, $MgCl_2$, and water)	Add retarders (boroglycerin, inert oils and waxes)

dimensions. It includes time for mixing, filling the tray and seating the impression in the mouth. It is 3–6 minutes for both types of pastes.

Final Setting Time

It is the time from the beginning of mixing until it gets maximum hardness, so that the impression can be withdrawn from the mouth with minimum distortion. It should occur within 10 minutes for type-I and 15 minutes for type-II.

Kreb's Penetrometer

It is used to find out the hardness of set material. Hardness is measured by noting the extent to which a loaded needle will penetrate on small specimens of set material (minimum depth of penetration). The hardness is expressed in terms of "millimeter" penetrated in a given time.

Thirty seconds after the start of mixing, the loaded needle (weight 100 gm) is lowered on to the surface of the specimen for 10 seconds and penetration is recorded to the nearest 0.1 mm.

Products with penetration values up to 0.5 mm are described as type I or hardset and products with values up to 0.9 mm or above are described as type II or softset. The hardest material sets faster (less than 10 minutes) compared to soft set material (less than 15 minutes).

Hardset materials have a more fluid consistency before setting and harder and more brittle after setting. Softset material is tougher and not as brittle, has a buttery consistency. It has a longer setting time of 15 minutes.

Consistency

Consistency is the amount of spreading of the material under a specified load when placed between the two glass plates immediately after mixing. Mixed paste should be homogeneous and it should flow uniformly against the tissues while the impression is being obtained. Otherwise, tissue displacement may occur. According to ADA specification number 16 it should be 30–50 mm for type-I and 20–45 mm for type II.

Dimensional Stability

The dimensional stability is quite satisfactory. A negligible shrinkage of less than 0.1% may occur during setting and there is no dimensional change after setting. The impression can be preserved indefinitely without a change in shape.

Rigidity and Strength

Strength is not critical requirement for this material since a tray supports it. The compressive strength of hardened ZOE paste may be as great as 7 MPa.

Manipulation

Selection of Materials

- Glass slab or oil impervious paper pad. Oil impervious paper pad is preferred to avoid cleaning a glass slab to which the material adheres firmly. Here the used paper is simply torn from the pad and thrown away after use.
- Stainless steel spatula.

Procedure

Manipulation stages of ZOE impression paste were shown in Figure 7.11. The proper proportion of two pastes is generally obtained by squeezing two ropes of pastes of the same length onto the mixing slab. A flexible stainless steel spatula is used for mixing. The reactor paste is first collected and applied over the base paste. It is now mixed with broad strokes in a sweeping motion until a uniform homogeneous color mix is obtained. Mixing time is approximately 1 minute.

Now the mix is collected and spread over the special tray and is placed in the mouth. The surface of the special tray should be dry since the material will not adhere to wet surfaces. Unfortunately, the mix will stick to the dried skin and instruments. So it is advisable to coat the patient's lips with petroleum jelly. This enables excess impression paste to be wiped away.

It is held firmly in position until the material has uniformly hardened.

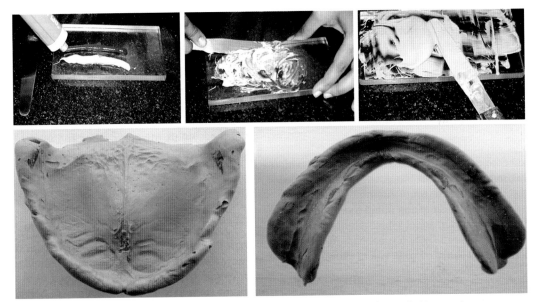

Fig. 7.11 Dispension, mixing, uniform consistency after mixing and recorded impression

Once the material has set, the impression is removed from the mouth. If the impression is not properly recorded another increment of a fresh mix can be placed over that and better impression can be obtained.

The impression is well-rinsed under running tap water for removal of any saliva or debris; disinfected and dried (to be shaken to dispose excess water).

Cast is made by pouring a mix of dental stone and water into the impression and allowing it to harden. No separating medium is required when making the cast.

The impression can be separated from the cast by immersing in hot water at 60°C for 5–6 min.

After use, the spatula blade can be cleaned by warming in a flame until it softens and the blade can be wiped clean with a paper towel. Solvents are also available for cleaning. They mainly contain naphtha, light cutting oils.

Advantages

- They are accurate, register details well and are quite stable dimensionally.
- They adhere well to dried surfaces of compound, resin and shellac bases.

- They require no separating medium before the cast is poured.
- They can be added and readopted if faulty.
- Easy to manipulate.
- Inexpensive.

Disadvantages

- It cannot be used when a slight undercut exists.
- Requires special tray for making impression.
- Some patients find the eugenol content unpleasant (may cause burning sensation or irritation to the oral tissues).
- Instruments are difficult to clean.

Uses

- Used for secondary or corrective wash impressions of edentulous arches.
- Temporary relining material and remodeling material.

Modifications

Surgical Paste

After gingivectomy (surgical removal of gingiva) an intraoral bandage such as a surgical ZOE paste may be placed over the wound to aid in the retention of a medicament and to promote healing.

Requirements

Should be/have
- Nontoxic, nonirritant, nonallergic to oral tissues.
- Soft and flexible.
- Strong enough to resist displacement during mastication.
- Bactericidal effect.
- Promote healing and aid in the retention of medicament.

Composition

The composition is same as that of the impression paste. However, these pastes are generally softer and slower setting (less amount of accelerator) in composition with impression paste. They contain more amounts of eugenol (weak antiseptic and sedative); fillers (to increase strength) and more amounts of plasticizers.

They are supplied as two pastes or powder and liquid system. The powder/liquid or two pastes are mixed together to form a paste like consistency. The mixture is formed into a rope and packed into the gingival wounds and interproximal spaces to provide retention to the dressing.

Drawbacks

- May cause chronic gastric disturbance, if it is worn for several weeks.
- May cause irritation and burning sensation.

Bite Registration Paste

The materials that are used for recording the occlusal relationship between natural or artificial teeth include impression plaster, impression compound, wax, resin and metallic oxide paste.

ZOE pastes are often used as recording material in the construction of complete denture and fixed or removable partial denture.

Composition

Supplied as two-paste system.

Composition is similar to conventional zinc oxide eugenol paste with slight modification. Plasticizers such as petrolatum are often added to reduce the tendency of the pastes to adhere to oral tissues.

Two pastes are mixed together and applied to register proper occlusion.

Properties

- Being brittle the paste will tend to fracture rather than distort on removal reducing the possibility of inaccurate registration.
- Offer almost no resistance to closing of mandible thus allowing a more accurate interocclusal relationship record to be formed.
- More stable than the one made in wax.

On the other hand the eugenol, if present, may be irritating effect to some patients.

Noneugenol Pastes (Substitutes for Eugenol)

Drawbacks of Eugenol

- Possible stinging or burning sensation caused by eugenol when it contacts soft tissues.
- Some patients find eugenol extremely disagreeable.
- Allergic response in some patients.
- Leaching of eugenol from surgical pack may cause the patient chronic gastric disturbance.

To cater for this type of patient, eugenol free zinc oxide pastes are available.

A material similar to the ZOE reaction product can be formed by a saponification reaction to produce an insoluble soap, if the zinc oxide is reacted with carboxylic acid (Ortho-ethoxy benzoic acid).

$$ZnO + 2\ RCOOH \rightarrow (RCOO)_2\ Zn + H_2O$$

Bactericides and other medicaments can be incorporated without interfering.

AQUEOUS ELASTIC IMPRESSION MATERIALS

The aqueous elastomeric impression materials are of two types: the reversible and irreversible hydrocolloids. The hydrocolloids are based on colloidal suspensions of polysaccharides in water. They exist in a form that is between that of a solution (individual atoms or molecules dispersed in a medium) and a suspension (aggregations of atoms or molecules dispersed in a medium). They may also be thought of as consisting of a dispersed particle phase (Agar) and dispersion medium phase (water). Dental hydrocolloids exist in two forms: a sol (a more or less viscous liquid) and a gel (an elastic solid). The impression material is introduced into the mouth as a sol and converts into a gel through either a chemical or a thermal process.

True Solution

If the size of the dispersed particles is small (less than 10^{-7} cm) and cannot be seen by naked eye or through a microscope, the system is termed as true solution, e.g. sugar solution.

Suspension and Emulsion

If the size of the dispersed particles is large (more than 10^{-4} cm) and can be seen by naked eye or through a microscope, the system is termed as suspension or emulsion.

Suspension: Solids dispersed in liquids, e.g. sand in water.

Emulsion: Liquids dispersed in liquids, e.g. oil and water.

Colloids

The term colloid is used to describe a state of matter in which the matter is divided into particles of size between 10^{-7} cm to 10^{-4} cm and distributed in another medium.

Colloids are often classified as fourth state of matter. It is an intermediate state between true solution and suspension. It contains two phases (heterogeneous system). They are:

Dispersed Phase

The substance, which is distributed in the form of colloidal particles, is known as dispersed phase. In a colloid the particles in the dispersed phase consist of molecules that are held together either by primary or secondary forces.

Dispersion Phase

The medium in which the colloidal particles are distributed or dispersed is known as dispersion medium.

HYDROCOLLOIDS

Hydrocolloids are the colloids that contain water as the dispersion medium.

Sol

A colloidal system in which the dispersed phase is a solid and dispersion medium is a liquid.

Gel

A heterogeneous biphasic system in which a liquid is dispersed in a solid dispersion medium is known as gel.

Gelation

Gelation is a process of conversion of viscous liquid sol into a semisolid jelly-like substance (sol → gel). It is a solidification process and brought about by either a physical change or a chemical reaction. The temperature at which a sol converts to a gel (in case of reversible hydrocolloids) is known as gelation temperature.

Mechanism of Gelation

The aggregates of molecules are dispersed within water when the material is in the sol form. By a reduction in temperature or by a chemical reaction the aggregates of molecules in a colloid can be made to join or agglomerate together to form a network of chains or fibrils or micelles. This fibril network encloses the dispersion medium, i.e. water (held in interstices between

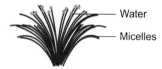

Fig. 7.12 Brush-heap structure

the fibrils by capillary attraction). These growing fibrils may branch and intermesh to form a "brush heap structure" (Fig. 7.12). After the molecules are joined together to form fibrils the consistency of the colloid becomes that of a jelly and it is in the gel form. Therefore the greater the concentration of gel the stronger will be the gel structure. In case of Agar the fibrils are held together by secondary forces, i.e. van der Waals forces and in alginates fibrils are held together by primary valency bonds, i.e. covalent bonds.

Reversible Hydrocolloids

If a colloid is changed from the sol state to the gel form and back again to the sol form, the material is known as reversible hydrocolloid. This process can be repeated several times, such a change in the state is brought about by a temperature change.

Gel to Sol

On heating, the gel converts to sol form. As the temperature raises, the kinetic energy of the molecules in the fibrils increases and they separate from each other to form sol.

Sol to Gel

When the temperature is reduced, by cooling, the secondary intermolecular forces once again come into play and molecules join together to form fibrils (gel). On heating the gel the secondary bonds are readily destroyed and broken and material returns to sol form.

Reversible hydrocolloid does not return to the sol state at the same temperature at which it is solidified (gelation temperature). The gel must be heated to a higher temperature known as liquefaction temperature to return it to sol condition. The temperature lag between the gelation temperature and liquefaction temperature of a gel is known as hysteresis.

Irreversible Hydrocolloids

Here the change from thick colloidal solution to a tough elastic gel is brought about by a chemical reaction. Once the gelation is completed the resultant gel cannot be converted back to its original sol state, such an impression material is described as irreversible hydrocolloid.

The molecules in the irreversible hydrocolloid are joined together by primary bonds. The bonds are very strong and cannot be affected by temperature change except temperatures at which decomposition takes place.

Sodium alginate + Calcium sulfate $\longrightarrow$ Calcium alginate + Sodium sulfate

General Properties

Dimensional Stability

They are dimensionally unstable because of syneresis and imbibition. They largely contain water (dispersion medium in sol and dispersed phase in gel), which is enclosed loosely within the gel fibrils. If the water content of the gel is reduced, the gel will shrink and if the gel then takes up water the gel will swell or expand. If these materials are used for obtaining impressions any change in dimension of impression after it has been removed from the mouth is a source of error.

Syneresis

Hydrocolloids will lose water content on standing in an atmosphere, which is not saturated with water vapor (dry atmosphere). The gel may lose water by evaporation from its surface or by exudation of fluid onto the surface of the gel. There also occurs the loss of some of more soluble constituents. Syneresis results in the formation of small water droplets of exudates on the surface of the hydrocolloids that is not pure water. It may be alkaline or acidic depending on the composition of the gel. Since the fluid is removed from the micelles of the gel by evaporation or syneresis, the gel shrinks. This effect is known as syneresis. This property is less in hydrocolloids containing a high concentration of dispersed medium.

Imbibition

If a hydrocolloid gel is placed in water it will absorb water by a process known as imbibition. The gel swells during imbibition thereby altering the original dimensions.

The reversible hydrocolloids will imbibe only water to replace that which they have lost by syneresis. Gel appears to exhibit memory in this respect (memory effect). However, some distortion of the gel may take place during syneresis and imbibition.

Irreversible hydrocolloids will continue to undergo imbibition if they are placed under water. They imbibe until their water content is much greater than that of the original gel.

Remedy

In order to ensure optimum accuracy the model should be cast as soon as possible. If it is not possible to pour it up immediately it can be stored in 100% relative humidity for not more than 1 hour. For shorter periods the surface of the impression can be covered with damp napkin.

Gel Strength

Hydrocolloid gels are relatively weak elastic solids, which are subjected to tensile fracture, i.e. tearing and flow. However, such a gel can support a sufficient level of stress without flow provided the stress is applied rapidly.

Factors Affecting Strength

1. Greater the density or concentration of dispersed phase in the sol greater will be the fibrils formed up on gelation and greater will be the strength.
2. Lower the temperature, stronger will be the gel strength for reversible hydrocolloids. As the temperature raises more of the fibrils may revert to the sol phage and strength decreases.

3. The manufacturers can control strength of the gel by adding appropriate amount of filler.
4. Faster loading or pressing causes greater resistance to deformation, i.e. it maximizes elastic recovery and minimizes permanent deformation. (Impression should be removed from the mouth with a single and sudden jerk).

AGAR IMPRESSION MATERIAL (REVERSIBLE HYDROCOLLOID)

Agar hydrocolloid impression materials are compounded from reversible Agar gels. When heated, they liquefy or go into sol state and on cooling they return to the gel state. Because this process can be repeated, a gel of this type is described as reversible.

Chemically, Agar is an organic hydrophilic hydrocolloid (polysaccharide) extracted from certain types of seaweed. It is sulfuric ester of a linear polymer of galactose.

ADA Specification Number: 11

Dispension

These materials are supplied in two forms:
a. *Tray material:* Supplied as gel in plastic or metallic types of disposable tubes.
b. *Syringe materials:* Supplied as gel in small cylinders of correct size to fit the syringe.

The only difference between two types is difference in color and greater fluidity in the syringe material.

Composition

Composition of Agar impression material is discussed in Table 7.6.

Gelation Mechanism

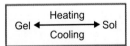

When the gel is heated, the kinetic energy of the fibrils will increase so that the interfibrillar

Table 7.6 Composition of Agar impression material

Ingredient	%	Functions
1. Agar	13–17	To provide the dispersed phase of sol and the continuous fibril structure.
2. Borax	0.2–0.5	To improve the viscosity of the sol and strength of the gel.
3. Potassium sulfate	1–2	Gypsum hardener – to counteract the inhibiting effect of borax and Agar on the setting of gypsum model material.
4. Alkyl benzoate	0.1	Preservative—to prevent the growth of mould in the impression materials during storage.
5. Diatomaceous earth (clay, silica, wax)	0.3–0.5	Filler – to control viscosity, rigidity and strength.
6. Water	85.5	To provide the continuous phase in the sol and second continuous phase of the gel, the amount controls the flow properties of the sol and the physical properties of the gel.
7. Thymol	Trace	Bactericide
8. Glycerin	Trace	Plasticizer
9. Coloring and flavoring agents	Trace	To improve the appearance and taste.

distance increases and the gel is converted to the sol because cohesion is less.

When the temperature of the sol decreases, the kinetic energy of sol particles decreases and fibrils will form and these form a brush heap structure. The fibrils are enclosed by weak van der Waals' forces. The water is enclosed loosely in the interstices between fibrils. When the gel is heated up to 100°C weak van der Waals forces disappear because of heat absorbed by fibrils and increase in their kinetic energy.

Liquefaction temperature of the gel, i.e. the temperature at which gel is converted to sol and gelation temperature, i.e. the temperature at which sol is converted to gel, both the temperatures are different for a hydrocolloid. This temperature lag or difference between liquefaction and gelation temperature is known as hysteresis, which makes the hydrocolloid to use in dentistry.

Properties

They are nontoxic, nonirritant to the oral tissues.

Viscosity of the Sol

After liquefaction the material is sufficiently fluid to record all the finer details. Agar is available in two viscosities, i.e. tray and syringe. Its low viscosity classifies it as a mucostatic impression material.

Gelation Time

Gelation time is a function of both temperature and time. It is approximately 5 minutes.

Gelation Temperatures

Gelation temperature should not be too high (may burn soft tissues) or too low (it is difficult to chill the material to form gel). According to ADA specification no. 11 gelation temperature should not be less than 32°C and should not be more than 45°C.

Gel Strength

According to ADA specification no. 11 the gel strength should not be less than 0.245 MPa. Strength depends on–

a. Concentration of dispersed phase
b. Temperature
c. Filler content.

Tear Strength

It is about 715 g/cm. It is very low. So use minimum thickness of 3–5 mm. It depends on the rate of loading, i.e. rapid removal is recommended to maximize tear strength and to minimize permanent deformation.

Flexibility

ADA requirement is 4–15%. Flexibility is measured as the amount of strain produced when a sample is stressed between 100–1000 g/cm². It is required for easy removal of the impression from undercuts.

Permanent Deformation

Agar impression materials are classified as elastic but they are not perfectly so. They undergo a small amount of deformation known as permanent set due to viscoelastic behavior.

Permanent deformation is measured as the percentage of deformation that occurs in a cylindrical sample after it is compressed 10% for 30 seconds.

According to ADA specification no. 11 it should be less than 1.5%.

Elastic recovery (ER)   = 100–1.5
                        = 98.5%

Permanent deformation is a time dependent property and is a function of:
 i. Percent compression
 ii. Time under compression
 iii. Time after removal of compressive load
 iv. Severity of undercuts.

Lower permanent deformation occurs when
 i. Percent compression is lower
 ii. Impression is under compression for shorter time
    (Remove the impression with a sudden jerk)
 iii. When the recovery time is long after removal.

If the thickness of the material is more between the tray and the teeth, the amount of compression is more, so more will be the deformation.

Dimensional Stability

Agar impression materials are dimensionally unstable due to syneresis and imbibition. So cast should be poured immediately after taking the impression.

Impression Trays

Water-cooled perforated trays are used for mechanical retention (Figs 7.13B and C).

Compatibility with Gypsum

Agar is compatible with die stone.

Electroplating

Agar impression material cannot be electroplated.

Disinfection

Agar impression can be disinfected by using iodopher bleach 'or' 2% glutaraldehyde.

Manipulation

Reversible hydrocolloids are normally conditioned prior to use, using a specially designed hydrocolloid conditioner (Fig. 7.13A). This consists of three temperature-controlled compartments containing water.
1. Liquefying component
2. Storage component
3. Conditioning 'or' tempering component.

Liquefaction of Gel (Gel to Sol)

The filled syringes and tubes are placed in one of the water baths of a hydrocolloid conditioner at 100°C for 10–15 minutes. This rapidly converts gel to sol. Insufficient boiling will lead to a granular stiff mass that will not reproduce the finer details.

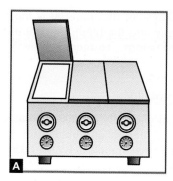 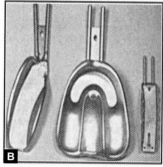 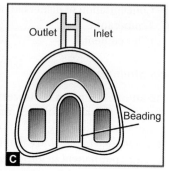

Figs 7.13A and B (A) Hydrocolloid conditioner (B) Water-cooled Rimlock trays
(C) Line diagram of water-cooled Rimlock trays

If the material is to be reliquefied after a previous use, approximately three minutes should be added to the boiling time, each time the material is reliquefied.

At higher altitudes, the temperature of water will not reach 100°C. In such cases a pressure cooker can be used or an agent such as "propylene glycol" can be added to the water until a temperature of 100°C is attained.

Storage of the Sol

After the Agar gel has been converted to sol, the tubes and syringes are then placed in storage bath, which is maintained at 63°C to 66°C. It can be stored at this temperature for several hours. Lower temperatures may result in some gelation and inaccurate reproduction of fine detail. The material in the syringe is never allowed to drop below this temperature. Otherwise, it will undergo gelation and it is then difficult to squeeze.

Conditioning or Tempering

The material that is used to fill the tray must be cooled or tempered. When the impression is to be taken, the stored Agar sol is squeezed in a perforated water cooled tray, a gauge pad 'or' glass is placed over the top of the tray and the tray is placed in conditioning bath at 43°–45°C for 5–10 minutes. The purpose is to:

i. Increase the viscosity of the sol so that it will not flow out of the tray.

ii. Reduce the temperature enough so that the material will not be uncomfortable to the patient.

The rate of gelation is influenced by the temperature at which the hydrocolloid is held. The lower the temperature the shorter should be the storage time in conditioning compartment.

Impression Making

In order to secure maximum detail, the prepared cavity is first filled by injecting the syringe material taken directly from storage bath. Before placing the tray material in the mouth, the water soaked outer layer of tray material is blotted with a dry gauge sponge. Failure to do so may prevent firm union between the tray and syringe material. The tray is immediately brought into position and seated with passive pressure.

Gelation

Gelation is accomplished by circulating cool water approximately 18–23°C through the tray for not less than 5 minutes. The coolest areas of the sol are converted to gel rapidly. So material in contact with tray sets more rapidly than in contact with oral tissues due to its lack of conductivity (tray to tissue side). Circulation of ice water will induce rapid gelation and more concentrations of stress in hydrocolloid, which is nearer the tray and distortion of impression may result.

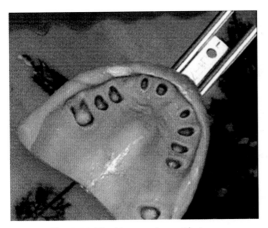

Fig. 7.14 Final impressing with Agar

Removal

After gelation, the impression is removed rapidly from the mouth with a single, sudden jerk in a direction parallel to the long axis of the tooth. Impression made with Agar gives accurate details (Fig. 7.14).

Washing

The impression is rinsed thoroughly with water and excess water is removed by shaking the impression.

Construction of Cast

Cast is poured immediately after recording the impression by pouring a mixture of water and suitable gypsum product. Improper manipulation techniques lead to failure of impression. Types of failures and their causes are discussed in Table 7.7.

Wet Field Technique

In this technique, the tooth surfaces and tissues are purposely wetted with warm water. Then syringe material is injected quickly in bulk to cover the occlusal and incisal areas. Then immediately tray material is seated over the syringe material. The hydraulic pressure of the viscous tray material forces the fluid syringe material into the areas to be recorded.

Table 7.7 Types of failures occur in Agar impressions

Type of failure	Causes
Grainy material	i. Inadequate boiling ii. Storage temperature too low iii. Storage temperature too long
Separation of tray and syringe material	i. Water soaked layer of tray material is not removed ii. Premature gelation of either syringe or tray material
Tearing	i. Inadequate bulk ii. Premature removal from the mouth iii. Syringe material partially gelled when tray is seated
External bubbles	Gelation of syringe material preventing flow
Irregular shaped voids	Material too cool or grainy
Rough and chalky stone material	i. Inadequate cleansing of impression ii. Excess water or potassium sulfate left in impression iii. Premature removal of die iv. Improper manipulation of the stone v. Air drying the impression before pouring
Distortion	i. Impression not poured immediately ii. Movement of the tray during gelation iii. Premature removal from the mouth iv. Improper removal from the mouth v. Use of ice water during initial stages of gelation

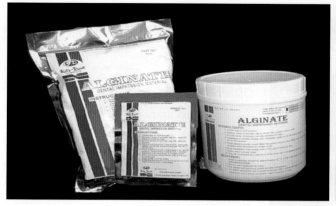
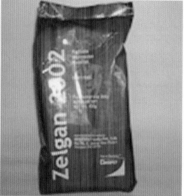

Fig. 7.15 Alginate impression materials

Theoretically, there is less chance that these materials will tear when the impression is removed from the mouth.

Uses of Agar

- For dentulous impressions.
- For crown and bridge impressions to a limited extent.
- For model duplication.

Advantages of Agar

- Reproduces finer details.
- Used for model duplication.
- Sufficiently flexible.
- High elastic recovery.
- Can be reused.

Disadvantages of Agar

- Dimensional instability.
- Impression cannot be electroplated.
- Low tear strength.
- Elaborated and expensive equipment is required for manipulation.

ALGINATE IMPRESSION MATERIAL (IRREVERSIBLE HYDROCOLLOID)

Dental alginate impression materials change from the sol phase to the gel phase because of a chemical reaction. Once the gelation is completed, the material cannot be reliquefied to a sol. These hydrocolloids are called "irreversible hydrocolloids" (Fig. 7.15).

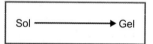

This material is based on alginic acid, which is prepared from brown seaweed (algae), which is a marine plant. Chemically, it is a linear polymer of anhydro – D – mannuronic acid of high molecular weight. Alginic acid is insoluble in water but the salts obtained with sodium, potassium, and ammonium is soluble. Sodium, potassium, and tri-ethanolamine alginates are used in dental impression materials.

ADA Specification Number: 18

Types

According to ADA specification number 18, alginate impression material is classified into two types:

Type – I: Fast set

Type – II: Normal set

Dispensing

Supplied as powder and available in two forms:
a. Bulk containers: Packaged in a sealed screw type plastic containers. It also contains a

plastic scoop for dispensing the powder and a cylinder for measuring the water (Fig. 7.15).

b. Small sealed packets or sachets (preweighed) constructed of plastic metal foil. This package prevents moisture contamination and extends the shelf-life of alginate (Fig. 7.15).

Fluoride is frequently also present (often as Na_2SiF_6) in concentrations ranging from 0.3–4% to improve the quality of the stone poured against the set alginate.

Composition of alginate

Discussed in Table 7.8.

Gelation

On mixing the powder with water a sol is formed and the alginate, the calcium salt, and phosphate begin to dissolve. Calcium sulfate rapidly reacts with soluble alginate to produce an insoluble calcium alginate gel in an aqueous solution. The production of calcium alginate is so rapid that it does not allow sufficient working time. Thus, a retarder, trisodium phosphate, is added to the solution to prolong the working time.

Trisodium phosphate reacts with calcium sulfate in preference to the soluble alginate to give a precipitate of calcium phosphate. This reaction delays the supply of calcium ions required for the gelation reaction and thereby increases the working time.

$$2\,Na_3PO_4 + 3\,CaSO_4 \longrightarrow Ca_3(PO_4)_2 + 3Na_2SO_4$$

When all the sodium phosphate has reacted the calcium ions begin to react with the soluble alginate to produce calcium alginate as a gel. As the reaction proceeds, the degree of cross-linking increases and gel develops elastic properties.

$$Na_n\,alginate + n/2\,Calcium\,sulfate \longrightarrow n/2\,Na_2SO_4 + Ca_{n/2}\,alginate$$

The set material is then a brush heap structure of fibrils of calcium alginate enclosing unreacted sodium alginate, excess water, filler particles and reaction byproducts.

Properties

Biological Properties

Alginate impression materials are nontoxic and nonirritant to the oral tissues.

Note: Alginate uses diatomaceous earth as filler. Diatomaceous earth contains finely divided silica

Table 7.8 Composition of alginate impression material

Ingredient	%	Functions
Soluble alginate (Na, K, NH$_4$ or tri-ethanol amine alginate)	15	Main reactive ingredient. Forms sol with water. Reacts with Ca ions to form a gel of calcium alginate.
Calcium sulfate dihydrate	16	Reactor – releases Ca ions to react with soluble alginate to form insoluble calcium alginate gel.
Trisodium phosphate	2	Retarder – to react preferentially with Ca ions and provides sufficient working time before gelation.
Diatomaceous earth	60	Filler—to increase strength and stiffness of the gel structure that is not tacky and controls the viscosity of the mix.
Zinc oxide	4	Filler—has some influence on physical properties and setting time of the gel.
Potassium titanium fluoride	3	Gypsum hardeners – to counteract the inhibiting effect of alginate on setting of die material and improve the surface of the stone model.
Flavoring agents (Winter green/peppermint)	Trace	To provide pleasant taste to make it more acceptable to the patient.
Color pigments	Trace	To provide characteristic color.

particles. Some of these particles are present in the dust, which rises from the tin or container after tumbling or fluffing or shaking. These silica particles are found to be a source of health hazard if inhaled.

Remedy: The tin or container is allowed to settle for a while after tumbling. Then hold the container away from the face when opened to avoid breathing the dust or use dust-free alginates.

Gelation Time

Gelation time is the time from the beginning of the mixing until the gelation occurs. It is measured as the time from the start of mixing until the material is no longer tacky or sticky when it is touched with clean and dry finger.

Based on gelation time there are two types of alginates:

Type-I: Fast set – 1 to 2 minutes.
Type-II: Normal set – 2 to 4.5 minutes.

Controlling of gelation time
1. By altering the W/P ratio or mixing time – not recommended.
2. By adding retarder to the material – controlled by the manufacturer.
3. By altering the temperature of water used for mixing. (Decrease in water temperature increases setting time).

Permanent Deformation

Alginate impression materials are classified as elastic but they are not perfectly so. They undergo a small amount of deformation known as permanent set due to their viscoelastic behavior.

Permanent deformation is measured as the percentage of deformation that occurs in a cylindrical specimen after it is compressed for 30 seconds. According to ADA specification no. 18, permanent deformation should be less than 3%.

Elastic recovery = 97% (100 – 3)

Permanent deformation is a time dependent property and is a function of:
i. Percent compression
ii. Time under compression
iii. Time after removal of compressive load
iv. Severity of undercuts.

Lower permanent deformation occurs when the:
i. Percent compression is lower
ii. Impression is under compression for shorter time
(Remove the impression with a sudden jerk)
iii. When the recovery time is long up to about 8 minutes.

If the thickness of the material is more between the tray and the teeth, the amount of compression is more, so more will be the deformation.

Gel Strength

According to ADA specification no. 18, the gel strength should not be less than 0.343 MPa.

Factors Affecting

1. Decrease in W/P ratio, within limits, increases strength.
2. Both under and over spatulation decreases strength.

Tear Strength

Tear strength varies from 300–700 gm/cm^2. It is very low. So use minimum thickness of 3–5 mm.

Flexibility

According to ADA specification no. 18, the flexibility should be 5–20%. It is measured as amount of strain produced when a sample is stressed between 100–1000 gm/cm^2. Most alginates have a typical value of 14%.

Dimensional Stability

Alginate impression materials are dimensionally unstable due to syneresis and imbibition. So cast should be poured immediately after taking the impression.

Impression Trays

Perforated trays (Fig. 7.16C) are used for mechanical interlocking of the material.

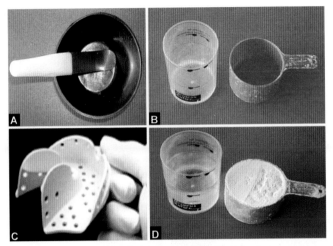

Figs 7.16A to D (A) Flexible rubber bowl and alginate spatula, (B) Alginate scoop and water measuring jar, (C) Perforated tray, and (D) Measured amount of alginate powder and water

Compatibility with Gypsum

Alginate is compatible with die stones.

Electroplating

Impressions cannot be electroplated.

Shelf-life

Alginate impression materials have a shorter shelf-life. They deteriorate rapidly at higher temperatures. Therefore, it is better not to stock the material more than one year and it should be stored in a cool and dry environment.

Manipulation

Instruments Required

Flexible rubber mixing bowl, alginate-mixing spatula with wide blade and perforated tray (Figs 7.16A to D).

Proportioning

The container of the powder should be shaken before use to get uniform distribution of constituents. The powder dispensing scoop is slightly over filled, tapped gently with spatula to fill the voids in the dispensing scoop and to ensure a reproducible volume of the powder is used in each mix. The blade of the spatula is then used to scrape off the excess from the top of the cup.

For maxillary impression: 2 scoops of powder + 1 measure of water by volume.

15 g of powder + 40 ml of water by weight.

For mandibular impression: 1 scoop of powder + ½ measure of water.

7.5 g of powder + 20 ml of water

The most accurate way of dispensing alginate is by weighing it; volumetric dispensing can differ from the recommended weight by 10–20%.

Mixing

The measured powder is shifted into premeasured water that has been placed in a clean rubber bowl. The powder is incorporated into water by careful spatulation.

Once the powder has been wetted, the material is mixed with a vigorous figure 8 motion with the mix being swiped or stropped between the blade of the spatula and sides of the mixing bowl with intermittent rotation of the bowl.

Mixing time is about 45 seconds. Both under spatulation and over spatulation should be avoided.

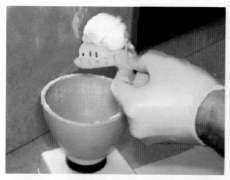
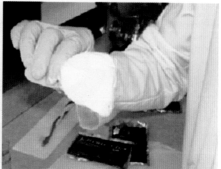

Fig. 7.17 Loading alginate material

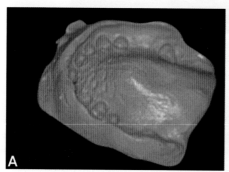
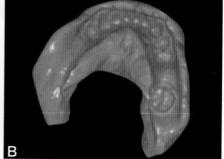

Figs 7.18A and B An alginate impression of (A) The upper arch; (B) Lower arch

Under spatulation
  i. Inadequate wetting and lack of homogeneity.
  ii. Mix will be grainy and poor recording of details.

Over spatulation
  i. Reduction in working time.
  ii. Reduction in strength due to destruction of gel fibrils as they form.

The final mix should be a smooth, creamy mixture that does not drip off the spatula when it is raised from the bowl.

Loading

The mixed alginate is transferred to a perforated tray by using mixing spatula and is generally added to the posterior portion of the tray and pushed towards anterior portion as shown in Figure 7.17.

Impression Making

The loaded tray is carried to the patient's mouth to record the impression. The posterior portion of the tray is usually seated first then the anterior part. The tray is held gently until the alginate sets (gelation starts from warmer tissue side to the cooler tray side).

Removal

After the seal between the impression and peripheral tissue is broken the tray and impression should be removed with a single sudden jerk to minimize permanent deformation.

Impressions made with alginate were shown in Figures 7.18A and B. One can make accurate impression when proper impression technique is followed. Types of failures in alginate impression were discussed in Table 7.9.

Table 7.9 Types of failures in alginate impressions

Types of failure	Causes
Grainy material	• Improper mixing • Prolonged mixing • Lower W/P ratio • Undue gelation
Tearing	• Moisture contamination • Premature removal from the mouth • Prolonged mixing • Inadequate bulk
External bubbles	• Undue gelation preventing flow • Air incorporation during mixing
Irregular-shaped voids	Moisture or debris on the tissue
Rough or chalky stone model	• Inadequate cleaning of impression • Excess water left in the impression • Premature removal of the model • Improper manipulation of stone
Distortion	• Movement of the tray during gelation • Premature removal from the mouth • Tray held in the mouth too long • Impression not poured immediately.

Washing

It should be washed under running tap water and excess water should be shaken off.

Disinfection

The impression can be disinfected by 10 minutes immersion or spray with sodium hypochlorite or glutaraldehyde or iodopher.

Construction of Cast

Cast should be poured immediately with a mix of dental stone and water, as they are not dimensionally stable.

Precautions

- The instruments must be absolutely clean. Small amount of gypsum left in the bowl will accelerate the reaction.
- Dust is raised due to tumbling of the powder, should not be inhaled.
- Correct W/P ratio as specified by the manufacturer has to be followed. Variation in W/P ratio affects setting time, permanent deformation, flexibility and strength.
- Air should not be incorporated during mixing.
- Both under and over spatulation should be avoided.
- The temperature of water used for mixing should be between 18°C– 23°C.
- At least 3–5 mm thickness of material should be present between the tray and the tissues.
- Tray should not be moved during gelation.
- Impression should be held in the mouth for at least 2–3 minutes after the material has gelled. Because strength and elasticity of the gel increases with time thus permitting superior reproduction of undercuts.
- Cast should be poured immediately. For shorter periods it can be stored in 100% humidity or its surface can be covered with damp napkin.
- Cast should not be left too long in the impression.

Advantages

- Reproduces excellent surface detail.
- High elastic recovery.
- Record undercuts.
- Comfortable to the patient.
- It is hygienic since fresh material is used each time.
- It is inexpensive.

Disadvantages

- Dimensionally unstable.
- Low tear strength.
- Cannot be electroplated.
- No proper storage medium.
- Cannot be added if faulty.

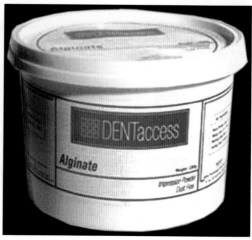

Fig. 7.19 Dust-free alginate

Uses

- Used for making the impressions of edentulous and partially edentulous mouths.
- To a limited extent in making the impressions of inlay, crown and bridges.
- In orthodontics, it is used to take the impression of the patient's mouth prior and during the treatment to construct study models.

Modified Alginates

Dust-free or Dust-less Alginates

It has been suggested that air-borne particles (dust) from alginate impression powders have the potential for causing respiratory problems. One study found that from 10–15% of these particles are siliceous fibers in the 3–20 micron size range; these dimensions are similar to those of asbestos and glass particles, which are known carcinogens.

Many materials have now been formulated which give off little or no dust particles avoiding dust inhalation. This can be achieved by coating the material with a dedusting agent such as glycerol to agglomerate the powder particles. This causes the powder to become denser than in the uncoated states (Fig. 7.19).

Siliconized Alginates

Alginates modified by the incorporation of silica particles have been developed. These are supplied as two pastes, which are mixed together. Tray and syringe consistencies are available. These materials have superior resistance to tearing when compared to unmodified alginates. However, dimensional stability is poor. These materials are considered as hybrids of alginates and silicone elastomer but their properties are closely related to those of alginates.

Alginates in the form of Sol

They are supplied as two-paste system. One contains the alginate sol while the second contains calcium reactor. They may be supplied in both tray and syringe viscosities.

Modified by the Addition of Chemical Indicators

The purpose is to indicate different stages of the manipulation, chemical reactions taking place and change in pH of the mix. The indicator incorporated gives a color change setting reaction proceeds.

For example, it shows violet color – during spatulation.

Pink color – ready to load.

White color – material has set.

Alginates Containing Disinfectants

Recently developed alginates contain disinfectant in the material itself that destroy the microorganisms. This eliminates the disinfection of the impression by immersing in or spraying with disinfectant, which may lead to dimensional changes, e.g. quaternary ammonium salt.

- COE hydrophilic gel (GC America) is a dustless alginate that contains 1.0% chlorhexidine diacetate as an antimicrobial agent.
- Jeltrate Plus Antimicrobial Alginate (Dentsply/Caulk) contains 1.7% didecyl-dimethyl ammonium chloride and has exhibited an ability to markedly reduce the number of bacteria present.
- Identic dust-free (Cadco) contains a proprietary antimicrobial agent.
- Blueprint Asept (de Trey) contains didecyl-dimethyl ammonium chloride and has been found to be effective in reducing bacterial counts.

Laminate Technique

In this technique, the Agar material is injected onto the prepared teeth and alginate in an impression tray positioned over it. Alginate gels by a chemical reaction whereas Agar gels by means of contact with cooler alginate rather than circulating water. The impression may be removed in about 4 minutes.

Advantages

- Cost of equipment is lower because only syringe needed to heat.
- Elimination of water-cooled trays.
- Records all the finer details.

Disadvantages

- Poor dimensional stability.

- The bond between alginate and Agar is not always strong.
- Highly viscous alginate may displace the Agar during seating.

Duplicating Materials

Duplicating materials are used to make an accurate replica of model or cast (Fig. 7.20). A duplicate refractory is used in the construction of prosthetic appliances (partial dentures) and orthodontic models. It is required for two reasons:

a. The cast on which the wax pattern of metal framework is to be formed must be made from a refractory investment, since it must withstand the casting temperatures.

b. The original cast is required for checking the accuracy of the metal framework and for processing the plastic portion of the denture.

ADA Specification Number: 20

Materials

Type I (reversible) It is of two types:

Class I (hydrocolloid) e.g. Agar

1. Reproduces excellent surface detail.
2. Can be reused.
3. Adequate strength and elasticity to duplicate undercut areas.
4. Not dimensionally stable.

Class II (nonaqueous) e.g. PVC gel.

They have high strength and chemical stability, which permits a large number of duplications before replacements.

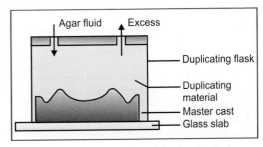

Fig. 7.20 Cross-section of duplicating flask

Type II (irreversible) It is also of two types:

Class I (hydrocolloid) e.g. Alginate
1. Does not require heating or storage equipment.
2. Cannot be reused.
3. Dimensionally unstable.

Class II (nonaqueous) e.g. polysilicones and polyethers.
• Very expensive.

Properties: According to ADA specification no. 20, duplicating materials (type-I and type-II) should have maximum of 3% permanent deformation.
  Flexibility = 4–5%

Duplicating procedure: Agar duplicating material is the most common type used in the dental laboratory technique for duplication, involves standing the cast on a glass slab surrounded by a metal duplicating flask. Agar gel is heated to 100°C to convert the gel to sol and then allowed to cool to 50°C before use. The fluid material is then poured through a hole in the top of the flask until it overflows through another hole as shown in Figure 7.20. When gelation is completed, the master cast is removed with a single sudden jerk to minimize permanent deformation. The duplicating cast should be poured immediately with refractory material (silica bonded or phosphate bonded) to avoid dimensional changes due to syneresis or imbibition.

NONAQUEOUS ELASTOMERIC IMPRESSION MATERIALS

Elastomers are a group of polymers that undergo very large reversible elongation at comparatively low stress.
  Or
  Elastomers are synthetic resin polymers with high elasticity due to their coiled structure.
  Or
  Elastomers are polymers which may be stressed in a manner similar to rubber and which will spring back to its original dimension when unstressed.

Elastomeric Impression Materials

The materials which will deform elastically while removing from the undercut areas and spring back to its original state after removing are called elastic impression materials.

ADA Specification Number: 19

Types

According to ADA specification number 19 for nonaqueous elastomeric impression material there are four types:
1. Polysulfide
2. Condensation polysilicone
3. Addition polysilicone
4. Polyether

Classification

1. *According to their chemical name-*
   a. Polysulfide
   b. Polysilicones
      i. Condensation
      ii. Addition
   c. Polyether
      i. Light activated polyether
      ii. Chemically activated polyether
2. *According to their viscosity-*
   a. Very high viscosity or putty elastomer (P)
   b. High viscosity or heavy body (tray consistency) – type I (H)
   c. Medium viscosity – regular body – type-II (R)
   d. Low viscosity – light body (syringe consistency) – type III (L)
   Polysulfides are available in – L, R, and H
   Condensation polysilicones – L,P
   Addition polysilicones – L, R, H, P
   Polyether – R + body modifier or L, H
3. *According to the method of polymerization-*
   a. Condensation polymerization, e.g. polysulfides and condensation polysilicones.
   b. Addition polymerization, e.g. addition polysilicone and polyether.
4. *According to the method of activation-*
   a. Chemical or catalyst activated, e.g. polysulfide, poly- silicones and chemical activated polyether

b. Light activated, e.g. light activated polyethers

5. According to the mode of dispensing–
   a. Single paste system, e.g. light activated polyether
   b. Two-paste system (Base + Reactor), e.g. polysulfides and polysilicones
   c. Single paste with reactor liquid, e.g. condensation polysilicones
   d. Three-paste system (Base + Reactor + Body Modifier) e.g. Chemically activated polyether

6. *According to their clinical application–*

Impression technique	Uses	Viscosities used
Double mix single impression or multiple mix technique	i. Cavity impressions of inlay and onlay ii. Impressions of crown	Light body + Heavy body
Double mix double impression	i. Cavity impressions of inlay and onlay ii. Impressions of crown iii. Impressions of partial dentures	Light body + putty body
Single mix single impression	i. Cavity impressions of inlay and onlay ii. Impressions of partial dentures iii. Impressions of full denture or edentulous mouths.	

Requirements

- Should be soft and flexible.
- Should exhibit reversible deformation.
- Should be a high polymer.
- Chain molecules should undergo uncoiling

and recoiling on application and removal of stress.

- They must be cross-linked so that–
  a. Chains do not slip under prolonged stretching.
  b. Chains will not go apart.
  c. Lower permanent deformation occurs.
- Should be amorphous.
- Glass transition temperature (Tg) should be below the room temperature.

POLYSULFIDE IMPRESSION MATERIAL

Alternative Names

1. Mercaptan impression material – by chemistry.
2. Thiokol – first manufacturing company.
3. Vulcanized impression materials – by processing technology.

Dispension

Supplied as two pastes in collapsible tubes (base and reactor).

Polysulfides are available in light, regular, and heavy body consistencies. May also be available in putty like consistency.

Composition

Composition of base and catalyst pastes are discussed in Table 7.10.

Setting Reaction

On mixing the two pastes, the terminal and pendant –SH groups of the polysulfide prepolymer are oxidized by lead dioxide to produce polysulfide rubber with the elimination of water as byproduct. During this reaction–

- Chain lengthening occurs due to the reaction of terminal –SH groups.
- Cross-linking occurs due to the reaction of pendant –SH groups.

Since the pendant –SH groups compose only a small percentage of available – SH groups, initially chain lengthening occurs which increases the viscosity of the mix.

Table 7.10 Composition of polysulfide impression material

Base

Ingredient	%	Functions
Moderately low molecular wt. polysulfide prepolymer with terminal –SH groups.	74-80	This is further polymerized and cross-linked to form rubber.
Moderately low molecular wt. polysulfide prepolymer with pendant –SH groups.	2	Undergoes cross-linking, which reduces permanent deformation during removal from the mouth.
Reinforcing fillers, e.g. TiO_2, chalk, lithopone ($BaSO_4$ + $ZnSO_4$)	16 (L)56 (P)	Paste former. Improves strength. Gives body and control viscosity. Modifies physical properties.
Plasticizer (Dibutyl phthalate)	0.5	To confer appropriate viscosity to the paste.

The base paste is normally white due to the filler and has an unpleasant odor caused by the high concentration of thoil (—SH) groups.

Reactor 'or' catalyst paste

Ingredient	%	Functions
Lead dioxide (PbO_2)	78	Oxidizing agent. Undergoes polymerization and cross-linking by oxidation of –SH groups. Gives characteristic dark brown color to the paste and has a bad smell.
Sulfur	3	To facilitate the reaction or as a promoter. Involved in the setting reaction.
Dibutyl phthalate	17	To form a paste with PbO2 and sulfur.
Inert oils (Stearic acid)	2	Retarder to control the rate of reaction.
Deodorants	Trace	To offset the unpleasant smell of PbO_2

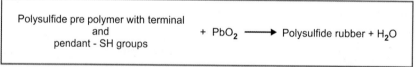

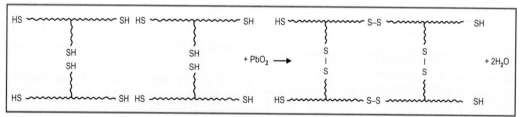

Polysulfide prepolymer with terminal and pendant –SH groups

Polysulfide rubber

The subsequent cross-linking links all the chains together in a three dimensional network which confers elastic properties to the material. This reaction is more effective in the presence of sulfur.

The polymerization of polysulfides is exothermic with a typical increase in temperature of 3–4°C. The reaction is sensitive to moisture and temperature and increase in either will accelerate the reaction.

During condensation process, water is formed as byproduct. Loss of even this small amount of water by evaporation will have a significant effect on the dimensional stability of the impression. Although the mix sets to rubber in about 10–20 minutes but the polymerization reaction continues for several hours.

Modifications

- One material avoids the use of PbO_2 and replaces it by an organic reactor such as cumene hydroperoxide or t-butyl hydroperoxide. However, this constituent is volatile and its loss by evaporation leads to shrinkage of the set mass.
- A recently developed polysulfide replaces the lead dioxide by inorganic hydroxide such as $Cu(OH)_2$.

Properties

- They are non-toxic and non-irritant to the oral tissues. It has a bad smell and odor due to the presence of PbO_2 and mercaptan groups.
  This problem can be avoided by using oxidizing agents such as cumene hydroperoxide or copper hydroxide.
- They are available in light; regular, heavy and putty body consistencies. The consistency is largely controlled by the amount of filler incorporated by the manufacturer. Availability in a range of viscosity will help the operator to choose the material with suitable flow property.

Working Time

The measurement of working time begins with the start of mixing and ends just before the impression material has developed elastic properties.

At the end of working time material is no longer capable of adequately registering necessary details. So the working time includes time for mixing, loading the tray and seating the impression in the mouth. It is measured at room temperature. The working time of polysulfide is about 3–6 minutes.

Setting Time

It is the time elapsed from the start of mixing until the material has polymerized sufficiently that it can be removed from the mouth with minimum permanent deformation. Setting time of polysulfide impression materials can be measured by:

- Vicat penetrometer
- Reciprocating rheometer.

Factors Affecting Setting Time

1. *Temperature:* Increase in the temperature accelerates curing rate and thereby decreases both working and setting time.
   Cooling is the practical method of increasing working time of the material. This can be accomplished by storing the material at a low temperature or by mixing on a chilled dry glass stab. But when the material is carried to the mouth, setting time is decreased due to the oral temperature.
2. By altering the base/reactor paste ratio: It is not recommended because mechanical properties can be adversely affected.
3. Adding a drop of water accelerates the curing rate.
4. Addition of retarder such as oleic acid increases working and setting time.

Flow After One Hour Setting

This property is very important because it relates to the amount of deformation of a polymerized impression material undergoes after being poured up with a gypsum product.

Flow after one hour setting is measured by determining the percentage of deformation of the sample after 1 hour setting, when it is subjected to a load of 100 g for 15 min. It is 1.5% more when compared with other elastic impression materials.

Permanent Deformation

Permanent deformation is measured as the percentage of deformation that occurs when the test sample is held under 12% strain for 30 seconds.

Permanent deformation of polysulfide impression material is 3%.

Elastic Recovery [ER] = $100 - 3 = 97\%$

Elastic properties improve with time. In other words, the longer the impression remains in the mouth, the greater the accuracy.

Elastic recovery is a function of:
a. Amount of strain (should be low)
b. Duration of strain (should be low).

Flexibility

Flexibility is the amount of strain produced when the sample is stressed between 100–1000 g/cm. It is approximately 5–10%.

Polysulfide is one of the least stiff or highly flexible materials, which allows the set material to be removed from the undercuts with minimum permanent deformation.

Tear Strength

Tear strength polysulfide is 4000 g/cm. They have highest resistance to tearing. But because of its susceptibility to distortion, it is possible that the impression may distort rather than tear. Rapid removal with a single sudden jerk increases the tear resistance.

Dimensional Stability

These materials are dimensionally unstable.

Reasons

1. Polymerization shrinkage during cross-linking.
2. Evaporation of volatile by product (water), formed during the reaction that causes shrinkage.
3. After removal from the mouth, incomplete recovery due to viscoelastic properties.
4. Thermal contraction that occurs when it is cooled from mouth temperature to room temperature and due to its large COTE of about 150 ppm/°C.
5. Although they are water repellent, they absorb fluids when exposed to water, disinfectant or a high humid condition.

Remedy: One way to minimize the polymerization shrinkage, loss of reaction byproducts and deformation associated with distortion, is to use a minimum amount of material.

The most accurate impressions can be made by using a custom or special tray (acrylic tray), because it ensures a uniform thickness of material.

Cast should be made within the first 30 minutes after removal of the impression from the mouth.

Hardness

Hardness is measured by shore-A-durometer. Hardness of polysulfide impression material is 30.

Disinfection

Polysulfide impressions can be disinfected by most of the antimicrobial solutions without adverse dimensional changes provided the disinfection time is short.

One recommended procedure is to immerse the impression for about 10 minutes in 10% hypochlorite solution.

Compatibility with Gypsum

These materials are compatible with die stones. Multiple dies can be poured but the successive dies are less accurate.

Impression Trays

Special tray needs to be fabricated.

Tray Adhesive

Tray must be painted with an adhesive to hold the impression material in place. This adhesive forms a tenacious bond between the rubber material and the tray. Tray adhesive for polysulfide contains *"Butyl rubber or Styrene acrylonitrile"* dissolved in a suitable solvent such as *"chloroform"*.

Electroplating

They can be electroplated to give metal-coated dies, which have greater resistance to abrasion than gypsum dies.

Shelf-Life

These materials have got adequate shelf-life.

Reproduction of Detail

These materials are capable of reproducing small lines of 0.025 mm width.

Advantages

- Longer working time.
- High tear resistance.
- High flexibility for easy removal from the undercut areas.
- Inexpensive.
- Long shelf-life.
- Impression can be electroplated.

Disadvantages

- Disagreeable taste and odor due to the presence of PbO_2 and – SH groups.
- Longer setting time.
- Dimensionally unstable due to the evaporation of byproducts.
- Need a special tray.
- Can stain the cloths.
- Second pour is less accurate.

Uses

- Impressions of crowns.
- Cavity impressions of inlays and onlays.
- Impressions of partially dentulous mouths.
- Impressions of complete dentulous mouths.

CONDENSATION POLYSILICONE IMPRESSION MATERIAL

These materials are also called as room temperature vulcanizing silicones.

Dispensing

They are supplied as–
- Two-paste system (Base paste + Reactor paste)
- Base paste + Reactor liquid.

Composition

Composition of base and catalyst pastes are discussed in Table 7.11.

Setting Reaction

On mixing the two components a reaction begins immediately in which the terminal hydroxyl groups of polysilicone prepolymer chains react

Table 7.11 Composition of condensation polysilicone impression material

Base	
Ingredient	Functions
1. Moderately low molecular weight polysilicone pre polymer with–OH terminal groups or hydroxyl terminal poly (dimethyl-siloxane)	It undergoes polymerization and cross-linking to form rubber.
2. Reinforcing fillers (35–75%) (Copper carbonate, Colloidal silica)	• As a paste former. • Increases strength of the set rubber. • Gives body and controls viscosity and modifies physical properties.
Reactor Paste	
Ingredient	Functions
1. Tri or tetra functional alkyl silicate or tetra ethyl ortho silicate. 2. Tin or stannous octoate [$Sn(C_7H_5COO)_2$]. 3. Reinforcing filler or thickening agents (Colloidal Silica). 4. Color pigments.	Acts as a cross-linking agent. Acts as a catalyst– • To form a paste. • To control the viscosity. To indicate uniform mix. To distinguish from the base paste.

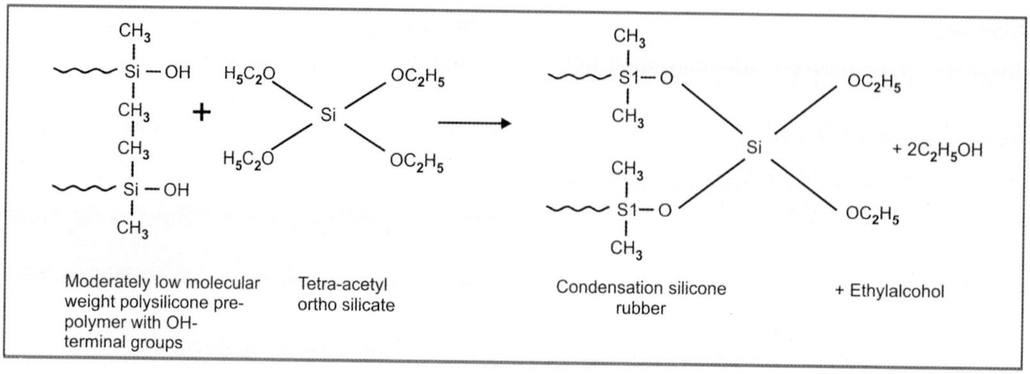

Fig. 7.21 Setting reaction of condensation polysilicone impression material

with cross-linking agent (tetraethylorthosilicate) under the influence of a catalyst (tin octate) (Fig. 7.21).

Each molecule of cross-linking agent may potentially react with up to four prepolymer chains causing extensive cross-linking. Cross-linking produces an increase in the viscosity and a rapid development of elastic properties.

Ethyl alcohol is a byproduct of the condensation reaction. Its subsequent evaporation probably accounts for much of the contraction during first 24 hours after setting in a set silicone rubber.

The multifunctional ethyl silicate produces a network of cross-linked structure that partly accounts for the low values of permanent deformation and flow values.

Setting time is 6–10 minutes.

Properties

- Silicone elastomers may be considered as nontoxic. But tin octate or stannous octate present in the reactor paste as catalyst when placed in direct contact with soft tissues found to be toxic. So care should be taken to mix the material well thus preventing the catalyst from coming in contact with the tissues.
- They are available in a variety of viscosities like light, regular, heavy and putty like elastomers and help the operator to choose the material with a suitable flow property and it also allows flexibility in choosing the correct impression technique.
- They are very hydrophobic and are repelled by water or saliva hence a dry field of operation is necessary. If not "*blow holes*" are likely to occur in the impression as it fails to dry away the residual moisture.

The contact angle with water is 98° indicating poor wettability and castability of die stone is 30%.

Working Time

Working time represents the maximum amount of time available to mix and handle the material before it is placed in the mouth. It is around 2–3 minutes.

Setting Time

Setting time is the time from the beginning of mixing until the material is sufficiently elastic so that it can be removed from the mouth without significant permanent deformation. Setting time is 6–10 minutes.

Both working and setting times are measured by Vicat penetrometer and Reciprocating rheometer.

Factors Affecting Setting Time

- Reaction is sensitive to temperature. Cooling the material or mixing on a cooler glass slab will increase working and setting times.
- By altering base/reactor ratio – Not recommended.

Elasticity

Condensation silicones are more ideally elastic than polysulfides. They exhibit minimal permanent deformation and recover rapidly when strained rapidly. Hence the impression must be removed rapidly with a single sudden jerk. Cross-linking reduces the permanent deformation of a set rubber. Prolonging the strain will increase the deformation because the polymer chains respond in viscous manner.

Permanent Deformation = 0.7%
Elastic Recovery = 100–0.7 = 99.3%

Flow After One Hour Setting

Flow after one hour setting is by determining the percentage of deformation of a cylindrical sample of 1 hour, when it is subjected to a load of 100g for 15 min. it is 0.1% and lower than polysulfides. It is low due to rapid setting reaction and highly cross-linked structure.

Flexibility

Flexibility is measured as the amount of strain produced when the sample is stressed between 100–1000 g/cm. Flexibility of condensation silicones is around 2–7%, not very stiff which means it is not very difficult to remove them from undercuts without distortion.

Tear Strength

Tear strength is lower (3500 g/cm) than polysulfides. But they do not tear as easily as hydrocolloids. The impression must be rapidly removed to maximize the tear strength.

Dimensional Stability

Dimensional stability is not good due to:
- Large polymerization shrinkage (0.6–1%) because the setting reaction continues even after the material is clinically set and the polymerization shrinkage continues.
- Loss of volatile reaction byproduct (ethyl alcohol), which produces a measurable weight loss (0.9%).
- Thermal contraction when cooled from mouth temperature to room temperature.

COTE = 190 ppm/°C

Thus, the most accurate model is obtained by pouring up the impression immediately (within first 30 min) after it is removed from the mouth.

Putty-wash technique is normally used to compensate for the poor dimensional stability.

Reproduction of Detail

These materials are capable of reproducing lines of 0.025 mm width.

Compatibility with Gypsum

These materials are compatible with die stone.

Electroplating

Dies can be electroplated with silver or copper. But because of their dimensional instability after setting, stone dies are more frequently made than metal.

Hardness

Hardness of condensation silicone is about 43. Hardness of these materials can be measured by shore A durometer.

Impression Trays

Disposable stock trays are normally preferred.

Tray Adhesive

Tray adhesive consists of poly (dimethyl siloxane) or other silicone that reacts with the impression material and ethyl silicate to create a physical bond with the tray.

Disinfection

Impression can be disinfected by immersing in most of available antimicrobial solutions for less than one hour.

Color Contrast

Base paste is colorless. Dyes are added to the colorless reactor paste to indicate the completion of mixing.

The different consistencies are in different colors or at least different shades of the same color so that they can be readily distinguished in an impression made by using putty wash technique.

Shelf-Life

Alkyl silicates are slightly unstable, particularly if they are mixed with a tin compound to form a single catalyst liquid. Thus, a limited shelf-life may result because of oxidation of the tin compound within the catalyst.

Shelf-life failure may also occur as a result of degradation of the base or cross-linkage of base during storage. Store the material in cool, dry environment.

Advantages

- Adequate working and setting times.
- Clean and pleasant odor and no staining.
- Adequate tear strength.
- Better elastic properties on removal.
- Available in complete range of viscosities thus allowing flexibility in choosing an impression technique.
- Less distortion on removal.

Disadvantages

- Poor dimensional stability.
- Adequate accuracy only when poured immediately.
- Need for a dry field of operation since it is hydrophobic.
- Poor shelf-life.

- Slightly more expensive.
- Putty wash method is technique sensitive.
- Liquid component of the reactor paste may be hazardous if not handled properly.

Uses

- Widely used for crown and bridge impressions.
- Cavity preparations of inlays and onlays.
- Occasionally used for partially dentulous mouth impression.

Modifications

A major modification of the condensation silicone material is a change in the setting mechanism. This modification has brought about a new family of impression materials, the addition reaction silicones.

ADDITION POLYSILICONE IMPRESSION MATERIAL

Addition polysilicones are often termed as polyvinyl siloxane or vinyl polysiloxane since they undergo vinyl polymerization or addition polymerization (Figs 7.22A to C).

Dispensing

Supplied as two-paste system and are available all four viscosities. Also available as single consistency called single phase or mono phase and can be used both as tray and syringe consistency due to its pseudoplastic nature.

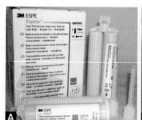 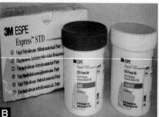 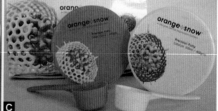

Figs 7.22A to C Addition polysilicone (A) Light body; (B) and (C) Putty body

Table 7.12 Composition of condensation polysilicone impression material

Base	
Ingredient	*Functions*
Moderately low molecular weight polysilicone prepolymer with silane terminal groups or poly (methyl hydrogen silicone).	Takes part in the polymerization reaction.
Reinforcing fillers (colloidal silica)	Controls viscosity and modifies the physical properties.
Reactor	
Ingredient	*Functions*
Moderately low molecular weight polysilicone prepolymer with vinyl terminal groups or poly (dimethyl vinyl siloxane) Reinforcing fillers (powdered silica)	• Main reactive ingredient. • Takes part in the polymerization reaction. • Paste former. • Increases strength. • Gives body and controls viscosity. • Modifies physical properties.
Chloroplatinic acid (H_2PtCl_6) Low molecular weight liquid polymer of the same type as the base polymer. Finely divided Pt or Pd Color pigments	As a catalyst– • Retarder. • Provides working and setting time. To absorb H_2 gas evolved or as a scavenger for H_2 gas. To distinguish it from base paste and for indicating completion of mixing.

Composition

Composition of base and catalyst pastes are discussed in Table 7.12.

Setting Reaction (Fig. 7.23)

On mixing the two pastes, a platinum catalyzed addition reaction occurs causing cross-linking between the two types of siloxane prepolymer. There are no byproducts (which result in minimum dimensional change) as long as the correct proportions of vinyl siloxane and hydride silicone are maintained and there are no impurities.

If the proportions are out of balance or impurities are present, then side reactions will produce hydrogen (H_2) gas. It is formed due to the reaction between residual silanol groups or moisture with hydrides of the base polymer.

Hydrogen gas that evolves from the set material can result in pinpoint voids in the stone cast that are poured immediately after removing from the mouth.

1. To minimize this, the present day silicones contain a noble metal such as platinum or palladium, which acts as a scavenger for the H_2 gas evolved.
2. Another method is to wait an hour or longer before pouring up the impression (until the H_2 gas is completely evolved). This delay does not cause detectable dimensional change.
3. Elimination of impurities.
4. Placing the impressions in the vacuum either before or after pouring the stone cast.

Cross-linking produces an increase in viscosity coupled with the increase in elastic properties. Increase in temperature increases rate of reaction and decreases working and setting times.

Setting time is about 6–8 min.

Properties

• They are highly biocompatible and cause less tissue reaction than condensation silicones. They do not possess an unpleasant taste or odor and are acceptable by the patient.

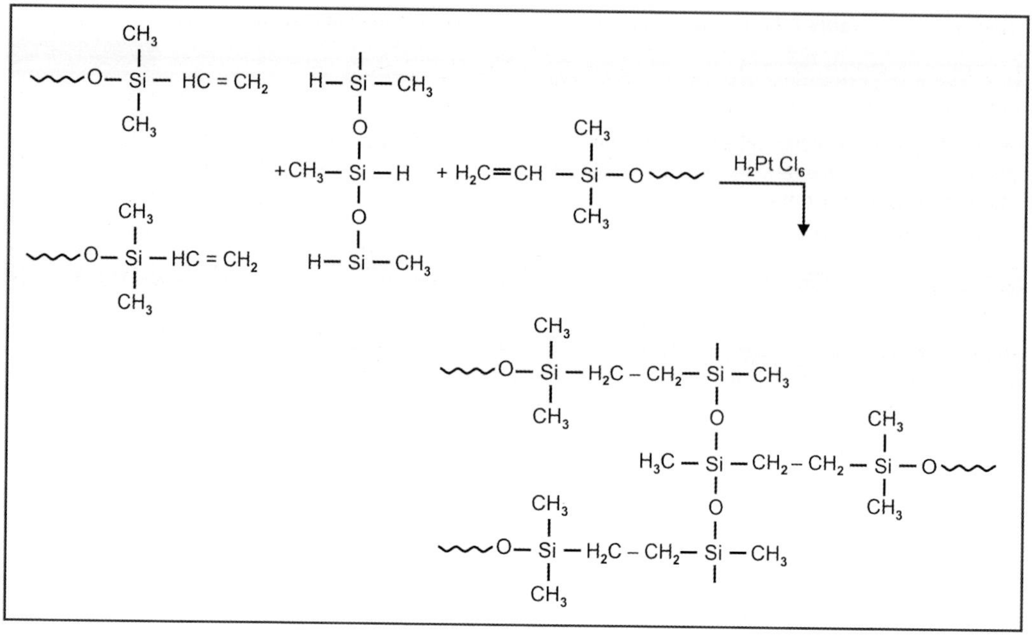

Fig. 7.23 Setting mechanism of addition polysilicone impression material

- They are available in complete range of viscosities, i.e. light, regular, heavy and putty body. It helps the operator to choose the material with suitable flow properties.
  For example, double mix double impression (putty + light)
  (Putty body – for preliminary impression Light body – secondary impression)
  The consistency is controlled by the amount of filler and molecular weight of the polymer.

Consistency

Light body:	36–55 mm.
Regular body:	30–40 mm.
Heavy body:	20–32 mm.
Putty body:	13–30 mm.

Pseudoplasticity

Addition polysilicones exhibit pseudoplastic property, i.e. viscosity gradually decreases as the shear stress increases. They are supplied as single consistency (single phase or mono phase). One mix is used on the tray (subjected to low shear stress) and another mix is loaded in a syringe (subjected to high shear stress). When syringed, the material flows readily and records the finer details.

Flow After One Hour Setting

Flow after one hour setting is measured by determining the percentage of deformation in a cylindrical sample of one hour old after it is subjected to a load of 100 g for 15 minutes. It relates to the amount of deformation after the impression being poured with a gypsum product. Flow after one hour setting for these materials is less than 0.05%, it is very low.

Working Time

The measurement of working time begins with the start of mix and ends just before the impression material has developed elastic properties.
The working time is about 2–3 minutes.

Setting Time

It is defined as the time elasping from the beginning of mixing until the curing has advanced sufficiently (becomes elastic) that the impression can be removed from the mouth with a minimum distortion. It is about 6–8 minutes.

Both working and setting times are measured by Vicat penetrometer and reciprocating rheometer.

Factors Affecting Setting Time

1. Increase in either temperature or humidity will decrease working and setting time.
2. Material can be refrigerated before mixing of the material on a cool dry slab to increase the working time and setting time.
3. Both working and setting times can be prolonged by the addition of retarder as supplied by the manufacturer.

Elasticity

Addition polysilicones are most ideally elastic of the currently available materials because the permanent deformation is very less that is about 0.07%.

Permanent deformation is measured as the percentage of deformation of that occurs when the test sample is held under 12% compression for 30 seconds. Amount of material and duration of strain affects the permanent deformation.

Elastic recovery = 99.93%

Tear Strength

Tear strength is adequate (3500 gm/cm) but if not handled correctly they will tear. They are highly viscoelastic, so using a rapid strain rate produces an elastic response.

Flexibility

Flexibility is the amount of strain produced when a sample stressed between 100–1000 gm/cm^2. It is very low (2–3%). Lower than any other rubber materials except polyether. So removal of the impression from undercut areas may be difficult because of its stiffness.

Dimensional Stability

Dimensionally stable because:

1. Clinically set material is so close to being completely cured so there is little polymerization shrinkage.
2. No volatile byproducts are released to cause the material to shrink.
3. Primary dimensional change comes from thermal shrinkage as the material cools from mouth to room temperature (COTE: 190 × 10^{-6} ppm/°C).
4. Impression does not have to be poured immediately. Most manufacturers claimed that pouring could be delayed up to 7 days.

The combination of superior elasticity and excellent dimensional stability means that multiple casts can be made from the same impression, all having the same accuracy.

Surface Reproduction

These materials are capable of reproducing lines of 0.025 mm width.

Hardness

Hardness is about 55. Hardness can be measured by shore A durometer.

Compatibility with Gypsum

Addition polysilicones are hydrophobic. So it is difficult to wet the surface of the impression by gypsum slurry. With these materials it is very difficult to get a bubble-free stone cast.

Remedy: There are a number of surfactants, sprays that reduce the surface tension, so that stone wets the surface of the impression.

Electroplating

Impressions can be electroplated with silver or copper to form electroplated dies.

Disinfection

Addition silicone impressions can be easily disinfected by 10–15 minutes immersion in 2% glutaraldehyde or 10% hypochlorite solution.

Impression Trays

Either stock or special trays can be used.

Tray Adhesive

Tray adhesive contains poly (dimethyl siloxane) or other silicone that reacts with the impression material and ethyl silicate to create a physical bond with the tray.

Color Contrast

It is supplied in two different pastes. Different viscosities of the same material are supplied in different colors. The base paste is usually colorless or white and the color pigments are added to the reactor to give a characteristic color.

Shelf-Life

It is about 2 years. Tubes or containers must be tightly closed when not in use and should be stored in a cool, dry environment.

Advantages

- Pleasant to handle (no disagreeable taste or odor).
- Excellent elasticity of 99.97%.
- Shorter setting time.
- Adequate tear strength.
- High dimensional stability.
- Impression can be stored for about 7 days without pouring.
- Impression can be electroplated.
- Available in complete range of viscosities.
- Produces a highly accurate impression.
- Easy to manipulate – Automatic device can be used.
- Stock or special tray can be used.
- Multiple accurate dies can be poured.

Disadvantages

- More expensive especially with automatic mixing device.
- Shorter working time.

- May release hydrogen gas on setting and produces pinpoint voids in the die.
- High surface tension causes difficulty in pouring the cast.
- Moisture incompatibility (hydrophobic).
- Low flexibility (stiff) value – difficult to remove from undercut areas.

Uses

- Most widely used for crown and bridge impressions.
- Cavity preparations of inlays and onlays.
- Impressions of partial and complete dentures.

Modifications

Hydrophilic Polyvinyl Siloxanes

High surface tension of polyvinyl siloxane causes difficulty in pouring the cast and moisture incompatibility makes it difficult to obtain good impression if saliva or blood is present in the mouth.

To compensate for these serious problems, a surfactant can be added to make the material hydrophilic. This surfactant reduces the contact angle, which improves wettability and thereby simplifies pouring the cast. There are a number of surfactant sprays, which reduce the surface tension. The most widely used surfactant is *"nonylphenoxy polyethanol homologues".*

- Pooling the spray or thick layer of wetting agent can affect the dimensional accuracy of the impression and cause the surface of the stone cast to be soft and porous.
- A dilute solution of soap is an effective surfactant but taste is rather offensive. So the commercial wetting agent may be preferred.

Drawbacks

1. Longer immersion in disinfectant solution will lead to the leaching of the surfactant and as a result the hydrophilic material becomes hydrophobic.
2. Addition of surfactant makes the preparation of electroformed dies difficult because the metallizing powder does not adhere well to the surface of the hydrophilic addition silicone.

POLYETHER IMPRESSION MATERIALS

Polyether impression material was introduced in Germany in late 1960's.

Dispension

They are dispensed as three-paste system (Base + Reactor + Body modifier) and are available in single consistency (heavy or regular body).

Composition

Base, reactor and body modifier paste's composition is discussed in Table 7.13.

Setting Reaction

When two pastes are mixed together a cationic, ring opening addition polymerization occurs. The ionized form of the sulfonic acid ester provides the initial source of cations and each stage of the reaction involves the opening of an epimine (aziridine) ring and the production of a fresh cation.

Distinct activation, initiation and propagation stages may be identified in the reaction. The reaction is of addition type with no byproducts being formed.

Since each prepolymer molecule has two reactive epimine groups, individual propagation reactions may produce simple chain lengthening and cross-linking.

As the reaction proceeds, the viscosity increases and eventually a relatively rigid cross-linked rubber is produced.

Imine terminated polyether prepolymer + sulphonic acid → polyether rubber.

Activation

Initiation

Table 7.13 Composition of polyether impression material

Base Paste	
Ingredients	*Functions*
Moderately low molecular weight polyether prepolymer with "imine" terminal groups.	Becomes cross-linked to form rubber.
Inert filler (Colloidal silica)	Gives body, controls viscosity and physical properties.
Plasticizer (glycol ether phthalate)	Aids in mixing.
Reactor	
Ingredients	*Functions*
Ester derivative of aromatic sulphonic acid (benzene sulphonic acid)	Cross-linking agent.
Inert filler (colloidal silica)	Gives body and controls viscosity.
Plasticizer (glycol ether phthalate)	To form paste.
Body Modifier	
Ingredients	*Functions*
Optyl pthalate and 5% methyl cellulose	• To reduce the stiffness • To reduce the viscosity of unset material • Provides more working time

Propagation

Properties

- The presence of aromatic sulphonic acid catalyst in the reactor paste sometimes causes irritation, hypersensitivity or contact dermatitis. Therefore direct contact of the skin with the reactor paste should be avoided. Thorough mixing should be done to prevent the reactor paste coming in contact with soft tissues. This material should be avoided for the patients with known allergic to this material.
- Originally polyethers are supplied as one viscosity. The pseudoplasticity allowed one mix to be used for both syringe and tray material.

  Manufacturers also supply an additional paste, body modifier that could be used to produce a thinner mix (added to the premixed material to render it more fluid for the purpose of injection).

  Recently, polyethers are supplied in low and heavy consistencies. The low viscosity is supplied with an automatic mixing device.

Working and Setting Time

The curing rate of polyether is less sensitive to temperature. Some modifications in base: accelerator ratio can be used to extend working time. Use of thinner or body modifier also extends working time with only a slight increase in the setting time. Also available for use with polyethers is a retarder that can extend working time without reducing the elastic properties or increasing polymerization shrinkage.

Mixing time: 30–45 seconds.
Working time: 2–4 minutes.
Setting time: 6–8 minutes.

Both working and setting time can be measured by:

1. Vicat penetrometer
2. Reciprocating rheometer.

Flow after one hour setting

Flow after one hour setting is measured by determining the percentage of deformation in a sample of one hour old after it is subjected to a load of 100 g for 15 minutes. The percentage of deformation is very low (0.03%), which is less than addition polysilicone. It is due to cross-linking and its high stiffness values.

Elasticity

Polyethers are slightly elastic. They have slightly higher permanent deformation values than addition polysilicones. Permanent deformation is about 1.1% and elastic recovery is 98.9%. Permanent deformation depends on the amount of material and duration of compression.

Flexibility

Polyethers are less flexible, 2%, (very stiff). So it is difficult to remove the impression from the undercut areas. Use of body modifier and minimum thickness of material (2 mm instead of 4 mm) will increase the flexibility.

Modified polyether has been introduced that has more flexibility and tear strength and working time. This material is identified by the addition of letter 'F' (flexible) following brand name.

Tear Strength

Tear strength is lowest (2700 g/cm – very low) of all the elastomeric impression materials. As a result thin strips of impression material may tear during removal.

Hardness

Hardness is about 84. It is measured by shore A durometer. It is high so more force is needed to remove the impression from the mouth.

Dimensional Stability

They are dimensionally stable because:
1. Polyether curing reaction produces no volatile byproducts.

2. Less polymerization shrinkage although residual polymerization continues beyond the clinical setting time for a much shorter period than polysulfides.

Theoretically, ring-opening reaction should produce a setting expansion rather than shrinkage. It is possible that thermal shrinkage offsets any polymerization expansion if it occurs.

Volume contraction: 0.4%.

Weight loss (after 24 hours): 0.02% - Due to the evaporation of water-soluble plasticizer.

COTE: 300 ppm/°C.

3. High stiffness of the material means that the force needed to remove the impression is greater for polyethers. Yet, the recovery is nearly complete because of excellent elastic properties. Thus, impressions can be poured immediately after removal, after several days and resulting casts will have same accuracy.

4. Polyethers exhibit the least amount of distortion from the loads imposed on the set material. Thus pouring up the impression and removing the cast several times does not alter the dimensional stability even though a fairly substantial force is needed each time the cast is removed from the impression.

One property that has a negative effect on the material is the absorption of water or fluids and simultaneous leaching of water-soluble plasticizer. So the impressions cannot be electroplated since electroplating bath contains water. However, there is no problem in this regard with the use of gypsum products. Thus, stored impressions must be kept in dry, cool environment to maintain its accuracy.

Surface Reproduction

Capable of reproducing 'v' shaped groove of 0.025 mm width.

Compatibility with Gypsum

Pouring the stone cast is easier. Polyethers are somewhat hydrophilic and form low contact angles with gypsum slurry and hence are easy to pour. But their high stiffness values make it difficult to remove the cast from the impression. Weaker stone cast may fracture during removal.

Impression Trays

Either stock or special trays can be used. It is important to use adequate amount of tray adhesive so that stress during removal does not dislodge the material from the tray.

Disinfection

Impressions can be disinfected by immersing in 2% glutaraldehyde solution for less than 10 minutes. If the immersion time is longer, they are susceptible to dimensional change because of their pronounced hydrophilic nature.

Shelf-Life

Shelf-life is adequate when stored under normal environmental conditions. Storing in a cool and dry environment prolongs the shelf-life. However, the chilled polyether becomes rigid and cannot be used. So it is necessary to allow the material to reach room temperature before using.

Advantages

- Faster working and setting times.
- Less hydrophobic – better wetting.
- Less distortion on removal.
- Good dimensional stability and excellent elastic recovery.
- Multiple dies can be poured with great accuracy.
- Pseudoplasticity.
- Long shelf-life.

Disadvantages

- More expensive.
- High stiffness values after setting.
- Low tear strength.
- Impressions are difficult to electroplate.
- Not available in complete range of viscosities.
- Poor dimensional stability under high humid conditions.
- Catalyst can be sensitizer.

Uses

- Mainly used for crown and bridge impressions.
- Impressions of cavity preparations of inlays and onlays.
- Impressions of partial and complete dentulous mouths.

Modifications

Reducing the stiffness and producing polyether in low and heavy body viscosities have been the major changes for this type of impression material.

LIGHT ACTIVATED POLYETHER IMPRESSION MATERIAL

Light activated polyether impression material was introduced in 1988.

Dispensing

Available as two viscosities.
1. Light body – Packed in disposable syringes.
2. Heavy body – Packed in tubes.

Composition

It contains–
  i. Visible light curing polyether – Urethane dimethacrylate elastomer resin.
  ii. Visible light cure photo initiator.
  iii. Photo accelerators.
  iv. Silicone dioxide as filler – It has a refractive index close to that of the resin, in order to provide translucency necessary for the depth of cure.

Properties

- Excellent elasticity.
- Very low dimensional changes upon setting. It can be poured immediately or up to two weeks.
- Polyether is very rigid (stiff). So undercuts should be blocked out for easy removal of the impression.

Manipulation

No mixing is required.

Light body material is syringed into the impression area. The tray is loaded with the heavy body material and placed in the patient's mouth. After the tray is seated in the mouth, both the viscosities are cured simultaneously using a visible light-curing unit having 8 mm or larger diameter probe. The curing time is approximately 3 minutes.

Advantages

- Command setting, i.e. infinite working time and shorter setting time.
- Excellent physical, mechanical and clinical properties.
- Simplification of the manipulation technique, i.e. no mixing is required.

Disadvantages

- Need for the special trays that are transparent to the visible light and are required to cure the material.
- Material should not be used in the patient's mouth with known allergy or sensitivity to urethanes or methacrylates.
- The material should be stored in a dark place, away from the light.

Measurement of Working and Setting Time of Elastomer

Working and setting time can be measured by:
1. Reciprocating rheometer.
2. Vicat penetrometer.

Reciprocating Rheometer

Wilson described reciprocating rheometer in 1966.

Principle: It is based on the motion of perforated tray through a mixed material and the tray is driven through a spring. As the time elapses, the viscosity of the mix increases and movement of the tray becomes restricted. Thus, a measurement of the movement of the tray gives information about the setting of the material.

Procedure: The material under test is mixed and placed on the perforated tray. The motor is switched on at 1.5 minutes after start of mixing. The movement of the tray is recorded on a rotating drum with the help of a pen assembly. As the time elapses from the start of mixing, the viscosity of the mix increases and resists the movement of the tray. The tray movement is restricted when resistance set by the material (due to increase in viscosity) is greater than that set up by the spring which drives the tray. The motor left running until the trace is completed.

Measurement: The total working is estimated as the time from the start of mixing until the tracing deviates from an initial parallel line as shown in Figure 7.24.

Setting time is taken to be that time when each side of the tracing is first deviated from the curve and becomes straight line as shown in Figure 7.24.

Advantages
- One instrument determines both working and setting time.
- The skill and time required to perform the test are minimal.
- Method is suitable for both elastic and nonelastic materials.
- Only a small amount of material is required.

Disadvantages
- Viscosity of the material cannot be measured.
- Working time obtained depends on the stiffness of the spring, which drives the performed tray.

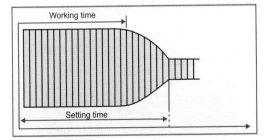

Fig. 7.24 Estimation of working and setting times by reciprocating rheometer

Vicat Penetrometer

It consists of rod weighing 300 g with a needle of 3 mm diameter. A metal ring of 8 mm height and 16 mm width is filled with freshly mixed material whose working time has to be measured and placed on the penetrometer base. The rod is lowered until it contacts the surface of the material and then the needle is released and allowed to penetrate the mix and it is repeated for every 30 seconds.

Initial set or working time is that time at which the needle no longer penetrates the specimen to the bottom of the ring.

Final set or setting time is the time of the first three identical nonmaximum penetrations reading (minimum depth of penetration).

Manipulation of Elastomers

1. Selection of materials.
2. Preparation of custom or special tray.
3. Adhesion to the tray.
4. Proportioning and mixing.
5. Impression techniques.

Selection of Materials

The selection of rubber impression material should be based on the clinical usage of the material and the properties required.

Preparation of a Special Tray

i. An impression of the patient's mouth using alginate (before cavity preparation).
ii. Stone cast.
iii. Covers the areas which are to be included in the final impression with one or two strips of base plate wax (acts as a spacer or relief).
iv. Resin dough is rolled into a sheet, adapted to the diagnostic cast and allowed to polymerize.
v. Wax sheet is removed from the tray. This tray provides a uniform bulk of material, minimal dimensional changes.

Adhesion to the Tray

Elastomers are nonadhesive to the trays. Adhesion can be achieved by the application of adhesive to the tray prior to the insertion of the impression material. The solvent from adhesive layer is then allowed to evaporate (otherwise the material will separate from the tray during removal from the mouth). The adhesive forms tenacious bond between the tray and the impression material.

Composition of tray adhesives

Polysulfides: Butyl rubber or styrene – acrylonitrile dissolved in a suitable volatile solvent such as chloroform.

Polysilicones: Poly (dimethyl siloxane) or similar reactive silicone, which acts as an adhesive for the rubber and ethyl silicate to create a physical bond with the tray.

In either case a slightly roughened surface of the tray will increase the adhesion. For putty elastomer, retention can be achieved by using perforated trays (mechanical retention).

Proportioning and Mixing

Two-paste system: Equal lengths of two pastes are squeezed onto a mixing pad or glass slab. Some manufacturers mark their pads at one-inch intervals as an aid for proportioning. The catalyst or reactor paste first collected with a stainless steel spatula and then distributed over the base, and the mixture is spread out over the mixing pad. The mass is then scraped up with the spatula blade and again smoothed out. The process is continued until the mixed paste is of uniform color with no streaks of the base or reactor appearing in the mixture. If the mix is not homogeneous, curing will not be uniform and distortion of impression will result.

Paste and reactor liquid: Certain length of the base paste is dispensed onto a mixing pad and liquid is placed inside the rope of the paste with a stated number of drops of liquid/unit length of the paste. The paste is picked up with spatula and smoothened. The mixing is continued until complete blending of material is obtained as indicated by an even color throughout the mass.

Two putty system: Putty elastomers are usually dispensed in a jar rather than in a tube. It is so viscous that it must be dispensed by volume using a scoop. It may be mixed with heavy spatula or kneaded in hands until the mix is free from individual color streaks.

Base putty and reactor liquid: Base putty is dispensed with a scoop. Depressions are made on the surface of the putty and the appropriate number of drops or length of accelerator is added. A stiff spatula is used to mix the putty and liquid reactor. Once the reactor is well-incorporated, mixing may be continued by hands for about 30 seconds. The final mix should mix free from individual streaks. Initial mixing by hands is not advisable since a high concentration of reactor contacts skin and may cause allergic response.

Automatic mixing: It is generally used for light viscosity and medium viscosity materials. It is used with addition poly-silicones and polyethers (Fig. 7.25).

Advantages

- There is a greater uniformity in proportioning and mixing.

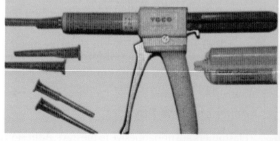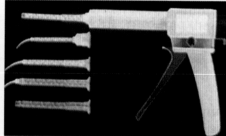

Fig. 7.25 Automatic mixing devices

- Very few air bubbles in the mix.
- Mixing time reduced.
- Possibilities for contamination of material are less.

Impression Techniques

Multiple Mix Technique

This technique is also called as *"double mix-single impression technique"* or *"syringe-tray technique".*

Consistencies
Heavy body – as a tray material.
Light body – as a syringe material.

Trays
- Special tray is required
- Can be used with polysulfides, polysilicones and polyethers.
  It is called multiple mix technique because two separate mixtures are required with two separate mixing pads and spatula.

Stages (Figs 7.26A to F)
1. Light body is mixed first and injected into the impression area.
2. Meanwhile the heavy body is mixed on a glass slab or paper pad, loaded on the tray and placed over the light body material.
3. The light and heavy body materials set together to give a single impression in which light body supported by heavy body and tray. Light body records all the finer details; whereas heavy body assures optimum accuracy and dimensional stability.
4. When both materials have set together, the impression is removed with a single sudden jerk to minimize distortion and is checked for the details.
5. Impression is cleaned under running tap water, excess water is shaken off and is disinfected.
6. A die is prepared by pouring high strength stone material and allowing it to harden.
   Pouring should not be delayed for polysulfides and condensation polysilicones because of their dimensional instability.

Advantages
- Less amount of material is required than with the stock trays.
- Sterilization of the tray is not required as it is used only once.
- Uniform thickness of material throughout the tray minimizes distortion resulting from curing shrinkage.
- Produces a dimensionally accurate and stable impression.

Drawbacks
- Construction of special tray is time consuming.
- Tray must be aged 24 hours to minimize further distortion before use.
- The monomer may be a sensitizer for some patients.

Uses
- Cavity impressions of inlays and onlays, crown and bridge impressions.

Reline Technique

This technique is also called as double mix-double impression technique or putty wash technique.

Consistencies
i. Putty elastomer – for primary impression.
ii. Light body – for secondary impressions.

This technique is most widely used with condensation and addition polysilicones.

Stages: Two stages are involved in this technique (Figs 7.27A to K).
1. *Preliminary impression:* Putty material is placed in a perforated stock tray (adhesive coated) and the impression is made before preparing the teeth. Space for the wash material is provided either by cutting away some of the putty material from the original impression or by using a spacer between the putty and the teeth when recording the preliminary impression. When the putty material has set, impression is removed and washed.

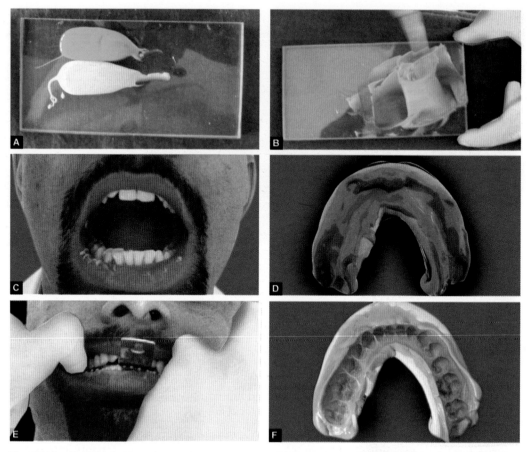

Figs 7.26A to F Multiple Mix technique (A) Dispension of light body material (B) Mixing of light body material (C) Loading some of the light body material onto the prepared tooth in the patient's mouth (D) Loading both heavy and light body material into an impression tray (E) Making the impression (F) Final impression

2. *Secondary impression:* After cavity preparation, the light body is mixed and injected into the cavity preparation (sometimes even into the putty impression tray). The tray plus preliminary impression is reinserted (preliminary impression acts as a custom tray for light body) and held gently until the material sets. Then the impression is removed with a single sudden jerk, washed, dried and die is prepared.

Advantages
- Rapid curing of putty material – preliminary impression needs to be held in the mouth for only few minutes.

- Elimination of time and expense of fabricating special tray.
- Low polymerization shrinkage since they contain less amount of polymer and more filler.
- Overall thermal expansion or contraction is less than that of a polymer because the filler particles have low COTE values.
- Metal stock trays are rigid and are not susceptible to distortion.

Drawbacks
- Practically putty wash technique leads to a gross inaccurate impression, if a critical portion of preliminary impression is held

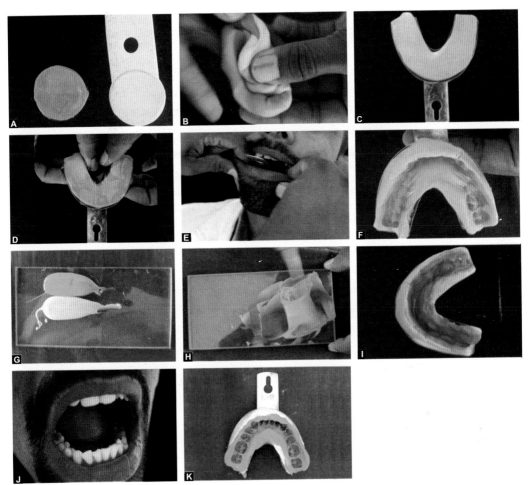

Figs 7.27A to K Reline technique (A) Dispension of putty material (B) Kneading of putty material (C) Loading putty impression materials onto a perforated stock tray (D) Placement of spacer, which provides space for light body material (E) Recording preliminary impression with putty material (F) Preliminary impression with putty material (G) Dispension of light body material (H) Mixing of light body material (I) Loading of light body material onto the preliminary impression recorded with putty material (J) Loading some of the light body materials on to prepared teeth (K) Final impression

under pressure while the wash material is setting, this leads to elastic deformation.
- Inadequate relief for wash material.
- Metal trays must be sterilized.
- Putty is quite expensive.
- More impression material is required.

Uses
- Impressions of crowns and bridges.
- Impressions of cavity preparations for inlays and onlays.

Single Mix-single Impression Technique

Consistency: Single consistency (regular or heavy) having pseudoplastic property (monophasic material).
- Used with addition polysilicones and polyethers as they have pseudoplastic property.
- This technique requires special tray.

When subjected to a low shear rates during spatulation or while an impression is made in a

Table 7.14 Types of failures and causes in elastomeric impressions

Failure	Causes
Rough or uneven surface	1. Incomplete polymerization caused by premature removal from the mouth.
	2. Contamination of the mix or oils or organic material on the teeth.
	3. Too rapid polymerization caused by high humidity or high temperature.
	4. Very high accelerator: base ratio for condensation polysilicones.
Bubbles	1. Too rapid polymerization preventing flow.
	2. Air incorporated during mixing.
Irregularly-shaped voids	Moisture or debris on the surface of the teeth.
Rough or chalky stone cast	1. Inadequate cleaning of impression.
	2. Excess water left on the impression.
	3. Excess wetting agent left in the impression.
	4. Premature removal of cast.
	5. Improper manipulation of the stone.
	6. Failure to wait at least 20 minutes before pouring.
Distortion	1. Continuing polymerization shrinkage of special tray caused by inadequate aging.
	2. Lack of adhesion of rubber to the tray caused by too few coats of adhesive.
	3. Filling the tray soon after the application of adhesive.
	4. Using wrong adhesive.
	5. Lack of mechanical retention for those materials where adhesive is ineffective.
	6. Development of elastic properties in the material before the tray is seated.
	7. Excessive bulk of the material.
	8. Insufficient relief for the reline material.
	9. Continued pressure against the impression material that has developed elastic properties.
	10. Movement of the tray during polymerization.
	11. Premature removal from the mouth.
	12. Improper removal from the mouth.
	13. Delayed pouring of polysulfide or condensation poly-silicone impressions.

tray they have high viscosity and possess body in the tray. The same material can also be used as a syringe material because at higher shear rates, as they pass through the syringe tip viscosity decreases.

A pseudoplastic mix becomes thinner when stressed more (shear thinning). A part of the mix is loaded on the tray and another part is loaded into the syringe and sprayed on the teeth. This thinned material has better flow. Tray is seated over the syringe material and held gently under pressure. After it sets, the impression is removed, washed and a die is made.

Uses

- Impressions of crowns and bridges.

- Impressions of cavity preparations for inlays and onlays.

Tube Impression Technique

Tray: A copper matrix band, which is short copper tube approximately 30 gauge in thickness with a length and diameter suitable for encompassing the particular tooth, involved.

Materials
- Green stick compound
  i. Used for recording preliminary impression.
  ii. Reinforces the band. Otherwise the impression will be squeezed by the fingers when it is removed from the tooth and distortion will occur.
- Light or regular body elastomer – secondary impression.

The adhesive is applied to the band. Green stick compound is softened and placed in a cylindrical copper band. The filled band is then passed over the tooth. The compound flows into the prepared cavity. After the compound has been cooled the impression is withdrawn from the mouth. The band is filled with previously mixed material. The prepared cavity is injected as usual with the syringe and filled band is pressed into the place (see Fig. 7.9).

Uses: In operative dentistry, it is used to obtain the impression of a single tooth in which cavity has been prepared.

Types of failures in elastomeric impressions are discussed in Table 7.14.

SUGGESTED READING

1. Abdullah MA. Effect of frequency and amplitude of vibration on void formation in dies poured from polyvinyl siloxane impressions. J Prosthet Dent. 1998;80:490-4.
2. Alejandro Peregrina, Martin F Land, Phillip Feil, Connie Price BA. Effect of two types of latex gloves and surfactants on polymerization inhibition of three polyvinylsiloxane impression materials. J Prosthet Dent. 2003;90:289-92.
3. Alex H Kang, Glen H Johnson, Xavier Lepe, John C Wataha. Accuracy of a reformulated fast-set vinyl polysiloxane impression material using dual-arch trays. J Prosthet Dent. 2009;101:332-41.
4. Baker PS, Plummer KD, Parr GR, Harry Parker M. Dermal and mucosal reactions to an antimicrobial irreversible hydrocolloid impression material: A clinical report. J Prosthet Dent. 2006;95: 190-3.
5. Balkenhol M, Haunschild S, Erbe C, Wöstmann B. Influence of prolonged setting time on permanent deformation of elastomeric impression materials. J Prosthet Dent. 2010;103:288-94.
6. Berg JC, Johnson GH, Lepe X, Adan-Plaza S. Temperature effects on the rheological properties of current polyether and polysiloxane impression materials during setting. J Prosthet Dent. 2003;90:150-61.
7. Blalock JS, Cooper JR, Rueggeberg FA. The effect of chlorine-based disinfectant on wettability of a vinyl polysiloxane impression material. J Prosthet Dent. 2010;104:333-41.
8. Boening KW, Walter MH, Schuette U. Clinical significance of surface activation of silicone impression materials. J Dent. 1998; 26:447-52.
9. Boraldi F, Coppi C, Bortolini S, Consolo U, Tiozzo R. Cytotoxic evaluation of elastomeric dental impression materials on a permanent mouse cell line and on a primary human gingival fibroblast culture. Materials. 2009;2:934-44; doi:10.3390/ma2030934.
10. Brent L Beyak, Winston WL Chee. Compatibility of elastomeric impression materials for use as soft tissue casts. J Prosthet Dent. 1996;76: 510-4.
11. Brosky ME, Major RJ, DeLong R, Hodges JS. Evaluation of dental arch reproduction using three-dimensional optical Digitization. J Prosthet Dent. 2003;90:434-40.
12. Caputi S, Varvara G. Dimensional accuracy of resultant casts made by a monophase, one-step and two-step, and a novel two-step putty/light-body impression technique: An in vitro study. J Prosthet Dent. 2008;99:274-81.
13. Chaimattayompo N, Park D. A modified putty-wash vinyl polysiloxane impression technique for fixed prosthodontics. J Prosthet Dent. 2007;98:483-5.
14. Chandur PK, Wadhwani Glen H Johnson, Xavier Lepe, Ariel J Raigrodski. Accuracy of newly formulated fast-setting elastomeric impression materials. J Prosthet Dent. 2005;93:530-9.
15. Chen SY, Liang WM, Chen FN. Factors affecting the accuracy of elastometric impression materials. J Dent. 2004;32:603-9.

16. Chun J, Pae A, Kim S. Polymerization shrinkage strain of interocclusal recording materials. Dent Mater. 2009;25:115-20.
17. Craig RG. Review of dental impression materials. Adv Dent Res. 1998;2(l):51-64.
18. Cynthia SP, Mary PW, Aisling MO, Paulette Spencer. Dimensional accuracy and surface detail reproduction of two hydrophilic vinyl polysiloxane impression materials tested under dry, moist, and wet conditions. J Prosthet Dent. 2003;90:365-72.
19. Elie E Daou. The elastomers for complete denture impression: A review of the literature. The Saudi Dent J. 2010;22:153-60.
20. Eriksson A, Ockert-Eriksson G, Lockowandt P, Linden L. Irreversible hydrocolloids for crown and bridge impressions: Effect of different treatments on compatibility of irreversible hydrocolloid impression material with type IV gypsums. Dent Mater. 1996;12:74-82.
21. Erkut S, Can G. Effects of glow-discharge and surfactant treatments on the wettability of vinyl polysiloxane impression materials. J Prosthet Dent. 2005;93:356-63.
22. Filiz Keyf. Some properties of elastomeric impression materials used in fixed prosthodontics. J of Islamic Academy of Sciences. 1994;7(1):44-8.
23. Finger WJ, Rie Kurokawa, Takahashi V, Komatsu M. Sulcus reproduction with elastomeric impression materials: A new in vitro testing method. Dent Mater. 2008;24:1655-60.
24. Gelson Luís Adabo, Elaine Zanarotti, Renata Garcia Fonseca, Carlos Alberto, dos Santos Cruz. Effect of disinfectant agents on dimensional stability of elastomeric impression materials. J Prosthet Dent. 1999;81:621-4.
25. Glen H Johnson, Xavier Lepe,Tar Chee Aw. The effect of surface moisture on detail reproduction of elastomeric Impressions. J Prosthet Dent. 2003;90:354-64.
26. Goldberg AJ. Viscoelastic properties of silicone, polysulfide, and polyether impression materials. J Dent Res Supplement. 1974; 53(4):1033-9.
27. Imbery TA, Nehring J, Charles Janus, Moon PC. Accuracy and dimensional stability of extended-pour and conventional alginate impression materials. J Am Dent Assoc. 2010;141:32-9.
28. Herbst D, Nel JC, Driessen CH, Becker PJ. Evaluation of impression accuracy for osseointegrated implant supported Super-structures. J Prosthet Dent. 2000;83:555-61.
29. Hiraguchi H, Kaketani M, Hirose H, Yoneyama T. The influence of storing alginate impressions sprayed with disinfectant on dimensional accuracy and deformation of maxillary edentulous stone models. Dent Mater J. 2010;29(3):309-15.
30. Johnson GH, Mancl LA, Schwedhelm ER, Verhoef DR, Lepe X. Clinical trial investigating success rates for polyether and vinyl polysiloxane impressions made with full-arch and dual-arch plastic trays. J Prosthet Dent. 2010;103:13-22.
31. Kanehira M, Finger WJ, Endo T. Volatilization of components and water absorption of polyether impressions. J Dent. 2006; 34:134-8.
32. Kess RS, Combe EC, Sparks BS. Effect of surface treatments on the wettability of vinyl polysiloxane impression materials. J Prosthet Dent. 2000;83:98-102.
33. Kimoto K, Tanaka K, Toyoda M, Ochiai KT. Indirect latex glove contamination and its inhibitory effect on vinyl polysiloxane polymerization. J Prosthet Dent. 2005;93:433-8.
34. Lepe X, Johnson GH. Accuracy of Polyether and addition silicone after long-term immersion disinfection. J Prosthet Dent. 1997; 78:245-9.
35. Lepe X, Johnson GH, Berg JC, Aw TC. Effect of mixing technique on surface characteristics of impression materials. J Prosthet Dent. 1998;79:495-502.
36. Livaditis GJ. Comparison of the new matrix system with traditional fixed prosthodontics impression procedures. J Prosthet Dent. 1998;79:200-7.
37. Lu H, Nguyen B, Powers JM. Mechanical properties of 3 hydrophilic addition silicone and polyether elastomeric impression materials. J Prosthet Dent. 2004;92:151-4.
38. Luthardta RG, Kochb R, Rudolpha H, Waltera MH. Qualitative computer aided evaluation of dental impressions in vivo. Dent Mater. 2006;22:69-76.
39. Magne P, Nielsen B. Interactions between impression materials and immediate dentin sealing. J Prosthet Dent. 2009;102:298-305.
40. Mandikos MN. Polyvinyl siloxane impression materials: An update on clinical use. Aus Dent J. 1998;43:(6):428-34.
41. Marafie Y, Looney S, Nelson S, Chan D, Browning W, Rueggeberg F. Retention strength of impression materials to a tray material using different adhesive methods: An in vitro study. J Prosthet Dent. 2008;100:432-40.

42. Marco Corso, Abdulhadi Abanomy, James Di Canzio, David Zurakowski, Steven M Morgano. The effect of temperature changes on the dimensional stability of polyvinyl siloxane and polyether impression materials. J Prosthet Dent. 1998;79:626-31.

43. María L Aguilar, Augusto Elias, Carlos E, Toro Vizcarrondo, Walter J Psoter. Analysis of three-dimensional distortion of two impression materials in the transfer of dental implants. J Prosthet Dent. 2009;101:202-9.

44. Maria de Pilar Rios, Steven M, Morgano R, Sheldon Stein, Lynda Rose. Effects of chemical disinfectant solutions on the stability and accuracy of the dental impression complex. J Prosthet Dent. 1996;76:356-62.

45. Markus Balkenhol, Bernd Wostmann, Masafumi Kanehira, Werner J Finger. Shark fin test and impression quality: A correlation analysis. J Dent. 2007;35:409-15.

46. Martin N, Martin MV, Jedynakiewicz NM. The dimensional stability of dental impression materials following immersion in disinfecting solutions. Dent Mater. 2007;23:760-8.

47. Martinez J, Combe EC, Pesun IJ. Rheological properties of Vinyl Polysiloxane impression pastes. Dent Mater. 2001;17:471-6.

48. Mats H Kronström, Glen H Johnson, Richard W Hompeschc. Accuracy of a new ring-opening metathesis elastomeric dental impression material with spray and immersion disinfection. J Prosthet Dent. 2010;103:23-30.

49. Matthew J German, Thomas E Carrick, John F McCabe. Surface detail reproduction of elastomeric impression materials related to rheological properties. Dent Mater. 2008;24:951-6.

50. Meththananda IM, Parker S, Patel MP, Braden M. The relationship between shore hardness of elastomeric dental materials and Young's modulus. Dent Mater. 2009;25:956-9.

51. Millar BJ, Dunne SM, Nesbit M. A comparison of three wetting agents used to facilitate the pouring of dies. J Prosthet Dent. 1995;74:341-4.

52. Millar BJ, Dune SM, Robinision PB. The effect of a surface wetting agent on void formation in impressions. J Prosthet Dent. 1997;77:54-6.

53. Millar BJ, Dunne SM, Robinson PB. In vitro study of the number of surface defects in monophase and two-phase addition silicone impressions. J Prosthet Dent. 1998;80:32-5.

54. Morgano SM, Milot P, Ducharme P, Rose L. Ability of various impression materials to produce duplicate dies from successive impressions. J Prosthet Dent. 1995;73:333-40.

55. Nathaniel C Lawson, John O Burgess, Mark S Litaker. Tensile elastic recovery of elastomeric impression materials. J Prosthet Dent. 2008;100:29-33.

56. Nishigawa G, Sato T, Suenaga K, Minagi S. Efficacy of tray adhesives for the adhesion of elastomer rubber impression materials to impression modeling plastics for border molding. J Prosthet Dent. 1998;79:140-4.

57. Pamenius M, Ohlson NG. Influence of dimensional stability of impression materials on the probability of acceptance of a prosthetic restoration. Biomoter. 1995;16:1193-7.

58. Pavel Bradna, Darina Cerna. Impact of water quality on setting of irreversible hydrocolloid impression materials. J Prosthet Dent. 2006;96:443-8.

59. Peregrina A, Land MF, Wandling C, Johnston WM. The effect of different adhesives on vinyl polysiloxane bond strength to two tray materials. J Prosthet Dent. 2005;94:209-13.

60. Raigrodski AJ, Dogan S, Manc LA, Heind H. A clinical comparison of two vinyl polysiloxane impression materials using the one-step technique. J Prosthet Dent. 2009;102:179-86.

61. Rajeev Butta, Christopher Jeremy Tredwin, Michael Nesbit, David R Moles. Type IV gypsum compatibility with five addition-reaction silicone impression materials. J Prosthet Dent. 2005;93:540-4.

62. Rentzia A, Coleman DC, O'Donnell MJ, Dowling AH, O'Sullivan M. Disinfection procedures: Their efficacy and effect on dimensional accuracy and surface quality of an irreversible hydrocolloid impression material. J Dent. 2011;39:133-40.

63. Rishi D Patel, Mathew T Kattadiyil, Charles J Goodacre, Myron S Winer. An in vitro investigation into the physical properties of irreversible hydrocolloid alternatives. J Prosthet Dent. 2010; 104:325-32.

64. Rodrigueza JM, Bartlett DW. The dimensional stability of impression materials and its effect on in vitro tooth wear studies. Dent Mater. 2011;27:253-8.

65. Sedda M, Casarotto A, Raustia A, Borracchini A. Effect of storage time on the accuracy of casts made from different irreversible hydrocolloids. J Contemp Dent Pract. 2008;(9)4:59-66.

66. Shaba OP, Adegbulegbe IC, Oderinu OH. Dimensional stability of alginate impression

material over a four hours time frame. Nig Ot J Hosp Med. 2007;17(1):1-4.

67. Shalinie King, Howard See, Graham Thomas, Michael Swain. Determining the complex modulus of alginate irreversible hydrocolloid dental material. Dent Mater. 2008;24:1545-8.

68. Siddiqui A, Braden M, Patel MP, Parker S. An experimental and theoretical study of the effect of sample thickness on the Shore hardness of elastomers. Dent Mater. 2010;26:560-4.

69. Sinal Shah, Geeta Sundaram, David Bartlett, Martyn Sherriff. The use of a 3D laser scanner using superimpositional software to assess the accuracy of impression techniques. J Dent. 2004;32: 653-8.

70. Srivastava A, Aaisa J, Tarun Kumar TA, Kishore G, Nagaraja Upadhya P. Alginates: a review of compositional aspects for dental applications. Trends Biomater Artif Organs. 2012;26(1): 31-6.

71. Stober T, Johnson GH, Schmitter M. Accuracy of the newly formulated vinyl siloxane ether elastomeric impression material. J Prosthet Dent. 2010;103:228-39.

72. Taylor RL, Wright PS, Maryan C. Disinfection procedures: their effect on the dimensional accuracy and surface quality of irreversible hydrocolloid impression materials and gypsum casts. Dent Mater. 2002;18:103-10.

73. Wu AY, Donovan TE. The use of vacuum-formed resin sheets as spacers for putty-wash impressions. J Prosthet Dent. 2007;97: 54-5.

74. Wu G, Yu X, Gu Z. Ultrasonically nebulised electrolysed oxidising water: a promising new infection control programme for impressions, metals and gypsum casts used in dental hospitals. J Hosp Infect. 2008;68:348-54.

Orthodontic Wires

8

The word 'orthodontics' is derived from Greek word 'Ortho' meaning 'right or correct', 'odonto' meaning tooth.

Orthodontics is the study of growth and development of the masticatory apparatus and the prevention and treatment of abnormalities of this development.

Orthodontic appliances are devices by which mild pressure may be applied to a tooth or group of teeth to bring about necessary changes.

CLASSIFICATIONS OF ORTHODONTIC APPLIANCES

Active

Active appliances exert a force on the teeth or supporting structures to bring about necessary tooth movement.

Passive

Passive appliances are mostly used to retain teeth, which have been moved into ideal location.

Orthodontic wires are one of the active components of fixed appliances. They can bring about various tooth movements through the medium of brackets and buccal tubes, which act as handles on the teeth.

REQUIREMENTS

- Should be nontoxic.
- Should be resistant to corrosion and tarnish.

- Modulus of elasticity should be high. It enables the wire to apply more force for tooth movement.
- Formability should be high so as to bend the wire into desired configuration without fracture.
- Spring back should be high which results in an increase in its range of action. Spring back is the measure of how far a wire can be deflected without causing permanent deformation. It is also called elastic deflection.
- Stiffness should be lower. It provides the ability to apply lower forces constantly for a lower time.
- Resilience should be high. It increases the working range.
- It should be soldered or welded.
- Ductility should be sufficient to allow fabrication of appliance.
- Should maintain the desirable properties for extended period of time after manufacture.
- Should provide least friction at bracket – wire interface. Otherwise it leads to undue strain, which limits the tooth movement.

CLASSIFICATIONS OF ORTHODONTIC WIRES

1. **Based on material used:**
   a. Stainless steel
   b. Co-Cr-Ni alloy
   c. β-Titanium alloys
   d. Ni-Ti alloys
   e. Gold alloys

2. **Based on cross-section:**
   a. Round
   b. Square
   c. Rectangular
   d. Multistranded
3. **Based on gauge size:**
   a. 0.018"
   b. 0.016"
   c. 0.07"

MATERIALS

Stainless Steel

Steel is an alloy of iron and carbon with up to 2% of carbon. Stainless steel wires are available in different gauges. The gauge indicates thickness of the wire. The stainless wire, which is shown in Figure 8.1 is the "19" gauge wire. In the solid state steel is able to adopt a variety of structures depending on the carbon content and temperature.

Austenitic steel is an interstitial solid solution of carbon in FCC iron. In this 2.1 wt% of carbon exists between 912– 1394°C. On slow cooling which gives a mixture of ferrite steel and cementite (Fe_3C). On rapid cooling or quenching which gives martensite steel.

Ferritic steel is a very ductile solid solution of carbon in BCC iron. This exists between room temperature to 912°C.

Martensitic steel is a solid solution of carbon in distorted BCC lattice of iron (Body Centered Tetragonal (BCT)). This results in increase in hardness and brittleness. Heating this from 200–450°C, reduces the brittleness, called tempering.

The term stainless steel is applied to all alloys of iron and carbon that contain Cr, Ni, Mn and others such as Si, P, S, Tantalum, Niobium, and Columbium.

Chromium renders the resistance to corrosion attack. When it is exposed to oxidizing atmosphere, it forms a thin, transparent but tough and impervious chromic oxide layer (Cr_2O_3). This protective oxide layer prevents further corrosion. This is called passivation. Chromium also reduces critical temperature at which austenitic structure breaks down on cooling.

Nickel reduces critical temperature and helps in corrosion resistance and also improves the strength.

Other elements in small amounts prevent the formation of carbides of iron and chromium (stabilizing agents). Molybdenum increases resistance to pitting corrosion.

Types (Table 8.1)

1. Ferritic stainless steel – little applications in dentistry.
2. Martensitic stainless steel – used for surgical and cutting instruments
3. Austenitic stainless steel – most widely used.
   In addition to chromium, nickel and carbon some other ingredients may also present in small amounts such as silicon, phosphorus, sulfur, manganese, tantalum, and niobium.

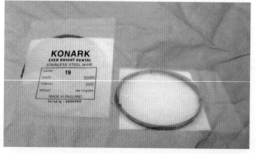

Fig. 8.1 Stainless steel wire

Table 8.1 Composition of three types of stainless steels

Types of stainless steel	Chromium	Nickel	Carbon
Ferritic (BCC)	11.5–27.0	0	0.20 max
Austenitic (FCC)	16.0–26.0	7.0–22.0	0.25 max
Martensitic (BCT)	11.5–17.0	0–2.5	0.15–1.20

Austenitic Stainless Steel (18-8 Stainless Steel)

Composition

Chromium – 18%
Nickel – 8%
Carbon – 0.25%
Si, P, Mn, Tantalum, Niobium, and Columbium – trace.

Austenitic stainless steels are proposed because–
- Greater ductility and ability to undergo more cold work without fracture.
- Substantial strengthening during cold working (some transformation to BCC).
- Greater ease of welding.
- Ability to fairly readily overcome sensitization.
- Less critical grain growth.
- Comparative ease of forming.
- Low cost.

Properties

They are obtained in three grades often referred to as soft (ductile), half hard and hard. The type of wire chosen according to the amount of bending, which must be carried out.

They have high modulus of elasticity (179 GPa) and therefore used to apply relatively high forces. Lower forces can be achieved by using a wire of smaller diameter. It is highly ductile which allows bending.

> Yield strength – 1579 MPa
> UTS – 2117 MPa
> Hardness – 600 KHN

Sensitization (Weld Decay)

The 18-8 stainless steel may lose its corrosion resistance if it is heated 400–900°C (during soldering); the exact temperature depends on the carbon content. At temperatures between 400–900°C, the small rapidly diffusing carbon atoms migrate to the grain boundaries from all parts of the crystal to combine with large, slowly diffusing chromium at the periphery of the grain where the energy is highest, and precipitates as chromium carbide (Cr_3C). This formation is most rapid at 650° C. This will lead to the depletion of grain boundary chromium and decrease in corrosion resistance since no chromium is available for passivation to occur. This is known as sensitization and results in intergranular corrosion and partial disintegration of metal and weakening the structure. This can be eliminated by:
1. Reducing the carbon content of steel (not economically feasible)
2. Stabilization.

Stabilization

The method employed most successfully is the introduction of some elements that precipitate as carbide in preference to chromium. If titanium, niobium, or columbium is introduced in amount approximately six times the carbon content, the precipitation of Cr_3C can be inhibited for shorter periods between 400–900°C. Stainless steel have been treated in this manner are said to be stabilized.

Soldering

Silver solders containing silver, copper, zinc, to which tin and indium are added to reduce fusion temperature and increase solderizability, can be used. Fluoride containing fluxes are used because ordinary solders cannot dissolve chromic oxide film. They can also be joined by soft welding.

During soldering, wires should not be overheated since this may cause recrystallization of the grain structure with subsequent lack of springiness. After soldering, it can be cleaned by pickling in warmed nitric acid.

General Causes of Corrosion

- Any surface inhomogeneity is a potential source of tarnish and corrosion.
- Severe strain hardening produces electric couples in the presence of saliva.
- Any surface roughness or unevenness (minimized by polishing).
- Incorporation of bits of carbon steel or similar metal in its surface during manipulation with pliers or during cutting with stainless steel bur.

- Soldered or brazed points leading to the formation of galvanic cell.

Cobalt-chromium-nickel Alloys (Elgiloy)

A cobalt-chromium-nickel alloy known as elgiloy is available in wire and band forms for various dental appliances. These alloys were originally developed for use as watch spring by ELGIU national company.

Composition

Cobalt	40%
Chromium	20%
Nickel	15%
Molybdenum	7%
Manganese	2%
Beryllium	0.04%
Carbon	0.16%
Iron	15.8%

Properties

Elgiloy wires are available in different tempers (amount of cold work) and usually color-coded. High spring temper (red), semispring temper (green), soft or ductile temper (yellow) are the different types available. They are easy to bend. They can be heat hardened (7 minutes at 482°C) after manipulation to relieve hardness (strength) approximately equal to that of stainless steel. Low cost. Tarnish and corrosion resistance is excellent. They can be soldered (fluoride fluxes are used) and welded.
- Proportional limit – 1610 MN/m^2
- Modulus of elasticity – 184 GPa
- Yield strength – 1413 MPa
- UTS – 1682 MPa
- VHN – 700 kg/mm^2.

Titanium Alloys (TMA Alloy)

Titanium-molybdenum alloy also known as β-titanium alloy, which was introduced in 1979 by Goldberg and Burstone. Pure titanium at temperatures lower than 885°C exists in a Hexagonal Close Packed (HCP) or α-crystal whereas at higher temperatures (above 885°C) the metal rearranges into a BCC or β-crystal lattice. Alloying elements are added to stabilize β-crystal lattice at room temperature that has better mechanical properties.

Composition

Titanium	78%
Molybdenum	11.5%
Zirconium	6%
Tin	4.5%

Properties

TMA has lower force magnitudes. Low elastic modulus (71.7 GPa). Lower yield strength (860 to 1170 MPa). Good ductility. High springable and highly formable. It can be highly cold worked. Mechanical properties can be altered by heat treatment that used α or β crystal lattice transformations, but it is not recommended. Excellent corrosion resistance. They can be welded by electrical resistance (true weldability).

Nickel-titanium Alloys (Nitinol)

A wrought Ni-Ti alloy known as Nitinol (Nickel-Titanium naval ordinance laboratory) was introduced in 1972. It is characterized by its high resiliency, limited formability, shape memory or thermal memory, and pseudoelastic or superelasticity.

Composition

Nickel	55%
Titanium	45%
Cobalt	0 to 2%

At higher temperatures a BCC lattice referred to as austenitic phase is stable, whereas appropriate cooling can induce transformation to HCP martensitic phase. This transformation can also be induced by the application of stress. There is a volumetric change associated with transition. This transformation results in two unique features. They are:
1. Shape memory
2. Pseudoelasticity or superelasticity.

Shape Memory

Shape memory is achieved by first establishing a shape at temperatures near 482°C if the appliance wire is then cooled and formed into a second shape and heated through a lower transition temperature range (TTR), the wire will return to its original shape. The cobalt content is used to control the transition temperature range, which can be near mouth temperature.

Superelasticity or Pseudoelasticity

Inducing the austenitic to martensitic transformation by stress can produce superelasticity, a phenomenon that is employed with Ni–Ti wires (Fig. 8.2).

Application of bending stress initially results in standard proportional stress-strain behavior (AB) as shown in Figure 8.2. However, at a stress sufficient to induce phase transformation (austenite to martensite) there is a significant increase in strain (BC) referred to as superelasticity or pseudoelasticity. This additional strain is caused by the volumetric change due to phase transformation. At point 'C', where the transformation is complete, the behavior reverts to conventional elastic and plastic strain with increasing stress (CD). Unloading results in the reverse transition and recovery. This results in lower forces and a large working range or spring back.

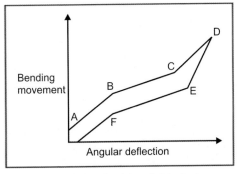

Fig. 8.2 Superelasticity of nitinol wire

Table 8.2 Properties of gold alloys

Material	Proportional limit	Tensile strength	Fusion temperature
PGP	552–1034 MPa	862–1241 MPa	1500–1530°C
PSC	690–793 MPa	965–1070 MPa	1050–1080°C

Properties

Modulus of elasticity   41.4 GPa
Yield strength   427 MPa
Ultimate tensile strength   1489 MPa
It has limited ductility and is not easy to bend without fracture. The alloy cannot be soldered or welded (joined by mechanical means).

Gold Alloys

Two types of gold alloys are available according to ADA No. 7.

Type I—noble or high noble— ≥ 75% of noble metal elements.

Type II—noble or high noble— ≥ 65% of noble metal elements.

There are also two other wires designated as PGP (Platinum–Gold–Palladium) and PSC (Platinum–Silver– Copper).

These wires are highly ductile, highly corrosion resistant. They can be heat hardened, can easily be soldered. Borax flux and gold solders are used for soldering. They have higher elastic modulus and therefore apply lower forces. The physical and thermal properties of 2 types of gold wires are given in Table 8.2. They are expensive. The high platinum and palladium contents increase the melting point and recrystallization temperature which ensures that the wires do not melt, recrystallize during soldering process. They also ensure a fine grain structure.

SUGGESTED READING

1. Burstone CJ, Liebler SAH, Goldberg AJ. Polyphenylene polymers as esthetic orthodontic archwires. Am J Orthod Dentofacial Orthop. 2011;139(4)Supple 1:e391-8.

2. Iijima M, Yuasa T, Endo K, Muguruma T, Ohno H, Mizoguchi I. Corrosion behavior of ion implanted nickel-titanium orthodontic wire in fluoride mouth rinse solutions. Dent Mater J. 2010;29(1): 53-8.

3. Kim H, Johnson WJ. Corrosion of stainless steel, nickel–titanium. Coated nickel titanium and titanium orthodontic arch wire. Angle Orthod. 1999;69:39-44.

4. Klump JP, Duncanson MG, Nanda RS, Curier GF. Elastic energy/stiffness ratios for selected orthodontic wires. Am J Orthod. 1994;106:588-96.

5. Kohl RW. Metallurgy in orthodontics. Angle Orthod. 1964;34: 37-52.

6. Krishnan V, Kumar JK . Weld characteristics of orthodontic arch-wire materials. Angle Orthod. 2004;74:533-8.

7. Krishnan V, Kumar JK. Mechanical properties and surface characteristics of three archwire alloys. Angle Orthod. 2004;74: 825-31.

8. Minick GT, Oesterle LJ, Newman SM, Shellhart WC. Bracket bond strengths of new adhesive systems. Am J Orthod Dentofacial Orthop. 2009;135:771-6.

9. Mistakidis I, Gkantidis N, Topouzelis N. Review of properties and clinical applications of orthodontic wires. Hellenic Orthodontic Review. 2011;14(1):45-66.

10. Ozturk Y, Firatli S, Almac L. An evaluation of intraoral molar distalization with Nickel-Titanium Coil Springs. Clinics in Dent Pract. 2005;3(4):15-20.

11. Talass ME. Optiflex archwire treatment of a skeletal Class HI open bite. J Clin Orthod. 1992;26:245-52.

12. Watanabe M, Nakata S, Morishita T. Organic polymer wire for aesthetic maxillary retainers. J Clin Orthod. 1996;30:266-71.

13. West AE, Jones ML, Newcombe RG. Multiflex versus super elastic; a randomized clinical trial of tooth alignmentability of initial archwires. Am J Orthod Dentofac Orthop. 1995;95:464-71.

14. Wilcock AJ Jr. Applied materials engineering for orthodontic wires. Aus Ortho J. 1989;11:22-9.

15. Zufall SW, Kusy RP. Sliding mechanics of coated composite wires and the development of an engineering model for binding. Angle Orthod. 2000;70:34-47.

Implant Materials

9

An implant is defined as a medical device made from one or more biomaterials that is intentionally placed within the body, either totally or partially buried beneath an epithelial surface.

BIOMATERIAL

The term biomaterial is defined as a nonviable material used in a medicinal device, intended to interact with biological systems. So generally stating implant is a device inserted into the body below the skin or oral mucosal membrane, which may penetrate for the purpose of modifying form and function of the jaws or face, usually by mechanical means.

Practicing dentists spend much of their time replacing partially missing tooth structure. However, researchers have now searched for improved methods of anchoring prosthetic material within the jaw to reconstruct an entire tooth either as a single restoration or as a support for a removable partial denture or a fixed partial denture.

Through the years, it has become obvious that this complex field of "dental implantology" would require the optimization of several important variables to enhance the chances of success. The variables are as follows:

i. Proper material selection and design.
ii. An understanding and evaluation of biologic interaction at the interface between the implant and tissue.
iii. An evaluation of quality of the existing bone.
iv. A careful and controlled surgical technique.

v. A joint approach between the various specialties to optimize patient selection.
vi. Implants spacing.
vii. Load distribution.
viii. Prosthodontic geometry.
ix. Follow-up care.

This knowledge has evolved at the expense of many failed implants, in part because clinical treatment often preceded controlled experimental studies in animals and humans.

For most of the period, they have been dominated by belief that success was predominately design related, although more recently the importance of the material of construction, aspects of their application were not, however, scientifically considered until recent decades.

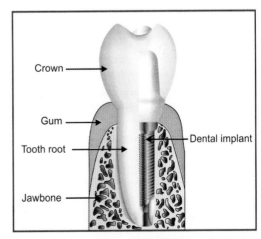

Fig. 9.1 Implant-supported replacement tooth that illustrates the bonding of tooth to the bone and implant to the bone

REQUIREMENTS

- They should promote osseointegration.
- They should be nontoxic and nonirritant.
- They should be chemically stable in the bone bed.
- They should be able to bear the masticatory forces.
- They should have mechanical properties similar to that of bone.
- It should be easy to manipulate, easy available and not expensive.

TYPES OF IMPLANTS

There are principally three types of devices used as follows:

Subperiosteal Implants

It is a framework that rests on the bony ridge but does not penetrate it. This has longest history of clinical trial. This type has been principally used in the atrophic mandible. They consist of a cast metal frame on which a prosthesis may be mounted (Fig. 9.2A).

The frame is usually made from cobalt-chromium alloy on a cast prepared from an impression of the jawbone. The technique can provide a very satisfactory result in the short-term. However, over periods in excess of fifteen years failures tend to become more common. The survival rate is 54% over 15 years.

Transosteal Implants

This penetrates completely through the mandible. Its use is limited to mandible (Fig. 9.2B). The survival rate of these implants is of 90% over an 8–16 year period. This type of implant typified by the ridge augmentation technique in which the highest of reabsorbed alveolar ridge was increased with an implant.

Various ceramics were popular for this, as well number of polymer based materials such as carbon-fiber composites.

Endosseous Implants

This is partially submerged and anchored within the bone (Fig. 9.2C). The endosseous implants

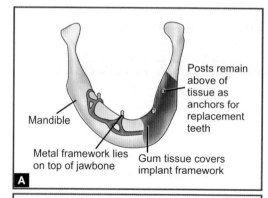

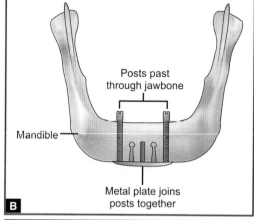

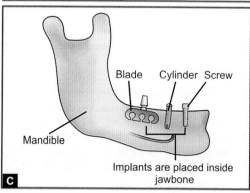

Figs 9.2A to C (A) Subperiosteal implant; (B) transosteal implant; (C) Endosseous implant

appear to offer the best solution interims of fewer clinical limitations and greater success. Reports suggest high success rate over a 15-year period for a specific type of cylindrical-shaped screw implant.

They have been manufactured as essentially blade, nail or screw-like devices inserted through the oral mucosa into the jawbone. They have been produced in a wide range of shapes and materials and until recently had an uncertain prognosis. The endosseous cylindrical design is now often thought of as being synonymous with dental implants.

Osseointegration

Bränemark observed the fusion of bone with titanium chambers when he had placed them into the femurs of rabbits. The word *"osseointegration"* is coined by him for such a phenomena, which is defined as the apparent direct attachment or connection of osseous tissue to an inert, alloplastic material without intervening connective tissue. During osseointegration, osteoblasts and mineralized matrix contacts the implant surface even when loads are applied. The first practical application of osseointegration was the implantation of new titanium roots in an edentulous patient in 1965 and the first ground breaking study was published 16 years later by Adell et al. in the *International Journal of Oral Surgery*. This is considered to be the beginning of the birth of modern implantology and its acceptance worldwide. Since then titanium and its alloys have been extensively used as implant materials for over 40 years due to their excellent biocompatibility, mechanical properties and high corrosion resistance. Biocompatibility of implants is very important with the physiological environment in which they are placed. Osseointegration provides a stable bone-implant connection that can support a dental prosthesis and transfer applied loads without concentrating stresses at the interface between the bone and the implant.

Osseointegration takes place when the bone is viable and space between the bone and implant must be less than 10 nm without any fibrous tissue. Both the aspects of osseointegration, maintenance of present bone (remodelling) and new bone formation (modelling), determine the fate of implant healing and implant stability. Before introduction of the Bränemark protocol, dental implants were commonly loaded at placement because immediate bone stimulation was considered to avoid crestal bone loss. Bränemark et al. in 1969 showed that direct bone apposition at the implant surface was possible and lasts under loading at the condition that implants were left to heal in a submerged way.

Implant Materials

1. Metals and alloys
2. Ceramics
3. Polymers
4. Composites.

METAL AND ALLOYS

Most commonly, metals and their alloys are used for dental implants.

Stainless Steel

Steel is an iron based alloy, which contains less than 1.2 percent of carbon. Stainless steel can be classified into three implant types based on its composition. They include ferritic, martensitic and austenitic steel.

Austenitic steel implants are the most commonly used material. The austenitic steel mainly contains 18% of chromium; provides corrosion resistance, 8% of nickel; stabilizes the austenitic structure, 80 percent iron and 0.05%–0.15% of Carbon.

Properties
- Nickel is considered as a potential allergenic agent.
- Austenitic steels have high strength and ductility so they are more resistant to brittle fracture.
- Tensile strength: 70–145 PSI.
- Elongation to fracture: 30%.
- Susceptible to pit and crevice corrosion.
- Direct contact with the dissimilar metal should be avoided as it results in galvanism.

Cobalt-Chromium-Molybdenum Alloys

They are used as cast and cast-annealed conditions. This permits custom fabrications of

Table 9.1 Composition of Co-Cr-Mo alloys

Component	Wt. %	Functions
Cobalt	63	• Increases MOE, strength and hardness.
		• Provides continuous phase for the basic properties.
Chromium	30	• Forms secondary phase.
		• Corrosion resistance.
Molybdenum	5	Provides strength and bulk corrosion resistance.
Carbon	Trace	Acts as a hardener.
Nickel	Trace	Forms the secondary phase.

alloys. Composition of these alloys is discussed in the Table 9.1.

Properties
• Excellent biocompatibility if properly fabricated.
• The amount of carbon greatly influences the mechanical properties of the alloy. For example, if the alloy contains more amount of carbon content, it reduces its ductility and vice versa.
• Co-Mo-Cr alloys have a high elastic modulus.

Advantages
• These alloys possess an outstanding resistance to corrosion and they have high modulus.
• Low cost and long-term clinical success.

Limitations: The cobalt alloys are least ductile and bending must be avoided.

Titanium and Titanium Alloys (Ti-Al-V alloys)

Titanium is the most popular implant material. Titanium exists in nature as a pure element with an atomic number of 22 in periodic table. For more than 25 years titanium has been used for both endosseous and sub-periosteal implants. Endosseous implants have taken the form of rods, posts, and blades made of either pure titanium or titanium alloys. Commercially pure titanium (Cp) is a very highly reactive metal. It oxidizes (passivates) on contact with air or normal tissue fluids. This reactivity is favorable to the implant devices because it minimizes biocorrosion. An oxide layer of 10Å thick on the cut surface of the titanium within a millisecond is formed. Thus any scratch in the oxide coating is essentially self-healing. Titanium can be further passivated by placing it in a nitric acid bath to form a thick, durable oxide coating. Cp titanium is available in four different grades such as Cp grade 1, Cp grade 2, Cp grade 3 and Cp grade 4. Cp titanium contains oxygen and minor amounts of impurities such as nitrogen, carbon, hydrogen, etc.

Titanium-Aluminum-Vanadium Alloys

Composition	
Component	Wt %
Titanium	90
Aluminum	6
Vanadium	4

Modulus of elasticity is slightly greater than Cp Ti and it is about 5.6 times that of compact bone. Although Ti is biologically compatible metal with high corrosion resistance, the titanium oxide surface does release some Ti ions at a low rate in the electrolytes such as those in blood and saliva.

Metal with Surface Coating

The new implant design used in titanium is plasma sprayed or coated with a thin layer of calcium phosphate ceramic or hydroxyl apatite to produce bioactive surface that promotes bone growth. The bond is chemical in nature as the bone integrates with the coated surface. In this, a porous or rough titanium surface has been fabricated by plasma spraying in a powder form of molten droplets at 1500°C temperature. The plasma sprayed layer is provided with 0.04 to 0.05 mm thickness after solidification.

Porous titanium surface from various fabrication methods may increase the total surface area (up to several times), produce attachment by osteoformation, enhance by increasing ionic interactions, introduce a dual physical and chemical anchor system and increase the load bearing capability from 25% to 30%. The coatings have been applied to a wide range of endosteal and subperiosteal dental implants with overall intent of improving implant surface biocompatibility profiles and implant longevities.

The Advantages of Coatings

- Tissue bonding.
- Components those are normal to physiological environments.
- Regions that serve as barriers elemental transfer, heat or electrical current flow.
- Control of color.
- Opportunities for the attachment of active biomolecules synthetic compounds.

Limitations

- Mechanical strength properties along the substructure to coating interface.
- Biodegradation that could adversely influence tissue stabilities.
- Tissue dependent changes in physical characteristics.
- Minimal resistance to scraping or scraping procedures associated with oral hygiene.
- Susceptibility to standard handling.
- Sterilizing.
- Placing methodologies.

Other Metals and Alloys

Many other metals and alloys have been used for dental implants device fabrication. Early spirals and cages included tantalum, platinum, iridium, gold, palladium, and alloys of these metals. More recently devices made from zirconium, hafnium and tungsten have been evaluated.

CERAMICS

Oxide ceramics were introduced for surgical implant devices because of inertness to biodegradation high strength and physical characteristics such as color, minimal thermal and electrical conductivity and wide range of elastic properties.

Ceramics are brittle and susceptible to flexible fracture but their outstanding feature of biocompatibility and inert behavior made them as an important implant material.

There are many types of ceramics out of which only two are well-developed and important.
1. Bioactive materials
2. Nonreactive family of ceramics.

Bioactive Material

Hydroxyapatite: They are rich in calcium phosphates in dental reconstructive surgery. It is the material with the formula $Ca_{10}(PO_4)_6(OH)_2$ that is similar to that of bone and teeth. It's mainly been used as an implant material for augmenting alveolar ridges or filling bony defects. These are produced in a block or granular form that is packed or fitted into site providing a scaffold for new bone growth.

Mixtures of particulates with collagen and subsequently with drugs and active organic compounds such as "*bone morphogenic proteins*" increased the range of application. The granular form of this material is difficult to keep it localized at the site of implantation. The material can be synthesized in either a dense or porous form, the later containing porosity 100–300 μm in size, which is adequate for bone in growth.

Advantages
i. Chemical composition of high purity and of substances that are similar to constituents of normal biological tissues.
ii. Excellent biocompatibility profiles within a variety of tissues when used as intended.
iii. Opportunity to provide attachments between selected calcium phosphate ceramics and hard and soft tissues.
iv. Minimal thermal and electrical conductivity plus capability to provide a physical and chemical barrier to ion transport.
v. Modulus of elasticity is more similar to bone than any other implant materials used for load bearing implants.

vi. Color is similar to bone, dentin and enamel.

Disadvantages
  i. Variation in chemical and structural characteristics for some currently available implant products.
  ii. Relatively low mechanical tensile and chemical strength under condition of fatigue loading.
  iii. Relatively low attachment strengths for some coating to substrate interfaces.
  iv. Variable solidities depending on the product and the clinical application.

Uses: Mainly for the endosteal and subperiosteal implants.

Bioglass

A dense ceramic material made from calcium oxide, sodium oxide, phosphorus pentoxide and silicon dioxide.

The strong bonding layer has been shown to be 100–200 μm thick roughly 100 times the thickness comparable layers formed by hydroxyapatite. The bond has been shown to be so strong that when tested to failure, fracture occurs within the bone or bioglass material leaving the interface intact.

Limitation: The brittle nature of bioglass becomes the limiting factors in its use as a stress bearing dental implant materials.

Nonreactive Family of Ceramics

High ceramics from Al, Ti, and Zr oxides have been utilized for root form endosteal blade and pin type dental implant. These are designed with either screw or blade shape and appear to work optimally when they are used as abutments for prosthesis in partially edentulous mouths.

The important ones are aluminum oxide, either as polycrystalline or as a single crystal (sapphire). It is not bioactive material since it does not promote the formation of bone as do the other ceramic materials.

Advantages
• Well-tolerated by bone.
• High strength.
• High stiffness.
• High hardness.

Carbon and Carbon Silicon Compounds

Carbon compounds are often classified as ceramics because of their chemical inertness and absence of ductility; however they are conductors of heat and electricity. Extensive applications for cardiovascular devices excellent biocompatibility profiles and moduli of elasticity close to that of bone have resulted in clinical trials of these compounds in dental and orthopedic prosthesis. Ceramic and carbon substances continue to be used as coatings on metallic and ceramic materials.

POLYMERS

Polymers have been fabricated in porous and solid forms for tissue attachment and replacement augmentation and as coatings for force transfer to soft and hard tissues.

Fiber Reinforced Polymers

They offer advantages in that they can be designed to match tissue properties, can be anisotropic with respect to mechanical characteristics, can be coated for tissue attachments and can be fabricated at relatively low cost.

COMPOSITES

Combination of polymer and other categories of synthetic biomaterials continue to be introduced. Several of the more inert polymers have been combined with particulate or fibers of carbon, aluminum oxide, and hydroxyapatite and glass ceramics.

Some are porous, while others are constructed as solid composite structural forms. In some cases, biodegradable polymers, such as polyvinyl alcohol (PVA), polylactides or glycolides, cyanoacrylates or other hydratable forms have been combined with biodegradable calcium phosphate particulate or fibers.

Limitations: Composites of polymers are especially sensitive to sterilization and handling technique.

   i. Most cannot be sterilized by ethylene oxide or steam.

   ii. Most are electrostatic and tend to gather dust or other particulate if exposed to semiclean air environments.

   iii. Tale or starch or surgical gloves, contact with a towel or gauze pad, or the touching of any contaminated area must be avoided for all biomaterials.

Advantages

   i. Long-term experience.

   ii. Excellent biocompatibility profiles.

   iii. Ability to control proper ties through composite structures.

   iv. Properties can be altered to suit clinical application.

SUGGESTED READING

1. Aronsson BO, Lausamaa J, Kasemo B. Glow discharge plasma treatment for surface cleaning and modification of metallic biomaterials. J Biomed Mater Res. 1997;35(1):49-73.

2. Ask M, Rolander U, Lausmaa J, Kasemo B. Microstructure and morphology of surface oxide films on Ti-6Al-4V. J Mater Res. 1990;5:1662-7.

3. Bowers KT, Keller JC, Randolph BA, Wick DG, Michaels CM. Optimization of surface micromorphology for enhanced osteoblast responses in vitro. Int J Oral Maxillofac Implants. 1992;7:302-10.

4. Browne M, Gregson PJ, West RH. Characterization of titanium alloy implant surfaces with improved dissolution resistance. J Mater Sci: Mater Med. 1996;7:323-9.

5. Browne M, Gregson PJ. Surface modification of titanium alloy implants. Biomaterials. 1994;15:894-8.

6. Buser D, Schenk RK, Steinemann S, Fiorellini JP, Fox CH, Stich S. Influence of surface characteristics on bone integration of titanium implants. A histomorphometric study on miniature pigs. J Biomed Mater Res. 1991a; 25:889-902.

7. Clark M Stanford. Advancements in implant surface technology for predictable long-term results–report". US Dentistry. 2006;30-2.

8. Cochran DL. Endosseous dental implant surfaces in human clinical trials. A comparison using meta-analysis. J Periodontol. 1999;70: 1523-39.

9. Faeda RS, Tavares HS, Sartori R, Guastaldi AC, Marcantonio E. Evaluation of titanium implants with surface modification by laser beam. Biomechanical study in rabbit tibias. Braz Oral Res. 2009; 23(2):137-43.

10. Gemelli E, Scariot A, Heriberto N, Camargo A. Thermal characterization of commercially pure titanium for dental applications. Mater Res. 2007;10(3):241-6.

11. Gotfredsen K, Wennerberg A, Johansson CB, Skovgaard LT, Hjørting-Hansen E. Anchorage of TiO_2-blasted, HA-coated and machined implants. An Experimental study in rabbits. J Biomed Mater Res. 1995;29:1223-31.

12. Guehennec LL, Soueidan A, Layrolle P, Amouriq Y. Surface treatments of titanium dental implants for rapid osseointegration. Dent Mater. 2007;23:844-54.

13. Guilherme AA Castilho, Maximiliano D Martins, Waldemar A, Macedo A. Surface characterization of titanium based implants. Braz J Phy. 2006;36(3B):1004-8.

14. Hsu S, Liu B, Lin W, Chiang H, Huang S, Cheng S. Characterization and biocompatibility of a titanium dental implant with a laser irradiated and dual-acid etched surface. Bio-Med Mater and Eng. 2007;17:53-68.

15. Iijima M, Yuasa T, Endo K, Muguruma T, Ohno H, Mizoguchi I. Corrosion behavior of ion implanted nickel-titanium orthodontic wire in fluoride mouth rinse solutions. Dent Mater J. 2010;29(1): 53-8.

16. Isabel De Monserrat Osorio Bernal, Ito Risa, Katagi Hiroki, Tsuboi ken-Ichiro, Yamada Naoko, Tanabe Toshi-Ichiro, Nagahara Kuniteru, Mori Masahiko. Dental implant surface roughness and topography: a review of the literature. J Gifu Dent Soc. 2009; 35(3):89-95.

17. Jan Eirik Ellingsen, Peter Thomsen, S Petter Lyngstadaas. Advances in dental materials and tissue regeneration. Periodontology. 2006;41: 136-56.

18. Kamachi Mudali U, Sridhar TM, Baldev Raj. Corrosion of bioimplants. Sadhana. 2003;28(3 and 4):601-37.

19. Kilpadi DW, Lemons JE. Surface energy characterization of unalloyed titanium implants. J Biomed Mater Res. 1994;28:1419-25.

20. Kim K, Ramaswamy N. Electrochemical surface modification of titanium in dentistry. Dent Mater J. 2009;28(1):20.

21. Larsson C, Thomsen P, Lausmaa J, Rodahl M, Kasemo B, Ericson LE. Bone response to surface modified titanium implants: studies on electropolished implants with different oxide thickness and morphology. Biomaterials. 1994;15(13):1062-74.

22. Larsson C, Thomsen P, Aronsson BO, Rodhal M, Lausmaa J, Kasemo B, et al. Bone response to surface modified titanium implants: studies on the early tissue response to machined and electropolished implants with different oxide thickness and morphology. Biomater. 1996;17(6):605-16.

23. Lee TM, Chang E, Yang CY. A comparison of the surface characteristics and ion release of Ti_6Al_4 and heat treated Ti_6Al_4V. J Biomed Mater Res. 2000;50:499-511.

24. Mendonça G, Mendonça DBS, Aragao FJL, Cooper LF. Advancing dental implant surface technology—from micron- to nanotopography—review. Biomaterials. 2008;29:3822-35.

25. Norton MR. The history of dental implants: a report. US Dentistry; 2006. pp. 24-6.

26. Nydegger BDT, Oxland T, Cochran DL, Schenk RK, Hirt HP, Snetivy D, et al. Interface shear strength of titanium implants with a sandblasted and acid-etched sur-face: a biomechanical study in the maxilla of miniature pigs. J Biomed Mater Res. 1999; 45(2):75-83.

27. Pan J, Thierry D, Leygraf C. Electrochemical and XPS studies of titanium for biomedical applications with respect to the effect of hydrogen peroxide. J Biomed Mater Res. 1994; 28(1):113-22.

28. Paramjit Singh. Titanium—"The wonder metal" of implant dentistry. The J Ind Prosthodont Soc. 2004;4(1):23-6.

29. Puleo DA, Nanci A. Understanding and controlling the boneimplant interface. Biomaterials. 1999;20:2311-21.

30. Pypen CMJM, Plenk H, Ebel MF, Svagera R, Wernisch J. Characterization of microblasted and reactive ion etched surfaces on the commercially pure metals niobium, tantalum and titanium. J Mater Sci: Mater Med. 1997;8(12):781-4.

31. Alla RK, Kishore G, Nagaraja U, Shammas M, Rama Krishna R, Ravi Chandra Shekhar K. Surface roughness of implants, trends. Biomater Artif Organs. 2011;25(3):112-8.

32. Rodríguez-Rius D, García-Saban FJ. Physico-chemical characterization of the surface of 9 dental implants with 3 different surface treatments. Med Oral Patol Oral Cir Bucal. 2005;10: 58-65.

33. Sean S Kohles, Melissa B Clark, Christopher A Brown, James N Kennedy. Direct assessment of profilometric roughness variability from typical implant surface types. The Int J of Oral and Maxil Implants. 2004;19(4):510-6.

34. Sergey V Dorozhkin. Calcium orthophosphates. J Mater Sci. 2007;42:1061-95.

35. Simon Z, Philip A Watson. Biomimetic dental implants—New ways to enhance osseointegration. J Can Dent Assoc. 2002;68(5): 286-8.

36. Sittig C, Textor M, Spencer ND, Wieland M, Vallotton PH. Surface characterization of implant materials c.p. Ti, Ti-6Al-4V with different pre-treatments. J Mater Sci: Mater Med. 1999; 10(1):35-46.

37. Sulekha G, Siddharth G, Alla RK. Titanium: A miracle metal in dentistry. Trends Biomater Artif Organs. 2013;27(1):42 6.

38. Stanford CM. Surface modifications of dental implants. Aus Dent J. 2008;53(1 suppl):s26- s33.

39. Tengvall P, Lundstrom I, Sjoqvist L, Elwing H, Bjursten LM. Titanium hydrogen peroxide interaction: A possible role in the biocompatibility of titanium. Biomaterials. 1989;10(2):118-20.

40. Tengvall P, Lundstrom I, Sjoqvist L, Elwing H, Bjursten LM. Titanium hydrogen peroxide interaction: Model studies of the influence of the inflammatory response on titanium implants. Biomaterials. 1989;10(3):166-75.

41. Thomsen P, Larsson C, Ericson LE, Sennerby L, Lausmaa J, Kasemo B. Structure of the interface between rabbit cortical bone and implants of gold, zirconium and titanium. J Mater Sci: Mater Med. 1997;8:653-65.

42. Tschernitschek H, Borchers L, Geurtsen W. Nonalloyed titanium as a bioinert metal – a review. Clinics in Dent Pract. 2005;3(4): 5-14.

43. Ulrich Joos, Ulrich Meyer. New paradigm in implant osseointegration. Head and Face Medicine. 2006;2:19.

44. Ulrich Joos, Andre Büchter, Hans-Peter Wiesmann, Ulrich Meyer. Strain driven fast osseointegration of implants. Head and Face Medicine. 2005;1:6.

45. Weerachai Singhatanadgit. Biological responses to new advanced surface modifications of endosseous medical implants. Bone and Tissue Regeneration Insights. 2009;2:1-11.

46. Wen HB, Liu Q, de Wijin JR, de Groot K, Cui FZ. Preparation of bioactive porous titanium surface by a new two-step chemical treatment. J Mater Sci: Mater Med. 1998;9(3):121-8.

47. Wennerberg A, Albrektsson T, Johansson C, Andersson B. Experimental study of turned and grit-blasted screw-shaped implants with special emphasis on effects of blasting material and surface topography. Biomaterials. 1996;17(1):15-22.

48. Wennerberg A, Albrektsson T, Lausmaa J. Torque and histomorphometric evaluation of c.p. titanium screws blasted with 25- and 75-microns- sized particles of Al_2O_3. J Biomed Mater Res. 1996;30(2):251-60.

49. Wieland M, Chehroudi B, Textor M, Brunette DM. Use of Ti-coated replicas to investigate the effects on fibroblast shape of surfaces with varying roughness and constant chemical composition. J Biomed Mater Res. 2002;60:434-44.

50. William R Lacefield. Materials characteristics of uncoated/ceramic-coated implant materials. Adv Dent Res. 2007;13:21-6.

51. Winter W, Krafft T, Steinmann P, Karl M. Quality of alveolar bone - Structure-dependent material properties and design of a novel measurement technique. The Mechanical Behavior of Biomedical Mater. 2011;4:541-8.

52. Yukari Shinonaga, Kenji Arita. Surface modification of stainless steel by plasma-based fluorine and silver dual ion implantation and deposition. Dent Mater J. 2009;28(6):735-42.

SECTION | 3

Laboratory Dental Materials

Gypsum Products

10

GYPSUM

Gypsum is a naturally occurring mineral found in many parts of the world. Chemically, it is $CaSO_4.2H_2O$ (Calcium sulfate dihydrate).

GYPSUM PRODUCTS

Gypsum products are the materials mainly obtained from gypsum, or the term gypsum product refers to various forms of calcium sulfate hydrous and anhydrous, manufactured by calcination of gypsum.

Gypsum products are the results of partial dehydration of gypsum, which produces calcium sulfate hemihydrate ($CaSO_4.1/2 H_2O$).

CLASSIFICATION OF GYPSUM PRODUCTS

1. *According to ADA specification number 25* gypsum products are classified into five types as given below:
2. *According to calcination* they are classified into two types:
   i. Calcium sulfate β-hemihydrate: Obtained by dry calcination, e.g. impression plaster (type I) and dental plaster (type II).
   ii. Calcium sulfate α-hemihydrate: Obtained by wet calcination, e.g. dental stone (type III), die stone with high strength (type IV) and die stone with high strength and high setting expansion (type V).

Calcium sulfate dihydrate $\xrightarrow[110°C–120°C]{\Delta}$ Calcium sulfate hemihydrate + Water

Types	Name	Applications
Type I	Impression plaster (β-hemihydrate)	For making corrective wash or secondary impressions (edentulous) in the construction of complete dentures.
Type II	Dental plaster/model plaster/ Plaster of Paris (β-hemihydrate)	1. Used for pouring casts or models of oral structures when high strength and abrasion resistance is not needed. 2. Used to fill the flask in denture construction.
Type III	Dental stone/hydrocal/ Class I stone (α-hemihydrate)	Used for construction of working casts in the fabrication complete dentures that fit soft tissues.
Type IV	Die stone with high strength/ Densite/Class II stone.	Used for making dies those are used for fabricating gold restorations, crowns, bridges, inlays, onlays, etc.
Type V	Die stone with high strength and high setting expansion/Class III stone/Crystocol.	Used for making very hard dies those are used for fabricating restorations, crowns, bridges, inlays, onlays, etc. with base metal alloys.

$$CaSO_4.\,2H_2O \xrightarrow{110°-130°C} (CaSO_4)_2+H_2O \xrightarrow{130°-200°C} \underset{\substack{\text{Hexagonal}\\\text{(Soluble)}}}{CaSO_4} \xrightarrow{>200°C} \underset{\substack{\text{Orhorhombic}\\\text{(Insoluble)}}}{CaSO_4}$$

MANUFACTURING

Gypsum products used in dentistry are formed by driving off part of crystallization from gypsum to form calcium sulfate hemihydrate.

Depending on the method of calcination different forms of the hemihydrate can be obtained.

Dry Calcination (β-Hemihydrate Manufacturing)

Produced by heating the gypsum mineral in an open kettle (vessel) at a temperature of about 110–120°C. The hemihydrate produced is called calcium sulfate β-hemihydrate (in absence of water). Such a powder is known to have somewhat irregular shape and is considered to be porous (sponginess) in nature.

Wet Calcination (α-Hemihydrate Manufacturing)

Different procedures can be used to obtain α-hemihydrate.
1. Calcined under steam pressure in an autoclave (in the presence of water vapor) at a temperature of 110–120°C. The powder particles of this product are more uniform in shape and denser than the particles of dental plaster. This is also called as autoclaved calcium sulfate hemihydrate or hydrocal (dental stone).
2. Produced by calcining finely divided ground gypsum in water with small quantity of organic acid or salt (sodium succinate) in an autoclave at 130°C. The product obtained is called crystocol (type V).
3. Produced by boiling or calcined in a 30% calcium chloride solution, after which the chlorides are washed away and the calcium

sulfate hemihydrate is dried and grounded to the desired fineness. The powder obtained by this process is densest of the three methods.

SETTING REACTION OR CHEMISTRY

$$CaSO_4.\,\tfrac{1}{2}H_2O+3H_2O \longrightarrow CaSO_4.2H_2O+3900\ cal\,/\,mol$$

When mixed with water, calcium sulfate hemihydrate combines with it to form the dihydrate by the exothermic reaction. Crystalline theory of setting is widely accepted theory. Others include colloidal theory.

CRYSTALLINE (DISSOLUTION-PRECIPITATION) THEORY OF SETTING

Process

Stage I: When a hemihydrate is mixed with water a suspension is formed, i.e. fluid and workable.

Stage II: The hemihydrate is sparingly soluble in water (0.9%). It dissolves until it forms a saturated solution.

Stage III: This saturated solution of the hemihydrate is supersaturated with respect to the dihydrate. So they later precipitate out at suitable nucleation sites in the suspension. (The solubility of dihydrate in water is 0.2%).

Stage IV: As the dihydrate crystallizes, more hemihydrate dissolves and the process continues until all the hemihydrate is converted to dihydrate. As the amount of gypsum forming increases it starts to liberate and the mass thickens and harder into a needle like crystals called spherulites.

Stage V: Finally intermeshing and entangling of crystals lead to a strong solid structure, which is the final set.

The reaction rate can be followed by the exothermic heat evolved.

PROPERTIES

W/P Ratio

It is the ratio of water to the powder usually expressed as the amount of water used per 100 gm of powder.

The w/p ratio is an important factor in determining the physical and chemical properties of the final gypsum product. To get good results water and powder should be proportioned properly by weight.

Theoretically, a ratio of 18.6 is required to satisfy the reaction. But in practice, however, more water than this is used when mixing plaster or stone to give a smooth workable mix. Thus water in excess is required for chemical reaction is called "excess water".

This excess water serves to wet the hemihydrate particle during mixing and does not react with hemihydrate crystals and can be seen by the presence of voids due to evaporation of excess water in the set product.

Type I   Impression plaster—60–70%
Type II   Model plaster—45–55%
Type III Dental stone—35–40%
Type IV   Die stone with high strength—22–26%
Type V   Die stone with high strength and high setting expansion—18–22%.

Effect of W/P Ratio on Properties of Gypsum Products

Low w/p ratio (less water, more powder): There will be more number of nuclei of crystallization per unit volume. These crystals are very close to each other, so they intermesh with one another during growth. This intermeshing gives strength and rigidity to final gypsum product.

Lower the w/p ratio shorter is the setting time, and more will be the strength and setting expansion.

High w/p ratio (more water, less powder): There will be very few numbers of nuclei per unit volume.

Higher the w/p ratio longer the setting time, and lesser the strength and setting expansion.

Setting Time

Setting time may be defined as the time elapsed from the beginning of mixing until the material hardens (gain certain rigidity) or the reaction completes.

Traditionally, two different setting times have been associated with the hardening of calcium sulfate dihydrate.

1. Initial setting time
2. Final setting time.

1. *Initial setting time:* During setting, viscosity of reactive mass begins to increase rapidly and at the same time the mass no longer flows into the fine details of the impression that means the material has reached its working time or initial set. At this point the material has reached initial setting time and should no longer be manipulated.

   Initial setting time must occur within 3 minutes from the start of mixing.

2. *Final setting time:* It is defined as the time at which the material is completely set and can be separated from the impression without distortion or fracture.

   According to ADA specification number 25, final setting times must occur within 12 ± 4 minutes from the start of mixing.

Measurement of Setting Time

1. Loss of glossy test or glass disappearance.
2. Penetration test.
3. Indentation test.
4. Exothermic reaction.

Loss of gloss: As the reaction proceeds some of the excess water is taken up in forming dihydrate by capillary action so that the mix loses its gloss. When loss of glass occurs further manipulation of gypsum mass should be avoided.

Penetration test: This test is conducted by using Vicat penetrometer. It consists of load weighing

300 gm with a needle of 1 mm diameter and 5 cm long. Ring container is filled with the mix setting time of which is to be measured (Fig. 10.1A). The rod is lowered until it contacts the surface of the material and then the needle is released and allows penetrating the mix.

When the needle fails to penetrate to the bottom of the container the material has reached Vicat setting time.

Initial setting time is defined as the time from the beginning of the mixing until the Vicat needle no longer penetrates the entire depth (5 cm) of a given mass of material.

Indentation test: In this, setting time tests are carried out by piercing the respective needle over the surface of the plaster/stone mix at fixed time intervals. The time at which the needle no longer indents the surface is considered as the setting time.

Small Gillmore needle is used to measure initial setting time of the gypsum product. This needle weighs 1/4 lb (113.4 g) and 1/12 inch in diameter (Fig. 10.1B). Setting time is defined as the time from the start of mixing until the smaller Gillmore needle fails to produce any indentation on the surface of the plaster mix.

Bigger Gillmore needle is used to measure the final setting time of gypsum products. This needle weighs 1 lb (453.6 g) and 1/24 inch in diameter (Fig. 10.1B). The setting time is defined as the setting time from the start of mixing until the bigger Gillmore needle fails to produce any indentation on the surface of the plaster mix.

Ready for Use

Technically, it may be considered at a time when the compressive strength is at least 80% of that obtained at 1 hour. Most modern products reach the ready for use state in 30 minutes.

Factors Affecting Setting Time

Theoretically, there are at least three methods by which setting time can be controlled.
1. Number of nuclei of crystallization can be increased or decreased.
2. Solubility of hemihydrate can be increased or decreased.
3. The rate of crystal growth can be increased or decreased.

Factors Controlled by the Dentist/Manufacturer

W/P ratio: Higher the W/P ratio slower is the rate of setting reaction and increases the setting time.

Particle size/fineness of particle: Smaller or finer the particle faster the rate of dissolution of

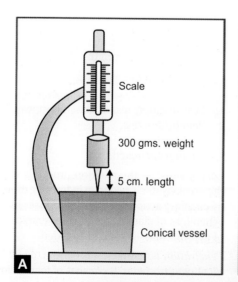
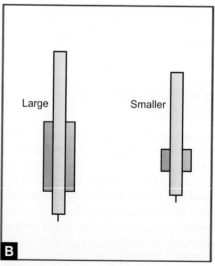

Figs 10.1A and B (A) Vicat penetrometer (B) Gillmore needles

hemihydrate, greater the number of nuclei of crystallization, which in turn accelerates rate of setting and decreases setting time.

Mixing time: Within practical limit an increase in amount of spatulation will shorten the setting time. The amount can be influenced by either speed or time of spatulation or combination of both. During spatulation the formed crystals are broken up by mixing spatula and are distributed throughout the mixture with the resulting formation of more nuclei of crystallization.

Impurity (uncalcined gypsum) or if the manufacturer adds gypsum, setting time will be shortened because the increasing number of nuclei of crystallization.

Hexagonal anhydrate – decreases the setting time.

Orthorhombic anhydrate – increases the setting time.

Humidity: The hemihydrate of gypsum is a hygroscopic material by nature. Initially, plaster takes up sufficient water vapor to start setting; first hydration produces a few crystals and these crystals act as nuclei of crystallization and increases the setting time.

Increased contamination by moisture produces sufficient dihydrate on the hemihydrate. Under these conditions the water penetrates dihydrate coating with difficulty and the setting time is prolonged. Therefore, gypsum product should be stored in a closed container and should be protected from the atmospheric humidity.

Temperature: As the temperature of mixing water increased from 20–37°C the rate of dihydrate formation increases and consequently setting time decreases.

As the temperature is around 40°C the rate of reaction decreases and the setting time is prolonged.

As the temperature of water exceeds 40°C, the solubility of the dihydrate increases. Near boiling point of water the solubility of dihydrate and hemihydrates are approximately equal (0.17). In this case, no reaction takes place and the plaster will not set to a harder mass of gypsum.

Addition of Chemical Modifiers

Accelerators: Accelerators are the chemicals that increase the rate of reaction so that the setting time is reduced to several minutes. An accelerator changes the hemihydrate to be much more soluble than dihydrate (increase the rate of dissolution of hemihydrate), thus accelerating the chemical reaction, e.g.

- Potassium sulfate appears to accelerate setting in any case, but particularly effective in case higher than 2% since the reaction product is syngenite ($K_2Ca(SO_4)_2.H_2O$), which crystallizes very rapidly.
- Na_2SO_4 – 3.4%, more than that acts as a retarder.
- NaCl – 2% in maximum cases.

Retarders: These are the chemicals that decrease the rate of reaction so that the setting time is increased.

Retarders generally act by forming an adsorb layer on the hemihydrate to reduce its solubility, e.g.

- Borax—it forms calcium borate as a reaction of it with calcium sulfate and subsequently deposited on the growing dihydrate crystal and thereby retards crystallization.
- NaCl—more than 2.0%
- Sodium sulfate—more than 12%
- Colloidal systems such as blood, saliva, and alginate and Agar impression materials, they retard rate of setting reaction by being adsorbed on crystals or calcium sulfate dihydrate nucleation sites and thus interfering hydration reaction.
- Citrates, acetates act by nuclei poison.

DIMENSIONAL CHANGES

Setting Expansion

As the setting of gypsum takes place, the growing crystals push each other and cause certain amount of expansion. This expansion ranges from 0.06–0.5% (linear expansion). This is the apparent or observed expansion.

But theoretically certain amount (approximately 7%) of contraction occurs. If equivalent volumes of hemihydrate, water and the reaction product (dihydrate) are compared, the volume of dihydrate formed is less than the equivalent volumes of hemihydrate and the water required.

The apparent volume is greater than the real volume due to the fact that as the material sets, the spherulites not only intermesh but also intercept each other during growth, i.e. if the growth of one crystal is interrupted by another, a stress is present at this point in the direction of the growth of the impinging crystals creating micropores. These micropores contain the excess water used for mixing. This excess water is lost on drying and the total empty space is greatly increased.

Greater the w/p ratio, greater is the porosity because the number of nuclei of crystallization per unit volume is decreased and less intermeshing of crystals of gypsum occurs.

When the plaster is poured to set in the impression mould any expansion is restricted or overcome by the frictional force between plaster and the mould surface. So during the initial set of plaster, apparent expansion is overcome by this friction.

Factors Affecting Setting Expansion

1. *Water/powder ratio:* If the w/p ratio is increased setting expansion is reduced because less number of spherulites per unit volume are formed, thus less outward thrust.
2. *Mixing time:* Longer time of mixing will break the spherulites and increases the setting expansion.
3. *Accelerators and retarders:* These decrease the setting expansion. Retarders either change the crystalline form of dihydrate or rate of crystallization is so rapid that growth is resisted. Expansion takes place after the induction period. But on addition of accelerator the rate of crystallization is so rapid that a rigid framework is formed before the crystallization is completed so setting expansion is reduced.

Two Types of Expansions

- Normal setting expansion
- Hygroscopic setting expansion.

Normal setting expansion: Setting expansion that occurs under normal condition that is without water immersion is termed as normal setting expansion (Fig. 10.2A).

Hygroscopic setting expansion: Expansion that occurs under water is known as hygroscopic setting expansion. This setting expansion that occurs under water is greater than the normal setting expansion (Fig. 10.2B). This water is added during/after the initial set. Comparison between normal and hygroscopic setting expansions were discussed in the Table 10.1

For the preparation of models and casts, this setting expansion should be minimum. But when the dental stone is used as the binder in investment materials, large setting expansion is required. This is to compensate casting shrinkage.

Hygroscopic expansion is more, if
- Time of immersion in water is more.
- Less w/p ratio.
- Longer spatulation time.
- Fresh material.
- No chemicals are added.

MANIPULATION

The plaster or stone is usually mixed in a flexible rubber or plastic bowl using a stiff bladed spatula. The water is dispensed in the bowl first, the powder is then added and allows settling into the water for approximately 30 seconds. This technique minimizes the amount of air incorporated into the mix during the initial spatulation.

Mixing

Mixing is carried by stirring the mixture vigorously and at the same time wiping the inside surface of the bowl with the spatula to be sure that all the powder is wet and mixed uniformly into

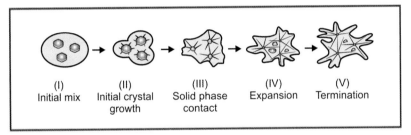

Fig. 10.2A Normal setting expansion

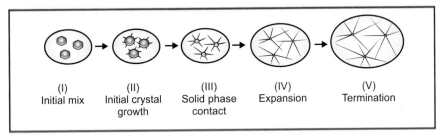

Fig. 10.2B Hygroscopic expansion

Table 10.1 Comparison of normal and hydroscopic setting expansion

Normal setting expansion	Hygroscopic setting expansion
Stage 1:	
The particles of hemihydrate surrounded by water	Same as in normal setting condition
Stage 2:	
• The dihydrate crystals begin to form. • Amount of water is reduced by hydration. • The particles are drawn more closely together.	• The setting takes place under water. • The water of hydration is replaced. • The distance between the particles remains the same.
Stage 3:	
• Dihydrate crystals grow in size. • Water around the particles is again decreased and particles more closely but contraction is opposed by the outward thrust of growing crystals.	• Water around the particles is replaced from outside. • The distance between the particles is further increased as the crystals grow.
Stage 4:	
The crystals become intermeshed and entangled. Thus the crystal growth is inhibited.	Crystals grow much more freely
Stage 5:	
The crystal growth is inhibited by lack of excess water so the crystal grows and expands to a limit	Water added during setting expansion provides more room for longer crystal growth. Therefore, greater setting expansion.

the water. The mixing is continued until all the mixture is smooth and homogeneous in texture. Mixing time approximately 1 minute with the rate of spatulation has been approximately 2 revolutions per second. The mix is then vibrated until no more air bubbles came to the surface.

Construction of Cast

In one method, strips of a soft wax called boxing wax are wrapped around the impression to form a mold or container for the gypsum material. Generally, the wax is extended approximately ½ inch beyond the tissue side of the impression to provide a base for the model or cast. This process is called boxing. The mixture of stone or plaster and water is then allowed to run into the impression under vibration, in such a manner that it pushes ahead itself as it fills the impressions of the teeth and other irregularities. The cast should not be separated unless it has thoroughly hardened (45-60 minutes). The completed cast should be smooth, neat and accurate in every detail.

Precautions

- Instruments should be clean.
- Proper w/p ratio of the material should be followed.
- Do the enough vibration to eliminate the air bubbles.
- Impression should be properly washed to remove blood or saliva. Otherwise it will interfere with the setting reaction.
- Cast should be removed after 45-60 minutes.

IMPRESSION PLASTER (TYPE – I)

Uses

1. Used for corrective wash or secondary impression of the edentulous arches.
2. It is primarily used when excess saliva produced by the accessory palatine gland.

Impression plaster, to which modifiers have been added to regulate the setting time and to control the setting expansion.

Composition

- $CaSO_4$ β-hemihydrate: Main reactive ingredient.
- Accelerator (K_2SO_4): 4% increases the rate of setting reaction.
- Borax: 0.04% retarder (to counteract the accelerator).
- Alizarin: 0.04% color pigment (to distinguish impression plaster and model plaster).
- Potato starch: To render them soluble in water and permits rapid separation of the cast from the impression material.
- Flavoring agent: To offset the bad taste of plaster.

Accelerator, borax, and alizarin dissolved in water and form a solution, called as antiexpansion solution.

Due to the addition of potato starch in plaster it is also called as soluble plaster. The starch softens and swells in hot water and impression disintegrates, and its removal from the cast is facilitated.

Setting Reaction

$$CaSO_4 \cdot \tfrac{1}{2}H_2O + 3H_2O \longrightarrow CaSO_4 \cdot 2H_2O + 3900 \text{ cal / mol}$$

Properties

W/P ratio: 0.60-0.70
Setting time: 4 ± 1 minutes.
Setting expansion: Maximum 0.15%
Wet strength: 6 MPa

Manipulation

The impression plaster should be mixed with water or an anti-expansion solution in the ratio of 100 g to 60-70 ml. A thin layer of mix of impression plaster is placed in the special tray and then placed in the mouth for recording the impression. After the material has set it is removed from the mouth, washed free of saliva and then the surface of the impression is painted with a separating medium (e.g. alcoholic solutions of varnish). Failure to do so results in bonding the cast to the surface of the impression material.

Advantages

- It reproduces good surface detail.
- Rate of set is under the control of operator (4 ± 1 minutes).
- The amount of setting expansion is also less. Dimensionally stable and accurate if used with antiexpansion solution.
- Compatible with all materials commonly used for making casts.
- Stable on storage over long time if it is kept in a sealed condition.
- Relatively inexpensive and easy to manipulate.

Drawbacks

- Set impression is brittle and may fracture when removed from undercut areas.
- Bad taste and rough feel.
- Water absorbing nature of these materials often causes patients to complain about a very dry sensation after impression has been recorded.
- Exothermic heat is disliked by many patients.
- Requires a separator before pouring the cast in the lab, this may cause surface inaccuracy.
- It cannot be used for compressing the soft tissues.

MODEL PLASTER OR DENTAL PLASTER (TYPE – II)

Dental plaster is manufactured by heating the gypsum in an open vessel at a temperature about 110–120°C. Dental plaster contains calcium sulfate β-hemihydrate, accelerators and retarders.

Setting Reaction

$$CaSO_4 \cdot \tfrac{1}{2}H_2O + 3H_2O \longrightarrow CaSO_4 \cdot 2H_2O + 3900 \text{ cal/mol}$$

Properties

W/P ratio: 0.45–0.50 g/ml
Setting time: 12 ± 4 minutes.
Setting expansion: Maximum 0.30%

Wet compressive strength: 9 MPa
Dry compressive strength: 25 MPa
Surface hardness: 60 RHN

Advantages

- Very easy to trim the models.
- Least expensive of the gypsum materials.

Uses

- Used for pouring cast of oral structures when high strength and high abrasion resistance is not required and dimensional accuracy is not typical.
- Used for filling a flask in denture construction.
- Used for mounting stone models in the articulators.

Synthetic Plaster

Plaster manufactured from the byproducts or waste products of the manufacture of phosphoric acid. The synthetic product is much more expensive than that made from natural gypsum.

TYPE – III (CLASS – I STONE/ HYDROCAL/DENTAL STONE)

Dental stone is manufactured by heating the gypsum in an autoclave with steam at a temperature of about 120–130°C.

Dental stone is composed of calcium sulfate α-hemihydrate, accelerators, retarders and color pigments.

Balanced Stone

A stone with a setting time established by the proper additions of both accelerators and retarders is said to be balanced stone, which regulates setting time and reduces setting expansion.

Setting Reaction

$$CaSO_4 \cdot \tfrac{1}{2}H_2O + 3H_2O \longrightarrow CaSO_4 \cdot 2H_2O + 3900 \text{ cal/mol}$$

Properties

W/P ratio: 0.35–0.40
Setting time: 12 ± 4 minutes.
Setting expansion: Maximum 0.20%
Wet compressive strength: 21 MPa
Dry compressive strength: 64 MPa
Surface hardness: 82 RHN

Advantages

- It is inexpensive and easy to manipulate.
- Dimensional stability and accuracy are good.
- Ability to reproduce fine details and sharp margins of impressions.

Drawbacks

- Mechanical properties are not ideal.
- Fracture of teeth from stone casts can occur with careless handling.
- Low abrasion resistance.

Uses

- Used to pour the workable casts in the fabrication of complete dentures.
- Used to process the denture because the stone has adequate strength for that purpose and the denture is easy to remove after process.

DIE MATERIALS

Die

The term die is normally used when referring to a positive replica of single tooth or reproductions of multiple teeth with prepared cavities used in constructing restorations such as crowns, bridges inlays and onlays.

Requirements

- Should have good abrasion resistance so that the surface will not be damaged during the carving of a wax pattern.
- Should have good strength to reduce the likelihood of accidental breakage.

- Should have the ability to reproduce the fine detail and sharp margins of impressions.
- Should remain dimensionally stable under normal conditions of use and storage. (Contraction should be zero).
- Should give good color contrast with various waxes, which are often used to produce wax patterns.
- Should be compatible with other materials with which it comes into contact.
- Should be relatively inexpensive.
- Should be easy to manipulate.
- Should have good shelf-life.

Types of Die Materials

1. Type IV and V gypsum products.
2. Zinc-silico phosphate cement.
3. Silver amalgam.
4. Epoxy resins, polyesters, epimines, etc.
5. Metal sprayed dies (e.g. bismuth and tin alloy)
6. Electroformed dies/metal plated dies.

Type IV and V Gypsum Products

- Type IV: Die stone with high strength.
- Type V: Die stone with high strength and high setting expansion.

Manufacturing and setting reactions are described earlier in the same chapter. Properties of type IV and V gypsum die materials are discussed in Table 10.2.

Table 10.2: Properties of type IV and gypsum die materials

Property	Type IV	Type V
W/P ratio	22–26	18–22
Setting time	8-16 minutes	8-16 minutes
Setting expansion	0.10	0.26
Wet compressive strength	58 MPa	76.4 MPa
Surface hardness	92 RHN	100 RHN
Dry strength	126.4 MPa	145.2 MPa

The greater setting expansion of type V is used for compensation of relatively large solidification shrinkage of base metal alloys.

Die stones have low abrasion resistance; attempts have been made to increase the hardness of gypsum products by the incorporation of the set gypsum with methyl methacrylate that is allowed to polymerize. Polymerization of the monomer produces a polymer phase, which occupies many of the porosities in set gypsum and increases strength and hardness.

Incorporating of wetting agents, "ligno-sulfates" which can reduce the water requirement of a stone and enable production of harder, stronger, denser set gypsum.

Advantages

- Have the ability to reproduce fine detail and sharp margins.
- Compatible with all impression materials.
- Dimensional accuracy is considered to be adequate.
- Relatively inexpensive.
- Easy to manipulate.

Disadvantages

- Mechanical properties are not ideal.
- Susceptibility to abrasion during carving of the wax pattern.

Electroformed Dies

Dies are made or formed by the electrodeposition of metal (Fig. 10.3).

Advantages

- Tough and good strength.
- Good abrasion resistance, which allows satisfactory finishing and polishing of metal restorations on the die.
- Dimensionally stable, i.e. no expansion or contraction occurs in the electrodeposition of a metal.
- Detailed reproduction of a line 4 μm or less in width is readily obtainable, when a nonaqueous elastomeric impression is used.

Hydrophilic impression materials (hydrocolloids and impression plaster) cannot be electroplated because they imbibe electrolytic solution and undergo dimensional changes. Some impression materials can be electroplated, e.g. impression compound, addition polysilicone, can be copper plated and addition polysilicone and polysulfides can be silver-plated.

In a dental electroplating process the impression is made electrically conductive and becomes cathode (-ve), and the metal which is to be deposited is made as anode (+ve).

Types

1. Copper (Cu) plated
2. Silver (Ag) plated.

Copper Plated Dies

Metallizing: A surface of the impression is rendered conductive by coating it with fine

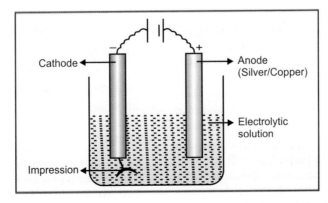

Fig. 10.3 Electrodeposition of metal on the impression in electroplating bath

particles of copper or graphite (because impression material is nonconductive). This process is called as "metallizing".

Selection of electrodes and type of battery: The coated impression is made the cathode (–ve) of plating bath with an anode of copper. The electrolyte is an acid solution of $CuSO_4$ together with organic ingredients (phenol or alcohol), which are believed to increase the hardness of the deposited metal. The electric current may be supplied by storage batteries of the dry cell type.

Procedure: As current is passed causing slow dissolution of the anode and movement of copper ions from anode to cathode so plating the impression. A current of 5–50 milliampere/cm^2 on cathode surface is applied for approximately 10 hours.

Dental stone is then cast into the plated impression when the stone has set the metal carved die can be removed from the impression.

Silver-plated Dies

Metallizing: A surface of the impression is rendered conductive by coating it with fine particles of silver or graphite.

Selection of electrodes and type of battery: The coated impression is made the cathode (–ve) of plating bath with an anode of silver. The electrolyte is an alkaline solution of AgCN together with KCN, and K_2NO_3. The electric current may be supplied by storage batteries of the dry cell type.

Procedure: As current is passed causing slow dissolution of the anode and movement of silver ions from anode to cathode so plating the impression. A current of 5–10 milliampere/cm^2 on cathode surface is applied for approximately 10 hours.

Dental stone is then cast into the plated impression when the stone has set the metal carved die can be removed from the impression.

Precautions: If any acid comes into contact with alkaline cyanide solution HCN gas will be raised, which is toxic and hazardous. Because of this raise, silver plating is not oftenly used.

Silver Amalgam Dies

Silver-tin or copper amalgams may be packed into rigid impression materials such as compound. The dimensional accuracy achieved depends upon the efficiency of condensation.

Disadvantages

- Condensation forces damage the thin sections of impression.
- Longer setting time.
- Difficult to locate the dowel into amalgam.
- Health hazardous due to the presence of mercury.

Metal-sprayed Dies

The fine particles of molten metal or alloy can be sprayed on to many impressions without burning. Metals and alloys can be melted with oxyacetylene or other flame.

The method is applicable to the elastomers and with care to impression compound. Slow spraying of molten metal or alloy can prevent softening of the impression compound.

Advantages

- Good accuracy.
- Dies can be produced within one hour.

Disadvantages

- Difficult to spray into deep recesses.
- Operator should wear the facemask to prevent inhalation of the fine spray of metal.
- Special equipment is required.

Silicophosphate Cement Dies

These cements may be used with all impression materials. They are vibrated and centrifuged into the impression.

Advantages

- Dies can be prepared within short period.
- These cement dies are hard and strong.
- Reproduce good surface details.

Disadvantages

- Brittleness.
- Chances of drying out of the die (should be stored in light oil).
- Dimensional instability.

SUGGESTED READING

1. Carlyle LW. Compatibility of irreversible hydrocolloid impression material with dental stones. J Prosthet Dent 1983; 49:434-7.
2. Gerrow JD, Price RB. Comparison of the surface detail reproduction of flexible die material systems. J Prosthet Dent 1998;80:485-9.
3. Gerrow JD, Schneider RL. A comparison of the compatibility of elastomeric impression materials, type IV dental stones, and liquid media. J Prosthet Dent. 1987;57:292-8.
4. Jack D Gerrow, Richard B. Price, comparison of the surface detail reproduction of flexible die material systems. J Prosthet Dent. 1998;80:485-9.
5. Sarma AC, Neiman R. A study of the effect of disinfectant chemicals on physical properties of die stone. Quint Int. 1990; 21:53.
6. Schelb E, Cavazos E, Kaiser DA, Troendle K. Compatibility of type IV dental stones with polyether impression materials. J Prosthet Dent. 1988;60:540-2.
7. Schelb E, Mazzocco CV, Jones JD, Prihoda T. Compatibility of type IV dental stones with polyvinyl siloxane impression materials. J Prosthet Dent. 1987;58:19-22.
8. Torrance A, Darvell BW. Effect of humidity on calcium sulphate hemihydrate. Aust Dent J. 1990;35:230.

Denture Base Resins

11

A complete denture may be defined as a removable dental prosthesis intended to replace the masticatory surface and associated structures of maxillary or mandibular arch such prosthesis is composed of artificial teeth attached to a denture base.

Denture base is the part of the denture that retains artificial teeth and rests on the soft tissues of the mouth. The denture base derives its support through intimate contact with underlying oral tissues.

The materials used for the fabrication of denture bases are called "denture base materials".

The materials used in the construction of denture bases may be divided into metallic and nonmetallic types. The non-metallic denture base materials are the polymer-based materials, which are discussed in this chapter. In general, they display excellent mechanical properties, and can be used in relatively thin sections. However, it is cheaper to construct appliances. In addition, the color and texture of these materials can be made to resemble natural gum tissue, thus making the appliances less conspicuous in the mouth. The artificial teeth are constructed either of porcelain or acrylic resin tinted to simulate the human teeth.

Many different materials have been used for denture bases. Historically, materials such as bone, wood, ivory, and vulcanized rubber were utilized and in addition to these other materials such as vulcanite, nitrocellulose, bakelite, vinyl plastics, porcelain, poly (methyl methacrylate) (PMMA), vinyl acrylics, polystyrene, epoxy resins, nylon, vinyl styrene, polycarbonate, polysulfone—unsaturated polyesters, polyurethane, polyvinyl acetate—ethylene hydrophilic polyacrylate, silicones, light activated urethane dimethacrylate, rubber reinforced acrylics, and butadiene reinforced acrylics.

So many materials have been developed to construct the removable complete or partial prosthesis. But PMMA remains the preferred material.

REQUIREMENTS OF DENTURE BASE MATERIALS

The ideal denture base material should possess several key physical attributes. Some of those properties are as follows:

Biological Requirements

i. In mixed or uncured state the denture base material should not be harmful to the technician involved in its handling.
ii. The denture base material should be nontoxic and non-irritant.
iii. Should not produce toxic fumes or dust during handling and manipulation.
iv. Should not support the growth of bacteria.
v. Should not be carcinogenic.

Chemical Requirements

A denture base material should chemically be inert, in the sense; it should be/should have—
i. Insoluble in oral fluids or any other fluids taken into the mouth.

ii. Impermeable and should not absorb water since this may alter the mechanical properties and cause the denture to become unhygienic.
iii. Good adhesion with artificial teeth and liners.

Mechanical Requirements

A denture base material should have–
i. High modulus of elasticity–
   a. To be rigid against masticatory deforming forces
   b. To achieve greater rigidity even in thin sections.
ii. High PL and EL: So that denture will not undergo permanent deformation when stressed.
iii. High compressive, tensile and transverse or flexural strength. To resist biting and chewing forces without fracture.
iv. High impact strength. To resist fracture under impact forces.
v. High fatigue strength–
   a. To resist fracture under repeated cyclic forces, which are common in the oral cavity.
   b. To have a long shelf-life to service.
vi. High resilience: To protect soft tissues by absorbing masticatory forces.
vii. High surface hardness–
   a. To prevent excessive wear of the material by abrasive denture cleanser or food stuff.
   b. Should take and retain a high polish.
viii. Low specific gravity–
   a. Denture should be as less weight as possible.
   b. This reduces the gravitational forces, which may act on an upper denture.
ix. Low surface energy: To prevent the deposition of food stuffs on the surface of denture.
x. Good dimensional stability
   a. In order to that the shape of the denture does not change over a period of time.
   b. Should neither expand nor contract nor warp during processing or during subsequent normal use by the patient.

Thermal Requirement

i. **Should have high thermal conductivity** to enable the denture wearer to maintain a healthy oral mucosa and retain a normal reaction to hot and cold stimuli.
ii. **COTE:** Should match with that of artificial tooth material.
iii. **Should have high softening temperature (Tg)** to prevent softening and distortion when hot foods taken into the mouth.
   a. Should ideally be above the temperature of boiling water for purposes of sterilization with evidence of wrapping.

Esthetic Requirements

A denture base material should be/should have–
i. Exhibit sufficient translucency so that it can be made to match the appearance of the oral tissues it is to replace.
ii. Capable of being tinted or pigmented.
iii. No change in colors or appearance of the material subsequent to its fabrication.

Other Requirements

A denture base material should be/ should have–
i. Radiopaque: Be capable of detection using normal diagnostic radiographic technique if accidentally swallowed.
ii. Relatively inexpensive
iii. Tasteless and odorless
iv. Long shelf-life
v. Easy to manipulation and fabricate without using expensive processing equipment.
vi. Possible to repair the resin easily and efficiently in case of unavoidable breakage.
vii. Easy to clean.

No known denture base material adequately fulfills all these requirements.

CLASSIFICATION OF DENTURE BASE MATERIALS

According to the Type of Materials

All denture base materials can be broadly classified into metallic and nonmetallic materials.

Nonmetallic denture base materials are widely used for the fabrication of dentures.

CLASSIFICATION OF DENTURE BASE RESINS

According to Development of Materials

a. Formerly used
   Example: Vulcanite, bakelite, cellulose nitrate, nylon, polyvinyl chloride, polystyrene, polycarbonates and epoxy resins.
b. Most widely used materials
   Example: Poly (methyl methacrylate) heat-cure and self-cure.
c. Recently developed
   Example: Fiber reinforced acrylics, high impact strength acrylics, vinyl acrylics, hydrophilic acrylics, fluid resins, radiopaque resins and light activated denture base resins.

According to the Method of Polymerization

a. Addition polymers, e.g. poly (methyl methacrylate), and polyvinyl chloride
b. Condensation polymers, e.g. nylon, bakelite.

According to the Method of Activation

  i. *Thermal*; e.g. poly (methyl methacrylate).
 ii. *Microwave*; e.g. poly (methyl methacrylate).
iii. *Catalyst*; e.g. poly (methyl methacrylate).
 iv. *Visible light activated*; e.g. poly (methyl methacrylate).

According to the Dispensing System

a. Power and liquid system, e.g. heat-cure and self-cure acrylic resins.
b. Sheets and ropes: (Single component system), e.g. light activated denture base resins.
c. Gel type, e.g. vinyl acrylics.

According to their Thermal Response

a. Thermoplastic, e.g. polyvinyl acrylics and polystyrene.
b. Thermosetting, e.g. PMMA.

In the beginning of 1900's polyvinyl chloride, vinyl acetate, modifications of bakelite, and cellulose plastics were used. The main disadvantages of these materials include difficult processing methods, lack of dimensional stability, brittleness, discoloration and expensive, recommended for suitable replacements. In 1937, Walter Wright introduced most useful resin to dentistry such as polymethyl methacrylate (PMMA) material, which proved to be the most satisfactory material tested up to that time. By the middle of 1940's almost all the dentures were fabricated with these acrylic resin materials.

The popularity of PMMA materials is based on its low cost, relative ease of use, and resilience on simple processing equipment. There are, however, significant differences in the chemistry among denture materials based on PMMA chemistry. Some materials are composed with high levels of cross-link resin and heat activated initiators to maximize the physical properties of processed materials.

These denture base materials are available, which polymerize either with or without the application of external heat. The former materials are called heat-cured polymethyl methacrylate and later is self-cured or chemically-cured materials.

HEAT ACTIVATED DENTURE BASE ACRYLIC RESINS

These materials are widely used for the construction of removable complete or partial dentures. In the heat-cured materials, polymerization is started by free radicals released from benzoyl peroxide.

Dispension and Composition

Heat-cured materials are available in the form of finely divided prepolymerized polymer powder and monomer liquid (Fig. 11.1).

Liquid is supplied in a dark brown colored bottle to avoid accidental polymerization when exposed to visible or UV radiation during transport a storage. Bottle should be kept closed to prevent evaporation and stored at the specified temperature recommended by the manufacturer. Composition of heat-activated acrylic denture base materials is discussed in Table 11.1.

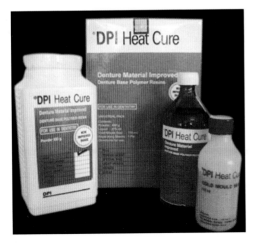

Fig. 11.1 Heat-cure acrylic resin

Setting Reaction

Whenever powder is added to the liquid and cured, the free radicals on activation, initiates polymer growth. In the presence of ethylene glycol dimethacrylate, a cross-linking agent, a rigid cross-linked poly (methyl methacrylate) is formed.

Properties

Properties of Methyl Methacrylate

Methyl methacrylate is a clear, transparent liquid at room temperature (Table 11.2).

Volatile liquid with distinct odor exaggerated by a relatively high vapor pressure at room temperature.

Other properties of methyl methacrylate are given in Table 11.2.

Properties of Poly (Methyl Methacrylate)

Poly (methyl methacrylate) is a transparent resin of remarkable clarity. It transmits light better than glass.

Biological Properties

Acrylic resin dentures contain methyl methacrylate as residual monomer. Residual monomer has the potential to elicit irritation, inflammation and allergic response of the oral mucosa. Further, residual monomer is capable of producing both stomatitis and an angular cheilitis.

Residual monomer present in heat-cure acrylic resin is 0.2–0.5% and in self-cure acrylic resin it is 2–5%.

Formaldehyde is another allergic agent in acrylic dentures responsible for mucosal injuries. Formaldehyde is formed as an oxidation product of the residual MMA monomer in inhibition layers and poorly polymerized resins. Formaldehyde formation was suggested to occur through the decomposition of the oxygen-methyl methacrylate copolymer or by the oxidation of methyl methacrylate. Formaldehyde is proved to be cytotoxic at much lower concentrations than methyl methacrylate. Formaldehyde is also a strong irritant to the mucous membranes even at low concentrations as low as 0.63 to 1.25 mg/m^3.

The allergic reaction occurs within a few to several hours after the mucosa is exposed to the resin. When allergic reactions were noted, they were described as white, necrotic lesions on the mucosa; either as small, multiple lesions or as large ulcers mimicking allergic stomatitis.

Chemical Properties

Solubility: Acrylic resins are soluble in aromatic hydrocarbons, ketones and esters. The solubility is around 0.04 mg/cm^2. Alcohol will cause crazing. Ethanol functions as a plasticizer and can reduce the glass transition temperature. Therefore, solutions containing alcohol should not be used for cleaning or storing the dentures. The water solubility of heat-cure acrylic resins is 0.02 mg/cm^2.

Water sorption: Water sorption of heat-cure acrylic resins is 0.69 mg/cm^2. The sorption of water changes the dimension of the denture when alternatively soaked in water and dried. This repeated drying and wetting incorporate stresses in the denture resulting in crazing.

Water absorption of heat-cured resins is 1.08×10^{-12} m^2/sec.

Table 11.1 Composition of heat-cure acrylic resin

Powder	
Ingredients	*Functions*
Prepolymerized poly (methyl methacrylate)	• Undergoes further polymerization. • Reduces the polymerization shrinkage.
Copolymers of PMMA (5%) e.g. ethyl or butyl methacrylates	• Increase the solubility of polymer in the monomer. • To produce a polymer somewhat more resistant to fracture by impact.
Initiator (0.2–1.5%) e.g. benzoyl peroxide or di-iso butyl azonitrile	Initiates the polymerization of the monomer liquid after being added to powder.
Plasticizer, e.g. Dibutyl phthalate	• Increases the solubility of polymer in the monomer. • Produces softer and more resilient polymer.
Color pigments, e.g. Mercuric sulfide—Red Cadmium sulfide—Yellow Ferric oxide—Brown Carbon black—Brown	Added to obtain the various tissue like shades.
Opacifiers, e.g. zinc or titanium oxides	Provides opacity.
Dyed synthetic fibers made from nylon or acrylic	To simulate the minute blood vessels in the underlying oral mucosa.
Inorganic particles, e.g. glass fibers, zirconium silicate, whiskers of alumina, SiC, boron nitride and carbon fibers.	• To improve the stiffness. • To decrease COTE.
Heavy metal compounds, e.g. barium, bismuth, etc.	• Imparts radiopacity.
Liquid	
Methyl methacrylate	Undergoes polymerization to produce PMMA.
Comonomers	Improves the properties of denture bases.
Inhibitor, e.g. Hydroquinone (0.003%–0.1%)	Prevents premature polymerization and prolongs the shelf-life of the liquid.
Plasticizers, e.g. butyl or octyl methacrylate and dibutyl phthalate	Producer softer and more resilient polymer.
Cross-linking agent, e.g. Ethylene glycol dimethacrylate	• Improves the physical properties of the denture. • Increases resistance to crazing.

Table 11.2 Properties of methylmethacrylate monomer

Property	Values
Melting point	-48°C
Boiling point	100.8°C
Density	0.945 g/cc at 20°C
Polymerization shrinkage	21%
Heat of polymerization	12,900 cal/mole

Adhesion: Chemically bonds to the acrylic teeth but not with the porcelain teeth.

Mechanical Properties

Modulus of elasticity: 3.8×10^3 Mpa.
Proportional limit : 26 Mpa.
Compressive strength: 76 Mpa
Tensile strength: 48–62 Mpa
Percentage of elongation: 1–2%
Impact strength: 0.98–1.27 J

Impact strength is very low. So dentures may break if dropped on a hard surface accidentally.

Surface hardness: 18–20 KHN

Density: 1.16–1.18 g/cc

Fatigue strength: 1.5×10^6 cycles at 17.2 MPa.

Thermal Properties

Thermal conductivity: The thermal conductivity of these resins is low, 5.7×10^{-4} °C/cm, this results in plastic denture bases serving as an insulator between the oral tissues and hot or cold materials taken into the mouth. In other words, patient will not feel the hot or cold sensation immediately.

Coefficient of thermal expansion: 81×10^{-6} /°C.

Heat distortion temperature: 71–91 /°C.

Glass transition temperature: 125°C.

Depolymerization temperature: 450°C.

Compression Molding Technique for the Fabrication of Complete Denture

The following are the steps involved in the fabrication of complete dentures using compression-molding technique:

1. Preliminaries
2. Flasking
3. Dewaxing
4. Separating medium
5. Proportioning and mixing
6. Trial closure
7. Final closure
8. Bench curing
9. Curing cycle
10. Bench cooling
11. Deflasking
12. Finishing and polishing.

Preliminaries: These are the steps involved from the making of preliminary impression to the arrangement of teeth in the occlusal rims. Actual steps involved are discussed in Flow chart 11.1.

Flasking

Dental flask is a device in which the wax denture model is invested and in which the denture is fabricated. Dental flask has three parts such as lower half, upper half and lid.

Procedure: Flasking is the process of investing the cast with waxed denture in a flask to make

Flow chart 11.1 Preliminary steps in compression molding technique

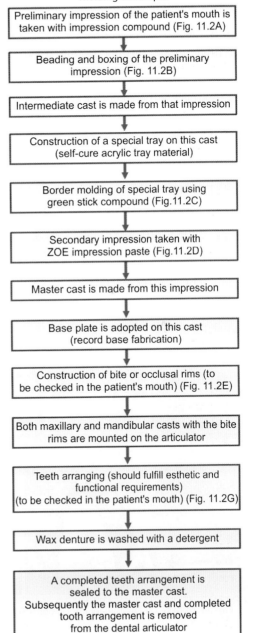

Preliminary impression of the patient's mouth is taken with impression compound (Fig. 11.2A)

↓

Beading and boxing of the preliminary impression (Fig. 11.2B)

↓

Intermediate cast is made from that impression

↓

Construction of a special tray on this cast (self-cure acrylic tray material)

↓

Border molding of special tray using green stick compound (Fig.11.2C)

↓

Secondary impression taken with ZOE impression paste (Fig.11.2D)

↓

Master cast is made from this impression

↓

Base plate is adopted on this cast (record base fabrication)

↓

Construction of bite or occlusal rims (to be checked in the patient's mouth) (Fig. 11.2E)

↓

Both maxillary and mandibular casts with the bite rims are mounted on the articulator

↓

Teeth arranging (should fulfill esthetic and functional requirements) (to be checked in the patient's mouth) (Fig. 11.2G)

↓

Wax denture is washed with a detergent

↓

A completed teeth arrangement is sealed to the master cast. Subsequently the master cast and completed tooth arrangement is removed from the dental articulator

a sectional mold used to form acrylic resin denture base.

i. The lower half is filled with freshly mixed dental stone. Center the cast in the lower half of the flask. Remove under cuts in the investment to facilitate dewaxing, packing and deflasking procedure (Fig. 11.3A).

ii. On reaching its initial set, the stone is coated with a separator (liquid soap or Vaseline or cold mold seal) to prevent the stone/plaster mix that is poured into the upper half of the flask from adhering to that in the lower half.

iii. A surface tension reducing agent is applied to exposed wax surface. Now place the upper half of the flask.

iv. The upper half can be filled in two ways:
1. It can be filled with one mix of plaster and the lid is placed as shown in Figure 11.3B.
2. As shown in Figure 11.3C, a mix of dental plaster is poured into the flask to cover all the surfaces of tooth arrangement and denture base but incisal and occlusal surfaces are minimally exposed. The plaster permitted to set and

subsequently coated with separator. Remaining portion of the flask is filled with the dental stone and lid of the flask is tapped into place, and it is allowed to set (capping or multiple pour tech) this facilitates the deflasking procedure.

v. Secure the flask in the clamp to ensure the metal halves of the flask are in contact.

Dewaxing

i. After flasking, place the flask in the boiling water bath for 5–10 minutes. This will soften the waxed denture base.

ii. The flask is then removed from the water bath and the appropriate segments are separated (Fig. 11.4A).

iii. The record base and softened wax remain in the lower half of the flask while the prosthetic teeth remain firmly embedded in the top of the flask (Fig. 11.4B).

iv. The record base and softened wax are carefully removed from the surfaces of the mold then flush the mold with clean hot water to which a detergent is added to remove residual wax.

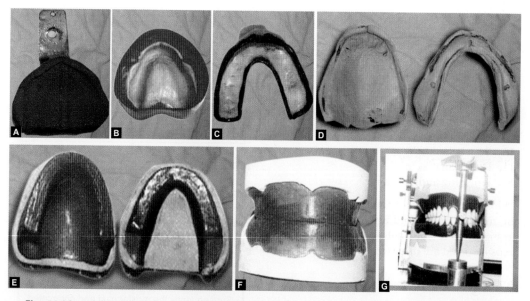

Figs 11.2A to G (A) Preliminary impression; (B) Boxing of impression; (C) Border molding of special tray; (D) Secondary impression; (E) Occlusal rims; (F) Sealing of occlusal rims; (G) Articulation of trial dentures

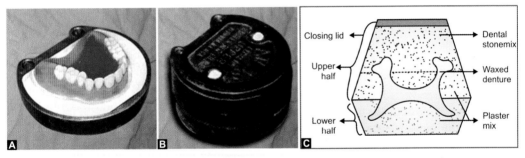

Figs 11.3A to C (A) Flasking; (B) After flasking; (C) Multiple-pour investing procedure

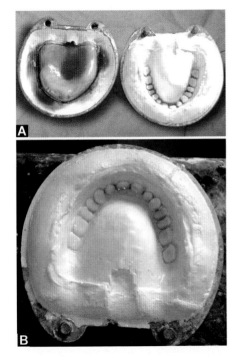

Figs 11.4A and B (A) Immediately after removing from the boiling water bath; (B) After dewaxing – Incisal and occlusal surfaces of acrylic teeth are firmly embedded in the stone/plaster

v. It is then allowed to get dried. When it is hot, it is applied with a thin coating of separating medium without trapping air bubbles.

Separating Medium

The next step in the denture base fabrication involves the application of an appropriate separating medium onto the walls of the mold cavity. This medium must prevent direct contact between the denture base resin and the mold surface.

One of the first widely used materials was tin foil. However, the process of the tin foiling is time consuming and difficult process causing dimensional inaccuracy and poor reproduction of details. So tin foil substitutes were developed, they include cellulose lacquers, solutions containing alginate compounds, soaps, evaporated milk and starch. The most popular separating agents are water-soluble alginate solutions. Composition of soluble alginate solution was discussed in Table 11.3.

Setting reaction: Soluble alginate solutions when applied to dental stone surfaces to produce a thin film of calcium alginate gel, which is water and organic solvent insoluble.

$$K_n \text{ alginate} + n/2 \text{ CaSO}_4 \rightarrow \text{Ca}_n \text{ alginate gel} + n/2 \text{ K}_2\text{SO}_4$$

Table 11.3 Composition of separating medium (soluble alginate solution)

Component	Wt %	Functions
K or Na alginate	2	Main reactive ingredient.
Di or tri sodium phosphate	0.7	• Improves flow property. • Decreases viscosity.
Glycerin	4	
Alcohol	7	
Esters of hydroxy benzoic acid	0.3	Preservative.
Water	86	

This film prevents direct contact of the denture base resin and the surrounding dental stone. Therefore, undesirable interactions between denture base resin and dental stone are eliminated.

Functions

i. To prevent the diffusion of water molecule from the mold (dental stone) into the unpolymerized packed dough.

If the water is permitted to pass from the mold surface into the denture base resin, it may affect the polymerization rate as well as the optical and physical properties of the processed denture.

The processed denture will craze readily because of the stresses incorporated by the evaporation of water during curing.

ii. To prevent the diffusion of monomer from the unpolymerized packed dough in the mold material.

If dissolved polymer/monomer is permitted to soak into the mold surfaces, portions of the investing medium may become fused to the denture base, after polymerization it will be virtually impossible to separate the investing material from the resin denture base. It produces rough surfaces with adherent mold material.

Application of separating medium: A small amount of the separator is dispensed into a disposable container. A fine brush is used to spread the separating medium onto the exposed surfaces of a warm, clean stone mold (Figs 11.5A and B).

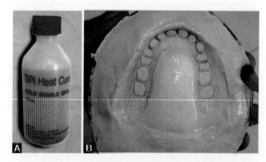

Figs 11.5A and B (A) Separating medium (B) Application of separating medium

Precautions

i. Coating must be given only when the flask can be held comfortably in the hand. Otherwise continuity of the film can be disrupted.

ii. De-waxing must be done thoroughly; otherwise any residual wax remaining on the mold surfaces will not permit the solution to contact and react with investment material. Thus, causing poor separation between the denture base material and the mold material.

iii. Coating must be thin and continuous without trapping air bubbles.

iv. Resin teeth surfaces should not be coated as it permits chemical bonding between the base material and the teeth.

Proportioning and Mixing

Polymer-monomer ratio: The main reason of adding polymer to monomer is to control the total quality of liquid monomer in a mix to be converted to polymer. If methyl methacrylate monomer alone, when polymerized, it undergoes a volumetric contraction of 21%. This would create significant difficulties in denture base fabrication and service.

To minimize volumetric shrinkage, manufacturers pre-polymerize a significant fraction of the denture base material (preshrinking). This polymerized material when mixed with monomer in the ratio of 3:1 by volume, the volumetric shrinkage may limit to 6% (0.5% linear shrinkage).

The amount of monomer in the mix must be sufficient to soften all the available polymer powder because it controls the workability of the mix.

The polymer/monomer ratio is usually 3–3.5:1 by volume or 2.5:1 by wt. this amount of monomer in the mix results in about 7% of volumetric contraction.

I. **If polymer/monomer ratio is too high:** (more polymer- less monomer)

a. Not all the polymer will wet by monomers and the cured acrylic resin will be granular.

b. Dough will be difficult to manage.

II. If polymer/monomer ratio is too low: (less polymer – more monomer)
   a. Polymerization shrinkage will be greater than 7%
   b. Dough forming time will be prolonged.
   c. There will be a tendency for porosity to occur in the denture.

Polymer-monomer interaction: The liquid monomer is first poured in a thick, clean glass jar and then the powder is added slowly to it. After all the powder has been added, the mix is stirred and vibrated thoroughly so that the mechanical mixed pigments and dyes are dispensed evenly throughout the material. On completing of stirring, a light lid must be placed on the glass jar to prevent evaporation of the monomer. The polymer will slowly dissolve in monomer, and the following physical changes could be observed:

1. *Wet standy stage:* At this stage the polymer settles in the monomer and forms a very liquid, incoherent uncontrollable mass. During this, little or no interactions occur on a molecule level. Polymer beads remain unaltered and the consistency of the mixture may be described as coarse or grainy.
2. *Stringy stage:* The monomer attacks the polymer. Monomer penetrates the polymer chains and softens. It is the polymer begins to dissolve in the monomer. This increases the viscosity of the mix. The stage is characterized by stringiness stickiness or adhesiveness when the material is touched or pulled apart.
3. *Dough or gel stage:* As the monomer diffuses into the polymer and the mass becomes more saturated with polymer in solution, it becomes smooth and dough like. It is no longer tacky, and it does not adhere to the walls of the mixing jar. When the mixture is in this stage, it is packed into the mold.
4. *Rubbery or elastic stage:* Monomer is dissipated by evaporation and by further penetration into remaining polymer beads. The mass loses its plasticity and becomes rubbery and is no longer suitable for molding. The mass rebounds when compressed or stretched.
5. *Stiff stage:* On standing for an extending period, the mixture becomes stiff due to the evaporation of free monomer. Mix appears very dry and is resistant to mechanical deformation.

Dough forming time: The time required for the resin mixture to reach dough-like stage is termed as the dough forming time.

ADA specification number 12 for denture base resins requires that this consistency be attained in less than 40 minutes from the start of mixing process. Most resins reach dough-like consistency in less than 10 minutes.

Factors affecting working and dough forming time
1. *Size of the polymer particle:* The smaller the particle size; more rapid is the dissolution and dough formation.
2. *Molecular weight of polymer:* Lower the molecular weight, faster the dough forming time.
3. *Plasticizers:* Plasticizers increase the solubility of the polymer in monomer thereby decrease the working time.
4. *Polymer-monomer ratio:* Higher the polymer-monomer ratio within the optimum limit, shorter is the dough forming time.
5. *Temperature:* Higher the temperature, shorter will be the dough forming time.

   The mixing jar can be placed on warm water bath (not above 50°C) to decrease the dough forming time. Similarly, the mixing jar can be kept in refrigerator to increase the dough forming time. When the mix is placed in the refrigerator, moisture contamination may be avoided by storing the resin in an airtight container. After removal from the refrigerator, the container should not be opened until it reaches room temperature.

Packing

Introduction of denture base resin into the mold cavity is termed packing (Fig. 11.6). It is essential that the mold cavity be properly filled at the time of polymerization.

Over packing: Introduction of too much material leads to a denture base that exhibits excessive thickness and resultant mall positioning of prosthetic teeth.

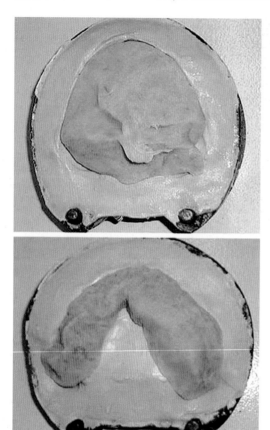

Fig. 11.6 Packing of acrylic dough into the mold

Under packing: Introduction too little material leads to noticeable denture base porosity.

To reduce the likelihood of over packing or under packing the mold cavity is packed in several steps. The powder-liquid mixture should be packed at the dough stage.

Too early packing: If it is packed at the sandy or stringy stage the material will be of too low viscosity to pack well and will flow out of the flask too easily. It may also result in porosity in the final denture base.

Delayed packing: If it is packed at the rubbery or stiff stage, the mix will be too viscous to flow under pressure and metal-to-metal contact of the flask halves will not be obtained. This may also result in loss of detail in the denture movement or fracture of the teeth.

Trial Closure

The resin dough from the mixing jar is rolled into a rope-like form, bent into a horseshoe shape and placed in the upper half (containing artificial teeth) of the flask (Fig. 11.6). A damp cellophane or polyethylene sheet is placed over the resin to prevent the adhesion of the resin to the lower mold surface when two halves of the flask is pressed together and to allow for easy separation of the flask halves during trial closure.

The flask is closed and the assembly is placed into a specially designed press (clamp) (Fig. 11.7A) and pressure is applied slowly to–

- Permit the resin dough to flow evenly throughout the mold space.
- Permit the excess or flash to flow out between the two halves of the flask.
- Remove air, which is incorporated within the dough during mixing.

Pressure is applied until the major portions of the flask closely approximate one another. Then the flask is opened, excess resin found on the relatively flat areas surrounding the mold called flash, is removed using a gently rounded instrument (Figs 11.7A and B).

A fresh polyethylene sheet is placed between the major portions of the flask and another trial closure is made. This trial packing procedure is repeated until the mold is filled and no flash is formed.

Final closure: During final closure, polyethylene sheet is removed and discarded. A mold-separating medium is applied to the surface of the investment and cast in the lower half of the flask. The flask is now closed in a clamp under pressure, which is maintained until the denture has been processed.

Bench Curing

Properly packed flasks should be allowed to stand for 30–60 minutes before beginning the curing cycle. This allows the monomer liquid to penetrate the powder thoroughly and uniformly. Otherwise, the sites containing more monomer will undergo more shrinkage and it will cause irregular voids in the processed denture base. It also provides longer flow period for the dough,

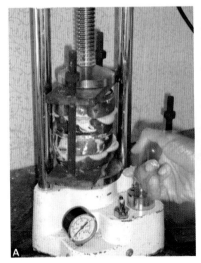 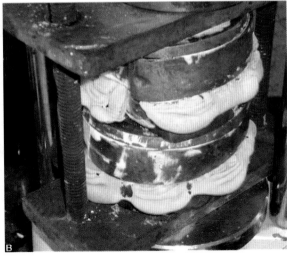

Figs 11.7A and B (A) Hydraulic bench press used for removal of excess flash; (B) Excess flash during trial closures

thus equalizing the pressure throughout the mold.

Curing

After bench curing, the flask is placed in a cold-water bath. It is then heated slowly. As the temperature of the water bath increases heat starts to conduct inside. When the temperature of acrylic dough reaches about 60°C, benzoyl peroxide (initiator) is decomposed to produce two free radicals. Each free radical rapidly reacts with an available monomer molecule to initiate polymerization.

The polymerization reaction propagates with the liberation of heat (12.9 kcal/mole) because the polymerization reaction is exothermic. If further heat is being added from the outside of the flask by conduction through plaster mold, the two sources of heat are complementary. The consequent rapid rise in temperature causes and further increases in the rate of polymerization, which again liberates more heat.

Since the acrylic resin and stone are poor thermal conductors of heat, the heat of reaction cannot be dissipated. Therefore, the temperature of the resin increases well above the temperatures

of surrounding materials and may increase to a value even up to about 120°C–130°C (Fig. 11.9A). This temperature is greater than the boiling point of monomer such as 100.8°C. So at these temperatures, residual monomer will boil and the monomer vapor enclosed by hard polymer and a porous structure will be created. This type of porosity will not be seen at the surface of denture base because exothermic heat can be conducted away from the surface of the denture into the investing medium and the temperature in thin region is not likely to rise above the boiling point of the monomer. These do not show gaseous porosity but their heat of reaction is passed onto the interior portions of dough. It is here the gaseous porosity is seen. In other words, it occurs away from the source of heat, i.e. at the center of a thick portion of denture when heat cannot be conducted away with sufficient rapidity and the temperature of the resin is likely to cross 100.8°C (Fig. 11.9A). The porosity can be seen in:

Lower denture: Lingual aspect in the premolar region (Fig. 11.8B).

Upper denture: Around the sloping sides of the palate (Fig. 11.8A).

Curing Cycle

The curing cycle is the technical name for the heating process employed to control the initial propagation of polymerization in the denture mold.

Or

The heating process used to control polymerization is termed as polymerization cycle or curing cycle.

Or

It is the procedure of polymerizing the acrylic resin dough by slowly raising the temperature until the curing starts, then by maintaining the temperature until the curing completes and then by slow cooling to room temperature.

For heat cure acrylic resins, the curing cycle used is of great importance in the quality of the final denture since the polymerization reaction is strongly exothermic. Ideally, this process should be well-controlled to avoid the effects of uncontrolled temperature rise such as boiling of monomer and denture base porosity. The following two methods have been suggested to obtain non-porous denture:

1. Slow curing cycle.
2. Fast curing cycle.

1. *Slow curing cycle*

It involves processing of denture base resin in a constant temperature water bath at 74°C for 8 hours or longer with no terminal boiling treatment.

- Lower the constant temperature, longer the time is needed for curing.
- If the bulk of the acrylic is more, better to cure at low temperature and longer time is required for curing.
- Slowly raise the temperature of water bath to about 74°C in about half an hour and maintain the temperature constant for 8 hours or more (Fig. 11.9B).

2. *Fast curing cycle*

Involves heating the resin at 74°C for approximately 1½ to 2 hours and then increasing the temperature of the water bath to 100°C and processing for one hour or more (Fig. 11.9C).

Slowly raise the temperature of the water bath to about 74°C in about half-an-hour and maintain the temperature constant for 1½ hours.

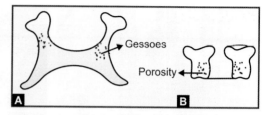

Figs 11.8A and B Porosity in (A) Maxillary denture around the slopes of the palate; (B) Mandibular denture at the lingual aspects of pre molars

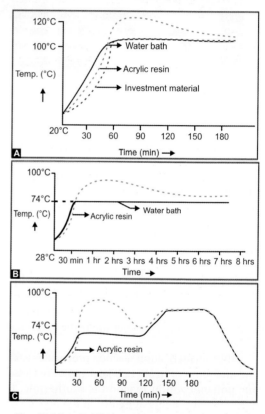

Figs 11.9A to C (A) Normal curing in boiling water; (B) Slow curing cycle; (C) Fast curing cycle

During this time, more than 95% of monomer is converted to polymer. In order to reduce the amount of residual monomer or to ensure the complete polymerization, the water in the bath can be boiled for about 1 hour. This technique enables a denture to be fabricated in a shorter time (Fig. 11.9C).

Bench Cooling

Following the completion of curing cycle, the denture flask should be cooled slowly to room temperature. During cooling process thermal shrinkage takes place due to the large COTE of acrylics. The magnitude of this shrinkage depends on the difference between the temperature at which the acrylic hardens and room temperature. Rapid cooling may result in warpage or distortion of the denture base because of differences in thermal contraction of acrylic resin and investing stone. Slow and even cooling of these materials minimizes potential difficulties. Hence, the flask should be removed from the water bath and bench cooled for 30 minutes. Subsequently, the flask should be immersed in cool tap water for 15 minutes.

Deflasking

After cooling completely, the flask is carefully opened and the denture is recovered by fracturing the plaster carefully. Otherwise, localized forces may fracture denture. The stone section is easily separated in one piece from the plaster, which is the cut away from the denture with knife.

Finishing and Polishing

The sticking plaster is removed and the thin excess projections are trimmed. It can be finished first with sand paper and then polished with pumice powder. Final glossy surface is obtained by polishing with French chalk using a cotton buff. The finished denture will have a smooth and shiny surface as shown in the Figure 11.10.

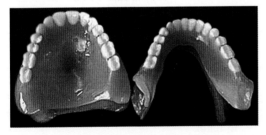

Fig. 11.10 Finished complete dentures

On completion of the finishing operation, the denture is stored in water to avoid drying and crazing until it is delivered to the patient.

Injection molding technique for the fabrication of complete dentures In addition to commonly employed compression molding technique, denture bases also may be fabricated via injection molding.

In this technique mold space is filled by injecting the resin under pressure before it hardens. To accomplish this, a specially designed flask is used.

One half of the flask is filled with freshly mixed dental stone, and the master cast is settled into the stone. The dental stone is contoured and permitted to set. Subsequently, sprues are attached to the wax denture base (Fig. 11.11A). The remaining portion of the flask is positioned and the investment process is completed. Wax elimination is performed and the flask is reassembled (Fig. 11.11B). Afterwards, the flask is placed into a carrier that maintains pressure on the assembly during resin introduction.

Acrylic resin is mixed and introduced into the mold via injection at room temperature. (The denture mold is connected to the injection cylinder by a sprue opening). The flask is placed into a water bath for polymerization of the denture base (Fig. 11.11C). As the material polymerizes, additional resin is introduced into the mold cavity, to compensate for the polymerization shrinkage. On completion the denture is recovered, adjusted, finished and polished.

In case of polystyrene resin, thermoplastic polymer is softened using heat and introduced into the mold while it is hot. Subsequently, the resin is permitted to cool and solidify. An advantage of this method is the reduced risk of monomer vapor inhalation.

Advantages
- Elimination of trial closures.
- Compensation for curing shrinkage.
- Control of pressure during polymerization, thus preserving the proper vertical dimensions.

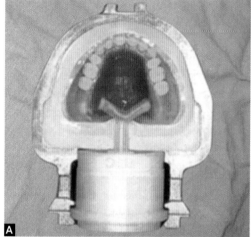

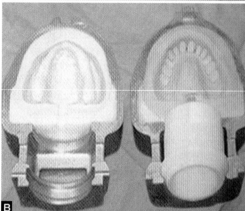

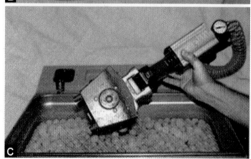

Figs 11.11A to C (A) Flasking (B) After dewaxing (C) Placing the flask in curing vessel

- Control of heat to minimize porosity in thick sections.

Drawbacks
- Inadequate spacing will lead to under filled molds.

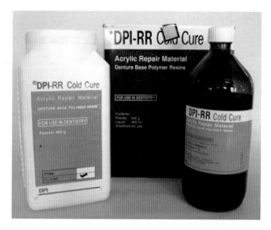

Figs 11.12 Self-cure acrylic resin

- Equipment cost.
- Injector is difficult to clean after dough has hardened.

CHEMICALLY ACTIVATED DENTURE BASE RESINS

The resin materials which polymerize without the application of heat or light are called chemically cured resins, i.e. polymerization reaction is initiated by a chemical (N, N– di methyl para toluidine) ingredient and the polymerization reaction completes at room temperature.

Dispension

These resins first used for dental purposes in Germany during World War-II and are known variously as self-cure or cold-cure or auto polymerizing resins. These are supplied as powder and liquid form (Fig. 11.12).

Composition

Powder

- Poly (Methyl methacrylate) or Copolymer beads.
- Benzoyl peroxide (maximum – 2.0%) – Initiator.
- Pigments
- Colored fibers (Nylon/acrylic) – added for esthetic effect.

Liquid

- Monomer – Methyl methacrylate.
- Ethyl glycol dimethacrylate – cross-linking agent.
- Hydroquinone – inhibitor.
- Dibutyl phthalate.
- Tertiary amine (Di Methyl Para Toluidine) – Activator (max. – 0.75%).

Setting Reaction

When polymer powder and monomer liquid are mixed together at room temperature, free radicals are produced from benzoyl peroxide by a reaction with dimethyl para toluidine which initiates the polymerization reaction. Chain reaction propagates with the liberation of heat until it is terminated. Except for the initiation stage other stages of polymerization are similar to heat cure acrylics.

The initiator is decomposed by incorporation of an activator in the form of a tertiary amine like N, N – dimethyl para toluidine.

The polymerization takes place at room temperature. The rate of polymerization is influenced by the particle size of the polymer, i.e. the smaller the particle, the more rapid is the polymerization.

Degree of polymerization is also less influenced by the type and concentration of both activator and initiator.

The reaction is exothermic and polymerization still results in a volumetric shrinkage, but the acrylic resin does not reach as high a peak temperature, since less external heat is added to the heat of polymerization.

Comparison between heat cure and self-cure is discussed in Table 11.4.

Properties

The polymerization of self-curing resins is never as complete as that of the heat curing type. 3–5% of self-curing resin is composed of free monomer. Free monomer may be released from the denture and irritate the oral tissues (potential irritant). Residual monomer will act as a plasticizer and make the resin weaker and more flexible (decreases transverse strength of the denture base).

The degree of polymerization achieved using chemically activated resin is not as complete as that achieved using heat activated systems. This indicates that there is a greater amount of unreacted monomer in the denture bases fabricated via chemical activation, hence inferior mechanical properties.

- Compressive strength – 65 MPa
- Tensile strength – < 60 MPa
- Impact strength – 0.78 J
- Surface hardness – 16–18 KHN
- Water sorption – 0.5–0.7 mg/cm^2
- Water solubility – 0.05 mg/cm^2

Chemically activated resins display slightly less shrinkage than their heat activated counterparts, because of a less complete polymerization. This imparts greater dimensional accuracy to chemically activated resins.

The color stability of chemically activated resins generally is inferior to the color stability of heat-activated resins. Tertiary amines present in the resin are susceptible to oxidation and accompanying color changes that may affect the appearance of the resin. Discoloration of these resins may be minimized via the addition of stabilizing agents that prevent such oxidation, called amine discoloration. Activators like organic acids produce products with improved color stability, but the compounds are not chemically stable.

The working time for chemically activated resin invariably is shorter than heat-cured materials. A lengthy initiation period is desirable, because this provides adequate time for trial closures. The initiation period can be prolonged by decreasing the temperature of the resin

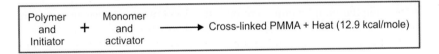

Table 11.4 Comparison between heat-cure and self-cure acrylic resins

Heat-cure	Self-cure
1. Method of curing Heat activated polymerization reaction starts only when heated up to 60°C.	Chemical or catalyst activated, starts soon after mixing.
2. Composition Monomer does not contain activator.	Contains activator (N,N – dimethyl para toluidine).
3. Residual monomer Less, i.e. 0.2–0.5%.	High, i.e. 3–5% (can cause irritation and act as plasticizer).
4. Degree of polymerization Higher, average molecular weight and hence better mechanical properties.	Lower, average molecular weight and hence inferior mechanical properties.
• Compressive strength: 75 MPa	• Compressive strength: 65 MPa
• Tensile strength: 60 MPa.	• Tensile strength: < 60 MPa.
• Impact strength: 0.98–1.27 J.	• Impact strength: 0.78 J.
• Surface hardness: 18–20 KHN.	• Surface hardness: 16–18 KHN.
5. Dough forming and working time Longer (only physical changes observed during mixing). 3 or 4 trial closures can be made.	Shorter due to simultaneous chemical and physical changes occurring in the mix. Only 1 or 2 trial closures can be made.
6. Color stability Good color stability	Not good due to subsequent oxidation of tertiary amine to form colored products.
7. Water sorption – 0.6 mg/cm^2 **Water solubility** – 0.02 mg/cm^2	0.7 mg/cm^2 0.05 mg/cm^2
8. Dimensional accuracy and stability Good but affected by thermal shrinkage, polymerization shrinkage, incorporation of processing stresses.	Greater dimensional accuracy due to less complete polymerization, thermal contraction, and hence better fit.
9. Internal porosity	
• Curing is to be done in water bath at temperature 70–80°C.	• Curing is to be done at room temperature under pressure.
• Peak temperature may rise about 120°C if curing is not done properly.	• Peak temperature may rise up to about 70°C (in thick regions due to the lack of conduction).
• Chances of getting porosity due to boiling monomer are more.	• Due to less peak temperature, chances of getting porosity due to boiling of monomer are less.
10. Uses Most widely used for fabricating complete, removable partial dentures, orthodontic appliances, to a limited extent for denture repair, relining, rebasing, etc.	To a limited extent for fabricating complete and removable partial dentures. Most widely used for preparing special trays, denture repair, relining, rebasing and removable orthodontic appliances. Can also be used as tooth colored restorative material.

mass by refrigerating the liquid component or mixing vessel prior to the mixing process. When the powder and liquid are mixed, the rate of polymerization process decreases. As a result, the resin mass remains in a dough-like stage for an extended period, and the working time is increased. Only one or two trial closures can be made.

Manipulation

Compression Molding Technique

The technique is similar to heat-cure acrylics, but after the final closure the dough is allowed to polymerize at room temperature rather than in a hot water bath. These materials start to polymerize as soon as the powder and liquid are mixed and proceed rapidly through the various consistency stages than the heat-cure acrylics.

The average time needed to reach the packing consistency is only 5 minutes. The increase in viscosity is a combination of physical and chemical changes occurring within mix. The denture mold is packed when the mix reaches the dough stage. Trial closures are made and the flash is removed. After final closure of the dental flask, pressure must be maintained throughout the polymerization process. Initial hardening of the resin generally occurs within 30 minutes of final flask closure. To ensure sufficient polymerization, the flask should be held under pressure for a minimum of 3 hours.

Advantages
- No porosity due to no boiling monomer is to be expected in the processing of a denture with the self-curing resins.
- Less thermal contraction, which results in better fit.
- Self-cure resins do not require hot water bath for curing since they can be cured at room temperature.

Disadvantages
- Low mechanical properties due to low degree of polymerization.
- Residual monomer content is more which can cause irritation to soft tissues.
- Color instability due to the oxidation of tertiary amines to form colored products.

Uses
- Quite oftenly used for fabricating complete dentures.
- For the construction of special trays.
- For denture repair, relining and rebasing.
- For removable orthodontic appliances.

Fluid Resin Technique (Pour Type Resins)

New innovations amongst chemically activated resins, these resins have powder particles that are much smaller, and when they are mixed with monomer the resulting mix is very fluid. A very fluid mix results from a much higher monomer-polymer ratio of about 1:2.5. They have low impact and fatigue strength, low transverse or bending strength, lower water sorption, higher solubility and higher residual monomer levels. Various steps involved in fluid resin technique have been given in Flow chart 11.2.

Advantages
- Simplification of the flasking, deflasking and finishing procedures.
- Elimination of trial closures.
- Smooth denture can be obtained.
- Shorter curing time (30–45 minutes).
- Agar may be reused.
- Reduced material costs.
- Decreased probability of damage to artificial teeth and denture bases during deflasking.
- Improved adaptation to underlying soft tissues.

Disadvantages
- Shifting of prosthetic teeth during processing.
- Air entrapment within the denture base material.
- Poor bonding between the denture base material and acrylic resin teeth.
- Dentures fabricated in this manner exhibit physical properties that are somewhat inferior to those of conventional heat-cured acrylic resins.

Polymerization by Microwaves

Poly (methyl methacrylate) resin also may be polymerized using microwave energy. This technique employs a specially formulated resin and a nonmetallic flask because metallic objects reflect microwaves. Fiber reinforced plastic flasks must be employed and the use of the desiccated gypsum for the mold is recommended to minimize water content and volume.

Flow chart 11.2 Various steps involved in fluid resin technique

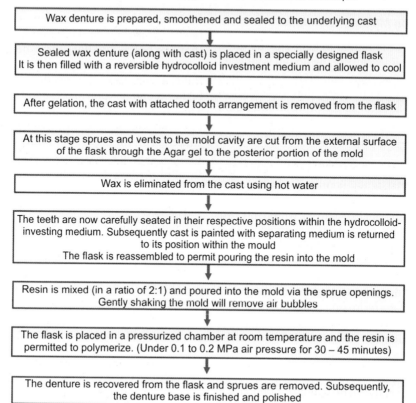

Wax denture is prepared, smoothened and sealed to the underlying cast

Sealed wax denture (along with cast) is placed in a specially designed flask. It is then filled with a reversible hydrocolloid investment medium and allowed to cool

After gelation, the cast with attached tooth arrangement is removed from the flask

At this stage sprues and vents to the mold cavity are cut from the external surface of the flask through the Agar gel to the posterior portion of the mold

Wax is eliminated from the cast using hot water

The teeth are now carefully seated in their respective positions within the hydrocolloid-investing medium. Subsequently cast is painted with separating medium is returned to its position within the mould. The flask is reassembled to permit pouring the resin into the mold

Resin is mixed (in a ratio of 2:1) and poured into the mold via the sprue openings. Gently shaking the mold will remove air bubbles

The flask is placed in a pressurized chamber at room temperature and the resin is permitted to polymerize. (Under 0.1 to 0.2 MPa air pressure for 30 – 45 minutes)

The denture is recovered from the flask and sprues are removed. Subsequently, the denture base is finished and polished

A conventional microwave oven used to supply the thermal energy (heat source) required for polymerization. This requires electromagnetically generated waves in the mega hertz frequency range. Typically, 2,450 MHz produces a wavelength of 120 nm. In this situation, methyl methacrylate molecules orient themselves in the direction of vibrating electromagnetic field, resulting in directional changes almost 5 billion times a second. Heat is rapidly generated within the monomer due to numerous intermolecular collisions.

As the degree of polymerization increases, the monomer content decreases proportionally, but the same quantity of energy is absorbed by less monomer as the reaction proceeds, thus increasing the activity of the remaining monomer. Theoretically, this could result in complete polymerization.

Advantages

- Short curing cycle (approximately 3 minutes).
- Have similar physical properties to conventional cures.
- Possess low residual monomer content and greater dimensional stability due to the excellent temperature control of the resin.

FABRICATION DEFECTS OF DENTURE

Rough/Irregular Surface

Various causes for rough/irregular surfaces in denture bases and their remedies to overcome surface irregularities were discussed in Table 11.5.

Internal Porosity

Various types of internal porosity and causes for those internal porosities in denture bases

Table 11.5 Causes and remedies for rough/irregular surface in denture bases

Causes	Remedies
Rough wax pattern.	Before flasking, it should be well-smoothened.
Improper wetting of wax pattern by plaster mix.	Should be polished with detergent to remove oily or greasy material.
Dry mix of plaster/stone – not all the plaster powder particles are wetted by water.	Use correct W/P ratio. • Dental stone: 30–40% • Dental plaster: 50–60%
Air bubbles trapped in the investing stone (may collect on the wax surface).	Should be removed by enough vibration.
Incomplete dewaxing (Residual wax prevents the reaction between separating medium and mould material).	Should be done thoroughly with boiling water so that there should not be any residual wax remaining on the mold surface.
Insufficient coating of separating medium. (Monomer diffuses into mold polymerizing there and producing rough surface)	Separating medium should be applied properly to the mold surface to get plaster free smooth surface. (Prevents diffusion of monomer into the mold).
Delayed packing (delayed evaporates).	Packing should be done when mix reaches full dough stage.
Lack of pressure and deficiency of material.	Excess material to be taken during trial closures and pressure should be applied and maintained until the curing completes.

and their remedies to overcome porosities were discussed in Table 11.6.

Dimensional Accuracy and Stability

Dimensional stability of the denture during processing and in service is important in the fit of the denture and the satisfaction of the patient. In general, if the denture is properly processed, the original fit and the dimensional stability of the various denture base plastics are good.

Changes in dimensions result from several conditions including coefficient of thermal expansion, polymerization shrinkage, and water sorption.

Greater the linear shrinkage, the greater is the discrepancy usually observed in the initial fit of the denture. Various causes for dimensional accuracy in denture bases and their remedies to maintain accurate dimensions were discussed in Table 11.7.

Water Sorption

When denture is put in water, due to the polar water of polymers water can enter and gradually get diffused inside which push the polymer chains resulting expansion of about 0.2%. The diffusion rate is higher at higher temperatures. For each 1% increase in the weight of the water absorbed, the acrylic resin expands linearly 0.23%.

This change in dimension with water absorption is important in the storage of dentures. Intermittent diffusion of water into and out of the denture base could release some of the internal stresses resulting permanent warpage. Once the denture has been processed, it is recommended that it is stored in water and not be allowed to dry out.

According to ADA specification number 12, water sorption of denture base materials should not be more than 0.8 mg/cm^2. Practically, the water sorption of heat-cure acrylic is 0.6 mg/cm^2 and for self-cure acrylic is around 0.5–0.7 mg/cm^2.

Water sorption can be determined by storing a dried plastic disk in distilled water at 37°C for 7 days and after which the increase in water is determined. (Dimensions of plastic disk are 50 mm in diameter and 0.5 mm in thick).

Table 11.6 Types of internal porosity, their causes and remedies

Type	Causes	Remedies
Shrinkage/under packing/contraction porosity:		
• Arises as a result of the reduction in volume of the dough which takes place on polymerization. • Appears as irregular voids throughout and on the surface of the denture. (Distributed uniformly throughout the material) • This type of porosity causes the resin to appear white. A pigmented resin may appear lighter in color for reason.	a. Inadequate pressure during polymerization b. Insufficient material in the mold during polymerization.	• Sufficient pressure must be applied during trial and final closures and the pressure should be maintained until the completion of curing. • Excess material is to be taken during trial closures so that the mold contains definite amount of material at the time of final closure and during polymerization.
Irregular voids		
• It is possible that some regions of the resin mass will contain more monomer than others. During polymerization these regions shrink more than adjacent regions and the liberated shrinkage tends to produce irregular voids.	a. Lack of homogeneity in the dough at the time of polymerization. b. Inadequate (in homogeneous) mixing of polymer powder and monomer liquid. Monomer rich areas undergo greater shrinkage during polymerization) c. Premature packing.	Can be eliminated by ensuring the greatest possible homogeneity of the resin. Bench curing provides time for more uniform dispersion of monomer throughout the mass of dough. During this monomer diffuses uniformly forming homogeneous dough. Use proper polymer-monomer ratio (2.5:1 parts by weight, and 3:1 by volume). Follow the well-controlled mixing procedure. The mix at the dough stage is more homogeneous than at the earlier stringy stage.
Gaseous or boiling monomer porosity		
Too rapid rate of heating and exothermic polymerization reaction. • Porosity occurs away from the source of heat or will not present at the surface of denture. • At the center of thick portion of denture where heat cannot be conducted away with sufficient rapidity.	Results from the vaporization of unreacted monomer and low molecular weight polymers, when the temperature of the resin reaches or crosses the boiling point of the monomer. a. Thicker sections of the denture base generate more exothermic heat than the thinner areas. b. Lack of conduction of heat.	Curing procedure should be well-controlled to avoid the effects of uncontrolled temperature rise such as boiling of monomer and denture base porosity. **Slow curing:** Processing the denture base resin at 74°C for 8 hours or longer with no boiling treatment. **Fast curing:** Processing the denture base resin at 74°C for 1½ hours to 2 hours and then rise the temperature of water bath to 100°C and processing for 1 hour or more.
Subsurface porosity		
• Can be seen in the center of a thick portion when heat cannot be conducted away with sufficient rapidity. • Temperature is likely to cross the boiling point of the monomer and as a result spherical voids are formed (below the surface) well inside the bulky portion of the denture.	Due to the partial conduction of heat from inside to outside. **Upper denture:** Running around the sloping sides of the palate. **Lower denture:** Thick lingual posterior area.	Proper curing cycle should be followed, i.e. slow curing/fast curing.
Air bubbles		
With fluid resins. If the air inclusions are not removed, voids may be produced in the resultant denture bases.	Caused by air inclusions during mixing and pouring procedures.	Careful mixing, spruing, and venting seem to help reduce the incidence of air inclusions.

Table 11.7 Causes and remedies for dimensional inaccuracy of denture bases

Causes	Remedies

Curing/polymerization shrinkage: When methyl methacrylate is polymerized the density changes from 0.945 to 1.19 g/cc. This change in density results in a volumetric shrinkage of 21% usually called polymerization shrinkage.
• Linear shrinkage: 2%.Curing shrinkage is large at the bulkiest portion. This causes slight decrease in curvature of palatal region.
	Can be minimized by–
	• Adding prepolymerized poly (methyl methacrylate) powder to methyl methacrylate monomer (2.5:1 by weight, 3:1 by volume). This ratio reduces the volumetric shrinkage of the dough during polymerization to about 3%.
	• Thermal expansion (81 ppm) of acrylic on heating is probably the main factor, which compensates for the polymerization shrinkage.
	• Inhibited to a large extent by friction within mold walls.
	• By the control of processing procedures such as–
	  a. Pressure on the dough during polymerization.
	  b. Flow of the resultant polymer at the curing temperature.

Thermal contraction or thermal shrinkage It is of about 0.4–0.5% occurs when fabricated denture cools from 80°C to 37°C due to large COTE (81 ppm) Linear shrinkage: 0.44%. The magnitude of the thermal shrinkage will depend on the difference between the temperature at which acrylic hardens and the room temperature. Total shrinkage: 2 + 0.44 = 2.44%	May be reduced to some extent by– • Curing the denture at low temperature as is reasonable. • Slow cooling which permits relief of these internal stresses by plastic deformation. • Inhibited by mold walls.

Processing (Internal) Stresses

Stresses are present within a polymer when the macromolecules are subjected to forces other than those of simple molecular attraction. In a stressed material, the molecular chains are uncomfortably arranged in relation to each other. Some degree of stress is always present in acrylic dentures. Whenever a natural dimensional change is inhibited, the affected material contains stresses. It may arise from several causes such as polymerization and thermal shrinkage, improper mixing and handling of the resin. The stresses present in the denture are related to its shape and size, the pressure applied during curing, the curing cycle used and the rate of cooling after processing. The stresses remaining with-in the denture are released at a later stage with a consequent warpage of the denture. Various causes for internal stresses in denture bases and their remedies to overcome them were discussed in Table 11.8.

Crazing

Crazing is the formation of very fine microcracks or flaws on the surface of a denture as shown in Figure 11.13. These cracks gradually become bigger and bigger (increase in depth, width and length) and can be seen under a microscope. Later the surface becomes hazy or foggy appearance (transparent resin) and finally it results in fracture.

Crazing is mainly due to the relaxation of internal stresses. Crazing may result from stress application or partial dissolution of a resin. It is believed that crazing is produced by mechanical separation of individual polymer chains on application of tensile stresses.

Site

Crazing generally begins at the surface of a resin and is oriented at right angles to tensile forces. Microcracks formed in this manner subsequently progress internally.

Table 11.8 Causes and remedies for processing stresses occur in denture bases

Causes	Remedies
Stresses due to differences in the COTE between porcelain teeth and acrylic denture base (1:10) (During the cooling process that follows polymerization, denture resin shrinks more than dental porcelain. As a result, axial/tangential tensile stresses are generated within the resin).	• Slow cooling to be followed after curing. • Use acrylic teeth for acrylic denture base.
Mechanical (tensile) stresses on repeated wetting and drying of the dentures causing alternate contraction and expansion.	Should be stored in water when not in use or service.
Crazing due to solvent action when a denture is being repaired some monomers come in contact with the resin and may cause crazing. Solvents reduce the molecular attraction between polymer chains and permit stress relief.	Development of improved acrylic resin teeth and cross-linked denture base resins have resulted in a decreased incidence of denture base crazing.
During polishing – If excessive heat is generated during polishing which can cause polymerization and produce sufficient surface, stresses in the denture cause crazing.	A wet polishing wheel and slurry of pumice and water should be used to avoid excessive local temperatures.
Minute cracks result from stresses produced by evaporation of water within the mold during curing.	Mold surface should be lined with a thin layer of separating medium to prevent the diffusion of water from the mold into the packed acrylic dough.
Dissimilar COTE and contraction of dental stone (investing medium) and acrylic denture base and plastic teeth. The stone with a different thermal coefficient creates residual stresses in the acrylic as it cools. These stresses may be released after the processed denture is deflasked and deformation or crazing (numerous small cracks) may result (sudden cooling).	Slow even cooling of these materials minimizes the effects of crazing.

Effects

Crazing has a weakening effect on a denture.
1. It reduces the strength (which can cause fracture).
2. Esthetic qualities of denture will be decreased.
3. Collects food debris and becomes unhygienic.

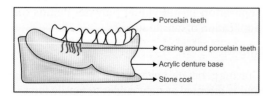

Fig. 11.13 Crazing in complete dentures

Fracture

1. Inadequate curing time—results in lowered strength and rigidity.
2. Excess grinding/polishing—heat may cause degradation of the resin. Molecules/depolymerization of poly (methyl methacrylate).
3. Chemically cured denture resins—undergo lesser degree of polymerization than do heat-cured types, and have lower strength values.
4. On impact forces—if dropped on hard surface.
5. Due to fatigue—from repeated bending of the denture in service.

Discoloration

Self-cure acrylic resins have a tendency to be less color stable than the heat-cured resins. Color stability is related to oxidation of the chemical activator (amine) left in the resin.

MODIFIED ACRYLICS

Rubber Reinforced Acrylics/High Impact Strength Materials

The impact strength of acrylic resins can be significantly improved by the incorporation of elastomers/rubbers. The elastomer is able to absorb energy on impact and thus protects the acrylic from fracture.

These materials are butadiene-styrene rubber reinforced poly (methyl methacrylate). The rubber particles are grafted to methyl methacrylate so that they will bond well to the heat polymerized matrix. These materials are supplied in a powder and liquid form and are processed in the same way as heat-cured methyl methacrylate materials.

These materials are practically useful for patients who have a history of breaking dentures during cleaning as a result of careless handling.

Advantages

- Better impact (2.1 J) and fatigue properties.
- Greater resistance to crack propagation.
- Small decrease in water sorption as a result of the incorporation of rubber.

Disadvantages

- Expensive.

Vinyl Acrylics

These materials supplied as powder and liquid.
- **Powder:** Vinyl and acrylic monomers are copolymerized resulting in a powder.
- **Liquid:** Methyl methacrylate monomer.

Advantages

- Impact strength for the polyvinyl acrylics is about twice that of poly (methyl methacrylate). (Better resistance to fracture when they sustain a sudden blow).
- Slightly stiffer than acrylic.

Hydrophilic Poly (Acrylates)

Poly (hydroxy ethyl methacrylate) has been used as a denture base material and a soft denture liner. Hydroxy substituted acrylics increase the water sorption and wettability of the copolymers by saliva, which enhances the denture retention.

Rapid Heat Polymerized Acrylics/Hybrid Acrylics

The hybrid acrylics can be polymerized in boiling water immediately after being packed into a denture flask. After being placed into the boiling water, the water is brought back to a full boil for 20 minutes. After the usual bench cooling to room temperature, the denture is deflasked, trimmed and polished in the conventional manner.

The initiator is formulated from both chemical and heat activated initiators to allow rapid polymerization without the porosity that one might expect.

Fiber Reinforced Acrylic

For example, Carbon fibers, ultra high modulus polyethylene, Kevlar (poly-P-phenylene terephthalamide), etc.
- They stiffen the denture base, reducing the possibility of fatigue fracture.
- Increases the flexural strength.

Disadvantages

- Must be placed in the part of the denture, which is under a tensile stress (positioning is critical).
- Bonding between the fibers and acrylic resin may be difficult to achieve (if no bonding is present—fibers weaken the denture).
- Difficult to construct dentures.
- Appearance of the denture is adversely affected because the carbon fibers are black.

Light Activated Denture Base Resins

Dispensing

Single component system, supplied in sheet and rope forms (having a clay-like consistency) packed in light proof pouches to prevent accidental polymerization.

Composition

Consists of urethane dimethacrylate matrix, microfine silica, high molecular weight acrylic resin monomers, and acrylic resin beads as organic filler, camphorquinone, and visible light initiator (camphorquinone).

Processing

Light activated resins cannot be flasked or invested in a conventional manner as it prevents passage of light (Fig. 11.14). Instead, teeth are arranged and the denture base is molded on an accurate cast. Subsequently, the denture is polymerized in a light chamber (curing unit) with blue light of 400–500 nm. The denture is rotated on a table in the chamber to provide uniform exposure to the light source. After polymerization, the denture is removed from

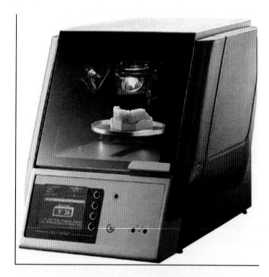

Fig. 11.14 Light curing chamber for light activated resins

the cast, finished and polished in a conventional manner.

Radiopaque Denture Base Resins

Acrylic resin is radiolucent. Several experimental approaches have been tried to solve this problem.

Examples for radiopaque additive–
  i. Metal/powdered metals—may weaken base and appearance is poor.
 ii. Inorganic salts such as $BaSO_4$ –
      • Low concentration—insufficient radiopacity.
      • High concentration—weaken the base.
iii. Comonomers containing heavy metals—polymers have poor mechanical properties, e.g. Barium acrylate
 iv. Halogen containing comonomers or additives, e.g. Tri- bromo phenyl methacrylate.
      • Additives may act as plasticizers.
      • Comonomers are expensive.

DENTURE REPAIR RESINS

The repair materials are usually acrylic resins of the powder-liquid type, similar to those used for denture bases. It may be light activated, heat activated or chemically activated. The material of choice will depend on the following factors:
1. Length of time required for making the repair.
2. Transverse strength obtainable with the repair of the materials.
3. Degree to which dimensional accuracy is maintained during repair.

Method

• The parts of broken denture are held together with sticky wax or wires.
• A stone cast is constructed in the denture base.
• The denture is removed from the cast, the wax is eliminated and the fractured joints are trimmed and smoothened to provide bulk for the repair resin.
• The cast is coated with a separating medium to facilitate subsequent removal of the

repaired denture and the denture parts are replaced (reassembled) on it.

- The fractured surfaces are first wetted with monomer using a brush. Increments of powder and monomer then added immediately (fluid consistency). It is then allowed to cure in a pressure chamber. The processed repair is finished by conventional procedures.

If a heat-cured acrylic resin is used, the denture should be completely flasked and curing should be carried out at temperatures not greater than 74° C for 8 hours or longer. This procedure minimizes the dimensional change of the denture base after deflasking.

Precautions

- The denture surfaces that are not directly involved in the repaired area should not be coated with monomer to prevent crazing.
- Joints with sharp angles should be avoided (V-shaped edges) to prevent concentration of stress.

Merits and Demerits of Denture Repair Resins

Merits	Demerits
Self-cured acrylic resins	
• Dimensional accuracy is not maintained because enough heat is present or liberated during polymerization to cause distortion from the release of stresses. • Flasking is not required. • Procedure is rapid and may be done while the patient waits.	• Lower transverse strength in the repaired area.
Heat-cured acrylic repair resins	
• Better transverse strength (80% of that of the original plastic).	• Longer curing time. • Curing temperature must be properly controlled. • Flask is required. • Tendency to distort curing processing.

Denture Rebasing and Relining

Dentures sometimes require adjustment of their fitting surfaces to accommodate changes in the contour of soft tissues. Due to partial resorption of underlying bone structure the denture may gradually lose retention. If the vertical dimension and occlusion of the denture have not been greatly altered, the retention may be regained by rebasing or relining.

Rebasing

Rebasing involves replacement of entire denture base. It is a process of refitting a denture by the replacement of the denture base without changing the occlusal relationships of the teeth.

Method

- An accurate impression of the soft tissues is obtained using the existing denture as custom tray.
- A stone cast is fabricated in the impression.
- Cast and denture are mounted in a specially designed device, reline jig, which will maintain the correct vertical and horizontal relationship between the cast and denture teeth.
- The teeth are set into plaster platform on the lower member. This platform will act as a reference into which the teeth may be placed and in which they will maintain their retention to the cast.
- After the teeth are thus indented for position, the denture is removed and the teeth are separated from the old denture base.
- The teeth are then assembled in the indent of the mounting device and held in their original relationship to the cast while they are waxed to the new base plate.
- A new denture is constructed using the same teeth as before.

Relining

Relining involves replacement of tissue surface of an existing denture. It refers to the process of adding base material to the tissue surface of the denture in a quantity to fill the space which exists between the original dental contour and altered tissue contour.

Classification

a. *Hard reline materials:* To improve the fitting surface of the denture.
b. *Soft lining materials:* Some patients are unable to tolerate a hard denture base and must be provided with a permanent soft cushion on the fitting surface of the denture.
c. *Tissue conditioners:* To act as a cushion, which will enable traumatized soft tissues to recover before recording an impression for a new denture.

Hard Reline Materials

These are used to improve the fitting surface of the denture (to ensure proper fit and function).

Method

• An impression of the soft tissues is obtained using the existing denture as an impression tray.
• A stone cast is constructed in the corrected denture.
• Cast with the attached denture is invested in a denture flask.
• After waiting for about 20 minutes the flask is opened and the impression material is removed from the denture. The tissue surface is cleaned to enhance bonding between the existing resin and the reline material.
• Then, an appropriate resin is introduced into the space left by the impression material and shaped using a compression molding technique. It is now allowed to polymerize.
• The denture is subsequently recovered, finished and polished.

Materials

1. *Self-cure acrylic resins*
   • A specialized mounting assembly, a reline jig, may be used instead of flasking.
   • Can be caused directly in the mouth.
   • Preferred because of low polymerization temperature which minimizes the distortion of the remaining denture base.

Drawbacks

• Many of these materials generate sufficient heat to injure oral tissue.
• Monomer can be leached out of the resin to irritate soft tissues. Direct reline materials should be considered as only a temporary measure.

2. *Heat-cure acrylic resins:* These materials are not widely used because significant heat may be generated and distortion of the existing denture base is more likely.

Conclusion: From the standpoint of denture stability, the rebasing process is preferred to the relining technique. (There is a tendency for it to distort or warp toward the relined side because of the diffusion of the monomer from the reliner before curing).

Soft Lining Materials/Resilient Liners

Resilient liners are the soft cushions like liners given to the denture base to absorb some of the energy produced by masticatory impact and to distribute the forces of mastication more evenly. They do not reduce the transmitted force but result in a smaller displacement of the oral mucosa.

The stiffness of the soft lining material is less than that of the oral mucosa and will absorb more of the energy and deform more. As the liner returns to its predeformed shape the absorbed energy is more slowly released. Hence a soft liner serves as a shock absorber between the occlusal surfaces of a denture and the underlying oral tissues. Such liners will protect the affected soft tissues from impact energies of mastication. Various soft lining materials were discussed in Table 11.9.

Indications

These materials are suggested for use:
• Patients who cannot tolerate a hard denture base. This problem generally arises if the patient has an irregular mandibular ridge covered by a thin and relatively low residual mucosa. In such cases soft lining on the denture will help to relieve the pain and increase patient acceptance of the denture.

Table 11.9 Soft lining materials

Material	Comments
1. Natural rubber (Cis 1, 4-polyisoprene cross-linked with sulfur).	• High water uptake caused distortion. • Very short intraoral life.
2. Vinyl resins plasticized poly (vinyl chloride) polyvinyl acrylate	• Plasticizers may leach out and harden the denture. • Not widely used.
3. Plasticized heat cure acrylic (P/L form) **Powder:** Acrylic resin polymer and copolymer (butyl methacrylate), initiator (Benzoyl peroxide), **Liquid:** Acrylic monomer and plasticizers (Di butyl phthalate).	• Plasticizers are not bound within the mass and therefore may be leached out of soft liners. As this occurs, soft liners become progressively more rigid. • Adhere well to the denture base. • May be considered as long-term soft liners.
4. Self-curing (room temperature curing) acrylics – polymerized by peroxideamine system.	• Curing can result in a high level of free monomer remaining in the materials. • The presence of free monomer can result in inferior mechanical properties and reduced biocompatibility.
5. Plasticized self-cure acrylics. **Powder:** PMMA + PEMA (Fig. 11.15). **Liquid:** 60–80% of plasticizer and ethylene glycol. Do not contain acrylic monomers.	• These liners are considered as short-term liners or tissue conditioners. • The distribution of larger plasticizer minimizes entanglement of polymer chains and they're by permits individual chains to slip past one another. This slipping motion permits rapid changes in the shape of the soft liner and provides a cushioning effect for the underlying tissues.
6. Hydrophilic acrylic monomers. Supplied as a gel or powder and monomer of hydroxy ethyl methacrylate (HEMA).	• Hard, brittle and becomes soft when exposed to saliva. • Dimensional instability due to rapid loss or gain of water.
7. Room temperature silicone rubber materials (two component system). **Base:** Hydroxyl terminated poly (dimethyl siloxane) + filler. **Reactor:** Tetra ethyl ortho silicate + Tin octate.	• Retain elastic properties for prolonged periods. • Lack of bonding to the PMMA denture base. • Support the growth of *Candida albicans*. • Adversely affected by denture cleansers.
8. Heat activated silicones (one component system)– Supplied as paste or gel. Poly (dimethyl siloxane) polymer with pendant or terminal vinyl groups + inert filler + peroxide initiator. *Adhesive:* Silicone polymer in a solvent	• High modulus of resilience and permanent resilience. • More resistant to aqueous environment (not affected by constituents of food and drinks). • Adequate bond strength to acrylic. • Provide good environment for the growth of the *Candida albicans*. • These adhesives serve as chemical intermediates that bond to both soft liners and denture resins.
9. Polyurethane and polyphosphazine.	

- Patients with irritation of denture bearing mucosa.
- Areas of severe undercuts or congenital or acquired defects of the palate.

Ideal Properties

- Biocompatibility – Should be nontoxic, nonirritant to the soft tissues.

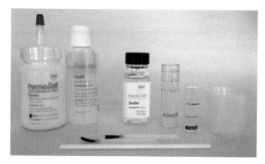

Fig. 11.15 Soft-lining materials

- Should not support the growth of harmful bacteria or fungus.
  Candida albicans – This is common yeast responsible for causing denture stomatitis, a common occurrence in denture wearers.
- Should be soft enough for the comfort of the patient (plasticizers should not be leached out of the material).
- Should be permanently resilient in order to give cushioning effect (high modulus of resilience) and prevent unacceptable distortion during service.
- Should adhere to the denture base and remain so in the mouth.
- Should have low water uptake—a similar level to that of the denture base is ideal (2–3%). A high uptake will cause distortion and may result in fouling of the lining due to ingress of bacteria.
- Should be wetted by saliva—a thin film of saliva is necessary for the retention of the denture and to act as a lubricant to prevent irritation of the mucosa.
- Should have sufficient mechanical properties—enough to withstand normal handling, brushing, etc.
- Should be easy to clean—not adversely affected by denture cleansers, not stained easy, etc.
- Should have good shelf-life.

Failures or problems with the use of soft lining materials

1. Inadequate bonding to the denture base, especially self-cure silicone rubbers.
2. Significant volume changes with the gain and loss of water–silicone liners and hydrophilic acrylics.
3. Hardening of liners due to the leaching of plasticizers from these materials. Hardening rates for these liners are associated with initial plasticizer content. As the plasticizer content increased, the probability for leaching also is increased. Hence, materials displaying high initial plasticizer content tend to harden rather rapidly.
4. Decrease in the denture base strength due to reduction in base thickness, solvent action of the silicone adhesive and the soft acrylic monomer (may cause partial dissolution of the accompanying denture base). The resultant decrease in base strength may result in fracture during clinical service.
5. Some lining split under stress/pull away from the denture base.
6. Difficult in trimming, adjusting and polishing of soft liners (specially for silicone surface due to its abrasive character).
7. Difficulty in cleaning—both oxygenating and hypochlorite type of denture cleansers will damage soft liners specially for silicone types.
8. Support the growth of the fungus, e.g.: *Candida albicans* specially for silicone rubbers—debris collected in the pores help myotic growth.
9. Disagreeable taste and odor.
10. There may be a change of color due to staining and deposits of calculus.

Tissue Conditioners

Tissue conditioners are soft liners used to treat an irritated mucosa supporting a denture.

Tissue conditioning materials are soft, resilient temporary relining materials which by reducing and evenly distributing stresses on the mucosa of the denture bearing area, have a rehabilitating effect on unhealthy tissue and allow affected tissues to return to normal status of health.

Relining the ill-fitting denture with a tissue conditioner allows the tissues to return to normal at which a new denture can be made.

Requirements

- Should have no irritant or toxic effect.
- Should massage the underlying tissue and stimulate blood circulation.
- Should be resilient in order that masticatory loads are absorbed without causing permanent deformation of the lining.
- Should be remaining soft during use in order to maintain a good cushioning effect on the underlying soft tissues.
- Must undergo viscous flow under load so that they change their form with the changing contours of the soft tissue, which allows good adaptation to the irritated denture bearing mucosa.

Materials

These materials are dispensed in the form of powder and liquid.
- *Powder:* Acrylic polymer/Copolymer.
- *Liquid:* Mixture of ethyl glycol + an aromatic ester (butyl glycolate or Dibutyl phthalate)

Manipulation

Both the powder and liquid are mixed, placed in the denture and seated in the patient's mouth. The ethanol swells the polymer beads and allows penetration by the ester plasticizer. As a result a gel is formed by polymer chain entanglement, the gel being essentially a solution of the polymer in the plasticizer. The resulting gel is viscoelastic in that it responds elastically to the rapid dynamic loading associated with mastication but will flow under constant loads.

These materials will conform to the anatomy of the residual ridge, gel in that position and continue to flow after application to fill the space between the denture base and the oral tissues. Thus they change their form with the changing contour of the supporting tissue, so that good adaptation of the denture to the tissue is maintained. In the mouth, first the ethanol and then the plasticizer is lost, resulting in hardening of the material. It is necessary that it should be replaced every 2–3 days during the treatment period. Repeated application of the material is therefore necessary to allow complete tissue recovery.

Special Uses

1. It is also useful after surgical removal of excess soft tissue over the denture bearing mucosa–the healthy areas should be covered by a layer of soft material, which reduces the stress on it.
2. Functional impression material – One that is applied to the fitting surface of a denture in order to secure an impression under functional stresses.

Problems of Leached Plasticizers

1. Can cause further irritation of traumatized tissues, specially in the high ethanol content materials.
2. Can also cause problems by plasticizing adjacent denture base materials. This will reduce rigidity and make the denture more prone to fracture.

Factors Affecting Gelation Rate of Tissue Conditioner

1. Molecular weight and particle size of polymer powder.
2. Amount of ethanol.
3. Type of plasticizer present.
4. Powder and liquid ratio.

Denture Cleansers

These are the agents used by the patients for cleaning artificial dentures. These include dentifrices, denture cleansers, soap and water, salt and soda, household cleansers, bleaches and vinegar. Various denture cleansing materials are discussed in Table 11.10.

Method

Either daily or overnight immersion in the agent or more generally brushing of the denture with the cleanser.

Table 11.10 Denture cleansers

Material	Ingredient	Drawbacks
Oxygenating cleansers For example, Alkyl perborate, which is available in the form of powder. This powder can dissolve in water. Perborate decomposes to form an alkaline peroxide solution. This decomposes again to liberate O_2 to clean the debris.	Alkaline perborate or peroxide, e.g. Sodium perborate. ($NaBO_2.\ H_2O_2.\ 3H_2O$)	• Do not easily remove hard deposits. • May be harmful to soft lining materials.
Hypochlorite solutions (alkaline hypochlorite)	Dilute sodium hypochlorite	• Can corrode stainless steel and Co – Cr alloys. • May leave an odor on the dentures (only for plastic dentures).
Dilute mineral acids	HCl or H_3PO_4	May corrode some alloys.
Denture cleansing powders (abrasive powder)	Abrasive agents ($CaCO_3$)	Can abrade denture base polymers and plastic teeth
Denture cleansing paste	Abrasive agents or acids	• Can abrade polymeric material. • It is difficult to remove paste completely from the denture.

Requirements

- Should be nontoxic, easy to remove and leaving no traces of irritant material.
- Should not be harmful to eyes, skin or clothing if accidentally splashed/spilled.
- Should be preferably bactericidal/fungicidal.
- Should attack/dissolve both the organic and inorganic portions of denture deposits.
  Soft deposits – These are removed by light brushing followed by rinsing.
  Hard deposits – These are more difficult to clean.
- Should be harmless all materials used in the construction of dentures, including denture base polymers, and alloys, acrylic and porcelain teeth, and resilient lining materials.
- Should have good shelf-life.

Precautions

- Household cleansers should not be used because these cleansers produce abrasion and leave a very rough surface. Their prolonged use can lead to deterioration of the fit and the esthetics of the appliance.

- Brushing with hard, stiff brushes should be avoided because these bristles produce scratches on the surface of the denture.
  The light brushing of a denture surface is an effective means of improving denture cleanliness.

Maxillofacial Materials

These are the materials used to correct facial defects (head and neck) resulting from cancer surgery, trauma, or developmental deformities. The replacement of a lost ear, nose, eye, other part of the head and neck requires the construction of a maxillofacial appliance, which allows the patients to lead a normal life. Various maxillofacial materials were discussed in Table 11.11.

Requirements

- Should not irritate the tissues with which it comes in contact and not produce any allergic reactions.
- Should be soft, pliable and capable of adapting to facial movements.

Table 11.11 Maxillofacial materials

Material	Merits	Demerits
Latexes	• Soft. • Inexpensive. • Easy to manipulate. • Forms life-like prosthesis.	• Finished products are weak. • Degenerates with age. • Color instability.
Synthetic latexes (Tri polymer of butyl acrylate, MMA, Methyl acrylamide).	More natural appearance.	Durability is not good.
Plasticized PVC PVC + Plasticizer + Cross-linking agent + UV stabilizers for color stability + color pigments.	Natural appearance.	Become hard with age due to leaching of plasticizers, UV stabilizers have an adverse effect. Requires complicated equipments.
Poly (methyl methacrylate)	Natural appearance when pigmented.	• Hard and heavy. • Does not move when the face moves. • Does not have the feel of skin.
Polyurethane Addition of di iso cyanate + polyol in the presence of initiator.	Life-like feel and appearance.	• Di isocyanates are toxic. • Susceptible to deterioration.
Room temperature vulcanizing silicones Hydroxyl terminated poly (dimethyl siloxane) + tetra ethyl ortho silicate fused silica + stannous octate.	Can be easily fabricated with simple equipment.	These are not stronger.
Heat vulcanized silicones	• Good strength. • Color stability.	Fabrication is very tedious.

- Should be light in weight so that it may be supported without fear of detachment during use.
- Should be skin like in appearance, soft to touch with such desirable qualities as translucence, skin color and texture.
- Should have ability to incorporate different color pigments to match skin color.
- Should be color stable as the finished prosthesis is subjected to sunlight, UV light, heat and cold.
- Should be resilient and have high resistance to tearing since edges of appliances are generally thin.
- Should not become hard or rigid during use by leaching of certain plasticizers.
- Should be easy to manipulate and require no complicated equipment.
- Should be easy to clean and manage by the patient, good shelf-life, less expensive, easily available, etc.

Method

An impression of the affected part is taken using elastic impression material. A stone cast is then fabricated. The artificial part is then carved in wax on the master cast. It is then invested and dewaxed. The mold is now ready to make the prosthesis.

Suitable color pigments are added to the matrix. At this stage patient should be present, so that pigments may be added to the material to give it a life like appearance and match the patient skin color. When color matching is achieved, the material is compression molded and processed. It is then finished in the conventional manner.

ARTIFICIAL TEETH

There are two types of teeth commonly used:
1. Acrylic or plastic teeth.
2. Porcelain teeth.

Acrylic Teeth or Plastic Teeth

Plastic teeth are made from acrylic and modified acrylic materials (Fig. 11.16). Different tooth colored pigments are used to produce the various tooth shades and a cross-linking agent is added to make it more resistant to crazing. They are produced in different shapes and sizes by either using compression molding or injection molding technique.

Requirements

- Good appearance: Should ideally be indistinguishable from natural teeth in shape, color and translucency. Good matching often requires that the shade and translucency of

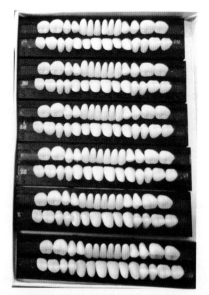

Fig. 11.16 Artificial acrylic teeth

the artificial teeth should vary from the tip of the crown to the gingival area.
- Should be a good attachment between the artificial teeth and the denture base.
    Small holes or metal pins are incorporated in the base of the porcelain teeth during their production to give mechanical retention to the denture base.
- Artificial teeth to be of low density in order that they do not increase the weight of the denture.
- Should be strong and tough in order to resist fracture.
- Should be hard enough to resist abrasive forces in the mouth and during cleaning, but should allow grinding with a dental bur, so that adjustments to the occlusion can be made by the dentist at the chair side.

Neither plastic nor porcelain is an ideal material for the fabrication of artificial teeth. The choice between plastic and porcelain teeth will depend on the application.

Precautions

- Acrylic teeth should not be flamed during the smoothening of the wax denture pattern because the resin teeth surfaces may be melted or burned. The resultant surface stresses induced during cooling may contribute to crazing in service.
- Acrylic teeth surfaces should not be coated with separating medium as it prevents chemical bonding between denture base and acrylic teeth.

Comparison of acrylic teeth with porcelain teeth have been discussed in Table 11.12.

RESIN IMPRESSION TRAYS AND TRAY MATERIALS

Resin impression trays are fabricated to fit specific arches. As a result, resin impression trays often are called custom trays.

Steps

- A preliminary impression is made using a stock tray with an appropriate impression material.

Table 11.12 Comparison of acrylic teeth with porcelain teeth

Acrylic teeth	Porcelain teeth
Biocompatible, insoluble in oral fluids, not have much resistance to organic solvents such as ketones and aromatic hydrocarbons which will attack noncross-linked plastic teeth.	Biocompatible, insoluble in oral fluids and more resistance to organic solvents.
Retention to the denture base is by chemical bonding if proper manipulation is observed.	Mechanical bonding by pins or under-cut holes.
Mechanical properties Not as brittle. Compressive strength: 75 MPa. Tensile strength: 60 MPa. Shear strength: 122 MPa. Modulus of elasticity: 2500 MPa. Density: 1.19 g/cc Proportional limit: 27 MPa. Poor abrasion resistance. Surface hardness: 18 KHN. Minimum abrasion of opposing dentition. Higher fracture toughness (soft but tough).	Brittle 330 MPa. 25 MPa. 111 MPa. 80,000 MPa. 2.35 g/cc. 250 Mpa. More resistant to abrasion. Surface hardness: 460 KHN. Abrades opposing natural teeth and gold surfaces. Low fracture toughness (hard and brittle).
Exhibit permanent deformation or cold flow under stresses below their elastic limit and their elastic limit and their dimension may be altered during use. Dimensional change with water absorption.	Show no dimensional change when stored in water and exhibit no permanent deformation from forces exerted on them in the mouth.
Easy to grind and polish.	More difficult to grind and difficult to polish. Grinding removes the surface glaze, which is impossible to regain.
More resistant to crazing if cross-linked.	Susceptible to crazing by thermal shock.
Thermal conductivity: 0.0006 units.	0.0025 units.
Thermal expansion same as acrylic denture base (81 ppm/°C).	Much lower than acrylic causes stresses in acrylic denture base.
Low heat distortion temperature.	High heat distortion temperature and are not affected by heat. However, sudden temperature changes may cause crazing or cracking of teeth.
Appearance: Can be excellent. Color slowly changes and difficult to match.	Can be excellent. Life like appearance and good color matching.
Natural feel. No clicking on contact with the opposing teeth (silent on contact).	Clicking occurs on contact with the opposing teeth. Sharp impact (click) sound.
In service considered transmitting less force to the mucosa.	Considered to transmit more forces to the mucosa.
Loss of vertical dimension.	Stable.
Indications for plastic teeth • In low stress bearing areas. • To oppose natural teeth or to oppose gold occlusal surfaces. • In patients with poor ridges and when limited inter-arch distance exists.	**Indications for porcelain teeth** • When patients have good ridge support. • Adequate inter-arch distance. • In those with maxillary and mandibular dentures oppose each other.

- A gypsum cast is generated.
- A suitable spacer is placed on the stone cast to provide the desired relief.
- A separating medium is painted onto exposed surfaces.
- Resin dough is formed by mixing an inorganically filled polymer and the appropriate monomer. The dough is rolled into a sheet approximately 2 mm thick, adapted to the diagnostic cast and allowed to polymerize.
- A resin impression tray may exhibit noticeable dimensional changes for 24 hours after fabrication and should not be used during this period. At the end of the prescribed period, the fit of the tray is evaluated intraorally and necessary modifications are made.
- Finally, the spacer is removed and a master impression is made using an appropriate elastomeric impression material.

Materials

Chemically activated poly (methyl methacrylate) resin.

Recently light activated urethane dimethacrylate resins also have been used in tray fabrication. Such resins are supplied in sheet and gel forms. Sheet forms are preferred for custom tray fabrication because of their favorable handling characteristics.

To facilitate tray fabrication, a diagnostic cast is made and one or more layers of wax relief spacer are placed. A separating medium is applied to exposed cast surfaces and a tray is fashioned using urethane dimethacrylate sheet material. The cast and the tray are placed in a light chamber and the resin is polymerized.

Trays fabrication using urethane dimethacrylate resins are dimensionally stable during polymerization stages. Nonetheless, these materials are brittle and release fine powder particles during grinding procedures.

STAINLESS STEEL AS A DENTURE BASE MATERIAL

Stainless steel has been occasionally used as denture base material since 1921. The austenitic steels represent the alloys used most extensively for dental appliances. The most common austenitic steel used in dentistry is 18 – 8 stainless steel.

The method used to form a stainless steel denture base is known as swaging technique.

Method

A thin sheet of 18 – 8 stainless steel (approximately 0.2 mm thick) is pressed between a die and a counter die. Dies and counter dies are made of low fusing alloys such as Zn, Cu – Mn – Al, Sn – Sb – Cu, Pb – Sb – Sn and Pb – Bi – Sn. The method of applying the pressure required for swaging may vary. Traditionally, a hydraulic press was used but modern techniques involve the use of sudden pressure wave, which adapt the sheet of alloy to the die very quickly.

The pressure wave may be generated by using controlled explosion (explosion forming) or a sudden controlled release of hydraulic pressure (hydraulic forming).

Advantages

- Very thin denture bases can be produced.
- Stainless steel is fracture resistant.
- The base is not heavy, because of the thinness of the material.
- Good corrosion resistance.
- Conducts heat rapidly, thereby ensuring that the patient retains a normal reflex reaction to hot and cold stimuli.

Disadvantages

- Possible dimensional inaccuracy, particularly if the contraction of the die material or alloy is not matched by expansion of the model.
- Loss of fine detail, since many stages are involved between recording the original impression and obtaining the final product.
- Dies and counter dies can be damaged under hydraulic pressure.
- It was difficult to ensure a uniform thickness of the finished plate.
- Uneven pressure on the die and counter die could cause wrinkling of the steel.

SUGGESTED READING

1. Amarnath GS, HS Indra Kumar, Byrasandra Chennappa Muddugangadhar. Bond strength and tensile strength of surface treated resin teeth with microwave cured and heat cured acrylic resin denture base: an *in vitro* study. Int Journal of Clinical Dental Science. 2011;2(1):27-32.

2. Azevedo A, Machado AL, Vergani CE, Giampaolo ET, Pavarina AC. Hardness of denture base and hard chair-side reline acrylic resins. J Appl Oral Sci. 2005;13(3):291-5.

3. Cao Z, Sun X, Yeh CK, Sun Y. Rechargeable infection-responsive antifungal denture materials. J Dent Res. 2010;89(12):1517-21.

4. Chai J, Takahashi Y, Kawaguchi M. The flexural strengths of denture base acrylic resins after relining with a visible-light-activated material. Int J Prosthodont. 1998;11(2):121-4.

5. Dinesh V, Tej Pal Singh A. Cyanoacrylate tissue adhesives in oral and maxillofacial surgery. J Ind Dent Assoc. 2002;73(10):171-4.

6. Ellis B, Faraj SA. The structure and surface topography of acrylic denture base materials. J Dent. 1980;8:102-8.

7. Goiato MC, Zucolotti BCR, dos Santos DM, Moreno A, Alves-Rezende MCR. Effects of thermocycling on mechanical properties of soft lining materials. Acta Odontol Latinoam. 2009;22(3):227-32.

8. Gosavi SS, Gosavi SY, Rama Krishna Alla. Local and systemic effects of unpolymerised monomers. Dent Res J. 2010;7(2):82-7.

9. Gupta A, Jain D. Materials used for maxillofacial prostheses reconstruction – a literature review. The J Ind Prosthodont Soc. 2003;3(1):11-5.

10. Gurbuz O, Unalan F, Dikbas I. Comparison of the transverse strength of six acrylic denture resins. OHDMBSC. 2010;9(1):21-4.

11. Harrison A, Magara JB, Huggett R. The effect of variation in powder particle size on the doughing and manipulation times and some mechanical properties of acrylic resin. Eur J Prosthodont Restor Dent. 1995;3:263-8.

12. Hirajima Y, Takahashi H, Minakuchi S. Influence of a denture strengthener on the deformation of a maxillary complete denture. Dent Mater J. 2009;28(4):507-12.

13. Hu X, Johnston WM, Seghi RR. Measuring the color of maxillofacial prosthetic material. J Dent Res. 2010;89(12):1522-7.

14. Huggett R, Bates JF, Packham DE. The effect of the curing cycle upon the molecular weight and properties of denture base materials. Dent Mater. 1987;3:107-12.

15. Jagger DC, Harrison A, Jandt KD. The reinforcement of dentures. J Oral Rehabil. 1999;26:185-94.

16. Katsumata Y, Hojo S, Hamano N, Watanabe T, Yamaguchi H, Okada S, et al. Bonding strength of autopolymerizing resin to nylon denture base polymer. Dent Mater J. 2009;28(4):409-18.

17. Kawaguchia T, Lassila LVJ, Tokuec A, Takahashi Y, Vallittu PK. Influence of molecular weight of polymethyl (methacrylate) beads on the properties and structure of cross-linked denture base polymer. J Mechanical Behavior of Biomedical Materials. 2011; 4:1846-51.

18. Kawara M, Komiyama O, Kimoto S, Kobayashi N, Kobayashi K, Nemoto K. Distortion behavior of heat-activated acrylic denture-base resin in conventional and long, low-temperature processing methods. J Dent Res. 1998;77(6):1446-53.

19. Kurt M, Saraç YS, Ural C, Duygu Saraç. Effect of pre-processing methods on bond strength between acrylic resin teeth and acrylic denture base resin. Gerodontology. 2012;29(2):e357-62.

20. Lee S, Morgano SM. Repair of posterior base of a maxillary complete denture by use of a cast of stone and resilient material. J Prosthet Dent. 1995;74:546-8.

21. McCabe JF. A polyvinylsiloxane denture soft lining material. J Dent. 1998;26:521-6.

22. Mohammed Sohail Memon, Norsiah Yunus, Abdul Aziz Abdul Razak. Some mechanical properties of a highly cross-linked, microwave-polymerized, injection-molded denture base polymer. Int J Prosthodont. 2001;14:214-8.

23. Naveen BH, Patil SB, Kumaraswamy K. A study on transverse strength of different denture base resins repaired by various materials and methods: An in vitro study. J Dent Sci and Res. 2003;1(1):66-73.

24. Prestipino V. Visible light cured resins: a technique for provisional fixed restorations. Quint Int. 1989;20:241-8.

25. Rama Krishna Alla, Suresh Sajjan MC, Ramaraju AV, Kishore Ginjupalli, Nagaraj Upadhya. Influence of Fiber Reinforcement on the Properties of Denture Base Resins. Journal of Biomaterials and NanoBiotechnology. 2013;4(1):91-7.

26. Shammas Mohammed, Rama Krishna Alla, Achut Devarhubli, Sunil Kumar MV. Changes in Fit of Denture Bases After Rebasing

with Different Techniques. Journal of Indian Prosthodontic Society, Supple; 2013.pp.71-6.

27. Stafford GD, Bates JF, Hugget R, Handley RW. A review of the properties of some denture base polymers. J Dent. 1980;8:292-306.

28. Vallittu PK, Narva K. Impact strength of a modified continuous glass fiber–poly(methyl methacrylate). Int J Prosthodont. 1997;10:142-8.

29. Vallittu PK, Ruyter IE, Buykuilmaz S. Polymerization time and temperature affects the residual monomer content of denture base polymers. Eur J Oral Sci. 1998;106:588-93.

30. Vojdani M, Sattari M, Khajehoseini Sh, Farzin M. Cytotoxicity of resin-based cleansers: an in vitro study. Iran Red Crescent Med J. 2010;12(2):158-62.

31. Vuorinen AM, Dyer SR, Lassila LV, Vallittu PK. Effect of rigid rod polymer filler on mechanical properties of polymethyl methacrylate denture base material. Dent Mater. 2008;24:708-13.

32. Whiting R, Jacobsen PH. Dynamic mechanical properties of resin-based filling materials. J Dent Res. 1980;59:55-60.

Dental Waxes

12

Waxes are one of the many essential materials used in dentistry. Fabrication of artificial restoration of soft and hard tissues of the oral cavity requires use of wax in one form or the other.

Waxes are organic polymers consisting of hydrocarbons and their derivatives. These are thermoplastic materials, which are normally solid at room temperature but melt without decomposition to form mobile liquids. Average molecular weight of waxes range from 400–4000.

A variety of natural resins and waxes have been used in dentistry for specific and well-defined purposes. In some instances, the most favorable qualities can be obtained from a single wax such as bees wax, but more often a blend of several waxes is necessary to develop the most desirable qualities. Waxes were first used in dentistry for the purpose of recording the impression of edentulous mouth.

APPLICATIONS

- Used in the formation of an inlay pattern.
- Used in the dental laboratory to box impressions prior to cast pouring with gypsum.
- Used as a base plate for the registration of jaw relationships.
- Used as a casting wax to establish minimum thickness to certain areas.
- Used as a utility wax to prevent distortion of impression materials.
- Used as a sticky wax to join fractured parts together.
- Used as a corrective impression wax to contact and register the detail of soft tissues.
- Used as a bite registration wax.

CLASSIFICATION

According to their Origin

According to their origin waxes are classified as:
- Natural waxes (Table 12.1)
- Synthetic waxes
- Other additives: Obtained as both natural materials and synthetic products.

Synthetic Waxes

Synthetic wax is a man-made wax synthesized from appropriate monomers. The synthetic waxes differ chemically from the natural waxes. The synthetic waxes have specific melting points and are blended with natural waxes. These are more often refined when compared to the natural waxes.

For example, polyethylene waxes, polyoxy ethylene glycol waxes, halogenated hydrocarbon waxes, complex N_2 derivatives of higher fatty acids, waxes derived from fatty acid ester of montan wax, a petroleum derivative.

According to the Application in Dentistry

- Used in the formation of an inlay pattern.
- Boxing wax: Used in the dental laboratory to box impressions prior to cast pouring with gypsum.
- Used as a base plate for the registration of jaw relationships.
- Used as a casting wax to establish minimum thickness to certain areas.

Table 12.1 Natural waxes

Type	Example	Source	Structure	Properties
Mineral	Paraffin wax	Obtained during the distillation of crude petroleum.	Straight chained hydrocarbon.	• Brittle at ambient temperature. • Crystalline in the form of plates or needles. • Softening temperature: 37–55°C • Melting range: 40–71°C
	Microcrystalline wax	Obtained from petroleum.	Branched chain hydrocarbon.	• Less brittle than paraffin wax due to their oil content. • Melting range: 60–80°C • Added to modify the softening and melting ranges of wax blends. • Less volumetric change during solidification
	Ozokerite		Contains both straight chain and branched chain hydrocarbons.	• It is earth wax. • Melting temperature: 65°C. • It is similar to microcrystalline wax.
	Ceresin	From natural and mineral petroleum.		• Added to increase the melting range of paraffin wax.
	Montan wax	Obtained by extracting lignites.	Mixtures of long chain esters.	• Melting temperature: 72–92°C.
Plant waxes	Carnauba wax		Composed of straight chain esters, alcohols, acids and hydrocarbons. Consists of 40–60% paraffin hydrocarbons.	• Melting temperature: 84–91°C. • Added to increase the melting range and hardness of paraffin wax.
	Candelilla wax			• Melting temperature: 68–75°C. • Added to harden paraffin waxes.
	Japan wax			• Tough malleable and sticky material. • Melts at 51°C. • Added to improve tackiness and emulsifying ability of paraffin wax.
	Cocoa butter			• Brittle substance at room temperature. • Used as a protector against dehydration of soft tissues.
Insect waxes	Bees wax			• Primary insect wax. • Less brittle. • Melting temperature: 63–70°C.
Animal waxes	Spermaceti wax	Obtained from the sperm of whale.		• Used as a coating in the manufacture of dental floss.

• Used as a utility wax to prevent distortion of impression materials.
• Used as a sticky wax to join fractured parts together.

• Used as a corrective impression wax to contact and register the detail of soft tissues.
• Used as a bite registration wax.

INLAY WAXES

Dental restorations such as inlays, crowns and bridges are formed by a casting process that utilizes the lost wax pattern technique. The type of wax used to fabricate the original of such restorations is known as inlay or casting waxes.

In the lost wax pattern technique, a pattern of the desired dental restoration is first made or constructed by wax that duplicates the shape and contour of the desired restoration. The carved wax pattern is then embedded in a mix of investment material to form a mold with a special channel for the entry of the molten metal into the mold.

ADA Specification Number: 4

Classification

According to ADA specification number 4, there are two types of inlay waxes.

Type I Medium wax or hard wax employed in direct technique.

Type II Soft wax used for indirect technique for inlays and crowns.

Dispension

Inlay waxes are manufactured in different color, size and shapes, e.g. deep blue, green or purple in sticks 3 inches long and ¼ inch in diameter and also dispensed in the form of small pellets or cones. Most common of all these is the stick form in purple color (Fig. 12.1).

Composition

Inlay waxes contain both natural and synthetic waxes. The detailed composition of inlay waxes is given in Table 12.2.

In some instances, Candelilla wax is also added either partially or wholly to replace the carnauba wax. It provides the same qualities as that of the carnauba wax but its melting point is lower and it is less hard than carnauba wax.

Table 12.2 Composition of inlay wax

Ingredient	Wt %	Functions
Paraffin wax	60%	• Main ingredient. • Used to establish melting point. • It is likely to flake while trimming • It does not give a glossy surface and hence modifiers are added.
Carnauba wax	25%	• Added to increase the melting range, decrease the flow at mouth temperature. • Contribute to the glossiness of the wax surface.
Ceresin	5%	Modifies the toughness and the general working and carving characteristics of wax.
Gum damar resin	3%	• Added to enhance smoothness of the surface. • Gives more resistance to flakiness or chipping. • Improves toughness of the wax.
Bees wax	5%	• Added to reduce the flow at mouth temperature. • Makes the wax less brittle at mouth temperature.
Synthetic resins	2%	Helps in stable flow properties.
Coloring agents	Trace	To impart the desired color.

Properties

Flow

One of the desirable properties of the type-I inlay wax is that it exhibits a marked plasticity or flow at a temperature slightly above that of the mouth. ADA specification number 4 provides

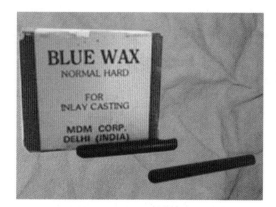

Fig. 12.1 Inlay casting wax

Table 12.3 Flow of inlay wax at various temperatures as per ADA specification no. 4

Type of wax	30°C Max.	37°C Max.	40°C Max.	40°C Min.	45°C Max.	45°C Min.
			Wax temperature			
Type I	—	1.0%	20%		90%	70%
Type II	1%	—		50%	90%	70%

certain requirements for the flow properties of inlay waxes at specific temperatures.

The flow is measured by subjecting cylindrical specimens to a load of 19.6 N for 10 minutes at specified temperature and measuring the percent of reduction in length. The maximum flow permitted for type-I waxes at 37°C is 1%. The low flow at this temperature permits carving and removal of wax pattern without distortion. In addition, both type-I and -II waxes must have a flow (minimal) of 70% at 45°C and a maximal flow of 90%, at approximately this temperature the wax is inserted (Table 12.3).

Thermal Properties

Thermal conductivity: Thermal conductivity of waxes is very low and sufficient time must be allowed during softening or hardening of inlay waxes for uniform softening and hardening of the wax mass. Due to uneven cooling or attempted manipulation in an inappropriately softened stage or carving wax not completely hardened, considerable amount of stresses may be generated within the body of the wax pattern with resulting distortion or warpage.

Coefficient of thermal expansion: The linear coefficient of thermal expansion of waxes is defined as the change in length per unit °C rise in temperature of waxes.

The inlay waxes have a very high COTE. The wax may expand as much as about 0.7% with

an increase in temperature of 20°C and may contract as much as 0.35% when it is cooled from mouth temperature to room temperature. The average linear COTE over such a temperature range is $360 \times 10^{-6}/°C$.

The inlay waxes have the highest thermal expansion coefficient when compared to other materials used in dentistry. According to ADA Specification Number 4, for type-I inlay wax the compensation for the shrinkage of about 0.4% that is experienced on cooling from mouth temperature to room temperature in direct technique.

For type-I wax, the maximum linear thermal expansion allowed between 25–30°C is 0.2% and 0.6% between 25–37°C range. However for type-II inlay waxes, thermal requirements are not specified.

Factors influencing co-efficient of thermal expansion
1. The amount thermal dimensional change may be affected by the previous treatment of wax.
2. Pressure.
3. Glass transition temperature: The temperature at which the change in rate occurs is known as the glass transition temperature. Some constituents of wax probably change their crystalline form, i.e. from plate-like to needle-like at this temperature and the wax is more plastic at higher temperature. Not all waxes exhibit transition temperatures.
4. Temperature of the die.
5. The method of applying pressure to the wax as it solidifies. However, these factors do not pose a serious problem in the indirect technique.

Manipulation of Inlay Waxes

In the process of manipulating inlay wax, dry heat is generally preferred to the use of water bath. The use of water bath can result in:
- Inclusion of droplets of water that could splatter on flaming.
- Distort the pattern during thermal changes.
- Leaching out of volatile, low melting point components into the surrounding medium.

Each of the types of inlay wax has different manipulating procedures involved that have to be undertaken carefully.

Direct Technique

- In the direct pattern forming procedure, the stick of inlay wax (type-I hard) is held well above the Bunsen flame and softened by heating and quickly rotated till the wax becomes soft and plastic.
- The wax should not be allowed to melt and must be softened to a uniform degree.
- Then the wax is kneaded thoroughly and inserted in the tooth cavity and held under pressure till it hardens.
- In order for the wax to be condensed easily and register accurate cavity details, the temperature of the insertion should be more than 45°C to ensure adequate flow and the wax held under pressure as it hardens.
- Pressure may be applied either with finger or by the patient biting the wax. It is not necessary to chill the pattern with cold water.
- Then it should be carefully withdrawn along the long axis of the preparation.
- A cold carving instrument must be generally used for direct patterns.

Indirect Technique

- Impression of the prepared cavity is taken with a suitable impression material, usually a rubber-based impression material.
- A die is prepared from that impression.
- The die is then coated with a lubricant in order to minimize or prevent the wax from sticking to the die. The lubricant should be

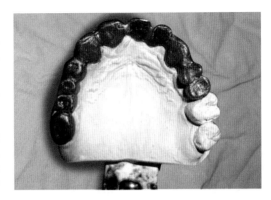

Fig. 12.2 Preparation of wax pattern by indirect technique

applied to the pattern in a film of minimal thickness. Any excess may prevent intimate adaptation of the wax to the die.
- The melted wax may be then added in layers with a wax spatula or an enamel hair brush onto the die, as shown in Figure 12.2.
- In the case of full cast or crown, the die may be dipped repeatedly into the liquid wax.
- The prepared cavity is over filled, and the wax is then carved to the proper contour. When the margins are being carved, extreme care should be taken to avoid abrading of the die.
- A silk cloth may be used for final polishing of the pattern.

Precautions

- The pattern should be touched as little as possible with the hands as it introduces thermal changes and leading to distortion or warpage.
- Wax pattern after removal should be checked for any cracks, or lack of marginal continuity and then washed and cleaned for any separating medium or saliva of the patient present.
- Over building and under building of wax must be avoided.
- For the best results, the pattern must be invested as soon as possible after it has been removed from the mouth or the die.

Wax Distortion

Distortion is one of the most serious problems faced when forming the pattern and removing it from the mouth or die specially in the direct technique.

Reasons for Distortion

- Thermal changes and from the release of internal stresses sustained by it during manipulation of the material. The stresses are induced from the natural tendency of the wax to contract on cooling, from occluded gas bubbles, change of shape during moulding and due to carving, etc. This can be illustrated by an experiment, elastic memory, as follows:
  — A piece of inlay wax softened over a flame, bent into a horseshoe shape and chilled. It is then floated in a pan of water at room temperature as shown in the Figure 12.3A. If it is permitted to remain in the position for a long period under the same temperature the horseshoe shape opens up reliving the internal stresses administered and thus distortion occurs (Fig. 12.3B). This is called elastic memory of waxes.
- According to the current theory of distortion, any method of manipulation that creates a structural integrity of the wax, involving localized variations in the intermolecular distance, may result in distortion of the pattern.

    Other factors which are under the control of operator, influence the distortion of the pattern are as follows.
- Uniform temperature.
- Uniform pressure.
- If the wax has to be melted and added to the pattern in order to repair some parts that were not accurately obtained, the added wax will introduce stress during cooling.
- *Carving*—During carving operation, some molecules of wax will be disturbed and the stresses will be introduced.
- Time and temperature of storage before investment may result in stress release.

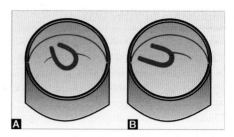

Figs 12.3A and B Elastic memory of waxes

- Distortion may also take place due to flow of wax under its own weight particularly at a higher temperature.

CASTING WAXES

The pattern for the metallic framework of removable partial denture and other similar structure is fabricated from the casting waxes.

The Federal Specification: U–W–140

Dispension

- Casting waxes are available in the form of sheets, usually of 28 and 30 gage (04 and 0.32 mm) thickness.
- Readymade shapes and in bulk.
- Readymade shapes are supplied as round, half round and half pear-shaped rods and wires of various gages of approximately 10 cm in length.

    Although casting waxes serve the same basic purpose as inlay waxes in the formation of patterns for metallic castings their physical properties differ slightly.

Composition

Paraffin wax – 60%
Carnauba wax – 25%
Ceresin – 10%
Bees wax – 5%.

Uses

- To establish minimum thickness in certain areas of the partial denture framework, such as the palatal and lingual bar.

- To produce the desired contour of the lingual bar.
- For postdamming of complete maxillary denture impressions.
- Used for checking high points of articulation.
- For producing over bites of cusp tips for the articulation of the stone cast, etc.

Baseplate Wax/Modeling Wax

It derives its name from its use on the base plate tray to establish the vertical dimension, the plane of occlusion and the initial arch form in the complete denture restoration.

Dispension

The base plate waxes normally supplied in sheets of dimension 7.6 × 15 × 0.13 cm in pink or red color (Fig. 12.4).

Composition

Base plate waxes may contain 70–80% paraffin base waxes or commercial ceresin, with small quantities of other waxes, resins and additives to develop the specific qualities desired in wax.

Typically the composition as follows:
Ceresin – 80%
Bees wax – 12%

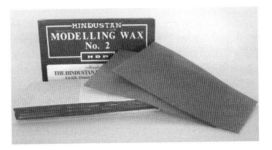

Fig. 12.4 Modeling wax

Carnauba – 2.5%
Natural and synthetic resin – 3.0%
Microcrystalline or synthetic waxes – 2.5%.

Classification

Type I: Soft
- Used in building contours and veneers.

Type II: Medium
- Used to make patterns in mouth.
- Specially used in temperate weather condition.

Type III: Hard
- Used to make patterns in mouth.
- Specially used in hot weather condition.

Properties Flow requirements of all three types of base plate waxes were given in Table 12.4.

Table 12.4 Requirements of base plate wax

Type	Temperature	Flow		Practical requirements
		Max.	Min.	
Type I	23°C	—	1.0	Softened sheets shall cohere readily without becoming flaky or adhering to fingers.
	37°C	45.0	85.0	
	45°C	—	—	
Type II	23°C	—	0.6	• No irritation of tissues.
	37°C	—	2.5	• Trim easily with a sharp instrument at 28°C.
	45°C	5.0	90.0	
Type III	23°C	—	0.2	
	37°C	—	1.2	
	45°C	5.0	50.0	

Uses

- Used on the base plate tray to establish the vertical dimension, the plane of occlusion, and the initial arch form in the technique for the complete denture restoration.
- May also be used to form all or portion of the tray itself.
- Serves as the material to produce the desired contour of the denture after teeth are set in position.
- Patterns for orthodontic appliances and prosthesis other than complete dentures, which are to be constructed of plastics, also are made of base plate wax.
- Also used to check the various articulating relations in the mouth and to transfer them to mechanical articulators.

PROCESSING WAXES

There are different types of processing waxes used in dentistry.
- Boxing wax
- Sticky wax
- Carding wax (Fig. 12.5B)
- Block out wax: Used to fill voids, undercuts for removable partial denture fabrication.
- White wax: Used for making patterns to stimulate a veneer facing.
- Utility wax.

Boxing Wax

To form a plaster or stone cast from an impression of edentulous arch, it is necessary first to form a wax box around the impression, into which the freshly mixed plaster or stone is poured and vibrated. This is important in order to develop a cast.

The terms carding wax and boxing wax appear to be interchangeably, although boxing wax is more correct according to usage.

Dispension

They are available in green or black in color.

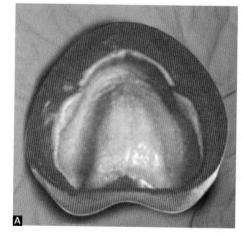

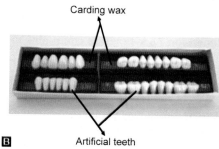

Figs 12.5A and B (A) Boxing of impression (B) Carding wax, arrangement of artificial teeth into carding wax

Boxing Process

The boxing operation usually consists of first adapting a long narrow strip of wax around the impression below its peripheral height, followed by a wide strip of wax, producing a form around the impression, as shown in Figure 12.5A.

Uses

- Used by the manufacturer to attach artificial teeth to the mounts on which they are supplied.
- Also used in the dental laboratory to box in impression prior to casting up.

Utility Wax

There are numerous instances in which an easily workable, adhesive wax is desired. A standard perforated tray for use with hydrocolloid for example, may easily be brought to a more desirable contour by such a wax. This is done to prevent a sag and distortion of impression material. A soft pliable adhesive wax may be used on the lingual portion of a bridge pontic to stabilize it while a labial plaster splint is poured.

Dispension

It is supplied in both stick and sheet form in a dark red or orange color.

Composition

It consists largely of bee's wax, petrolatum of other soft waxes in varying properties, exact composition is not known.

Uses

- Used with standard perforated tray for use with hydrocolloid.
- A soft, pliable, adhesive wax may be used on the lingual portion of a bridge pontic to stabilize it while a labial plaster splint is poured.

Sticky Wax

Sticky wax is also called as Model cement. A suitable sticky wax for prosthetic dentistry is formulated from a mixture of waxes and resins or other additive ingredient such a material is sticky when melted and will adhere closely to the surfaces upon which it is applied. At room temperature however the wax is firm and free from tackiness and is brittle.

Dispension

They are usually dispensed in the form of sticks (Fig. 12.6).

Composition

It is mainly made of bee's wax, which gives the sticky property to the wax and some naturally occurring resins. There are a number of formulas representing both high and low resin content.

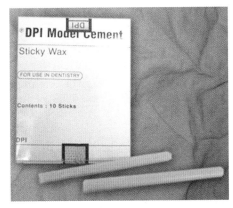

Fig. 12.6 Sticky wax

In addition to the rosin and yellow bees wax, which is major constituent, coloring agents and other natural resins such as gum damar may be present.

Uses

- To seal a plaster split to a stone model in the process of forming porcelain facings.
- Used to seal broken denture fragments prior to denture repair.
- Used to join metal fragments prior to soldering.

IMPRESSION WAXES

Impression waxes exhibit high flow and distort on withdrawal from undercuts. Waxes used for dental impression are limited to use in edentulous region of mouth.

Types

1. Corrective impression wax.
2. Bite registration wax.

Corrective Impression Wax

It is claimed that this type of impression material records the mucous membrane and underlying tissues in a functional state in which movable tissues are displaced to such a degree that functional contact with the base of the denture is obtained.

Composition: They are formulated from hydrocarbon waxes such as paraffin and ceresin and may contain metal particles.

Uses

• Used as a wax veneer over an original impression to contact and register detail of the soft mucosa.

Bite Registration Wax

They are the type of waxes, which distort if they are withdrawn from undercut areas and therefore limited use.

Composition: They are frequently made from 28 gage casting wax sheets or from hard base plate wax. But waxes identified as bite waxes appear to be formulated from bees wax or hydrocarbon waxes such as paraffin or ceresin.

Certain bite registration waxes contain aluminum or copper particles.

Uses

• They are used in edentulous portion of mouth.
• Used to articulate accurately certain models of opposing quadrants.

SUGGESTED READING

1. Farah JW, Powers JM. Bite registration materials. Dent Advis. 1998;15(4):1.
2. Iglesias A, Powers JM, Pierpont HP. Accuracy of wax, autopolymerized, and light polymerized resin pattern materials. J Prosthet Dent. 1996;5:201.
3. Ito M, Yamagishi T, Oshida Y. Effect of selected physical properties of waxes on investments and casting shrinkage. J Prosthet Dent. 1999;75:211.
4. Martin JW, Jacob RF, King GE. Boxing the altered cast impression for the dentate obturator by using plaster and pumice. J Prosthet Dent. 1988;59:382-4.
5. Morrison JT, Duncanson MG Jr, Shillingburg HT Jr. Wetting effects of surface treatments on inlay wax-investment combinations. J Dent Res. 1981;60:1858.
6. Nagda SJ. Laboratory section: waxes in fixed partial denture. The J Ind Prosthodont Soc. 2003;3(1):39.
7. Tan KM, Singer MT, Masri R, Driscoll CF. Modified fluid wax impression for a severely resorbed edentulous mandibular ridge. J Prosthet Dent. 2009;101:279-82.

Investment Materials

13

When a restoration or appliance is being made by a "lost wax" process, the wax pattern is embedded in an investment material. After the investment material has set, the wax is removed by burn out process, that creates a space in the investment called as mold space, which is filled by the material of which the restoration or appliance is to be made.

An investment material can be described as a ceramic material that is suitable for forming a mold into which a metal or alloy is cast.

IDEAL PROPERTIES REQUIRED FOR AN INVESTMENT

- Should not react with wax and alloys.
- Should be easily manipulated.
- The inner surface of the mold should not breakdown at higher temperature.
- At higher temperature, the investment must not decompose to give off gases that could corrode the surface of the alloy.
- The investment should have enough expansion to compensate for shrinkage of the wax pattern and the metal that takes place during the casting procedure.
- A dental casting investment should be porous enough to allow the air or other gases in the mold cavity to escape easily during the casting procedure.
- The investment should produce a smooth surface and fine detail and margins on the casting.
- Should have long shelf life.
- Should be inexpensive.

- Should have high compressive strength to withstand impact forces of molten alloy.

No single material is known that completely fulfills all of these requirements.

GENERAL COMPOSITION

Generally an investment is a mixture of the following materials:

Refractory Material

Refractory material is usually a form of silicon dioxide such as quartz, tridymite or cristobalite or mixture of these.

Contraction of gypsum during casting can be eliminated by using the proper form of silica in the investment. Silica exists in four allotropic forms such as quartz, tridymite, cristobalite and fused quartz. Among these quartz and tridymite are of dental interest.

On heating quartz (at 575°C), tridymite (between 117°C and 163°C or cristobalite (between 200°C and 270°C) change their crystalline structures from α-form to β-form. This change in crystalline structure results in decrease in density and increase in volume that causes rapid increase in linear expansion (Quartz-1.4%, tridymite-1.0% and cristobalite-1.8%), which helps in compensating the casting shrinkage. The amount of expansion is more for cristobalite and less for tridymite.

Combinations of different types of silica can also be used in dental investments (quartz or cristobalite). As per the type of silica is present in an investment it can be classified as *"quartz or cristobalite investment".*

Fused quartz does not change its crystalline form below its fusion point. It can be characterized as an amorphous and glass-like. Fused quartz undergoes very little expansion so its use is restricted in dental investments.

Binder Material

Binder materials are used to form a coherent solid mass with refractory material. Most commonly used binders in dental investments are α-calcium sulfate hemihydrate, phosphate, and ethyl silicate.

Other Chemicals

These include sodium chloride, boric acid, potassium sulfate, graphite, copper powder or/ and MgO; are added in a small quantity to modify some physical and mechanical properties of the investment.

In general, there are three types of investments. The choice of investment material on melting range of alloy and preference of clinician.

    i. Gypsum bonded investment (for conventional gold alloys)

   ii. Phosphate bonded investment (for metal ceramic restorations)

  iii. Ethyl silicate bonded investment (for casting of RPD with base metal alloy).

CLASSIFICATION OF INVESTMENTS

1. Based on type of binder present:
   a. Gypsum bonded investment: $CaSO_4$ α-hemihydrate
   b. Phosphate bonded investment: Mono-ammonium phosphate
   c. Silica bonded investment: Ethyl silicate.
2. Based on refractory material:
   a. Quartz investments
   b. Cristobalite investments
3. Based on temperature of casting:
   a. Low temperature investments
   b. High temperature investments.

GYPSUM BONDED INVESTMENTS

Gypsum

Gypsum is a mineral that is mined in various parts of the world. Chemically the gypsum that is produced for dental purposes is nearly pure calcium sulfate dihydrate.

ADA specification no. 2 for casting investments for dental gold alloys includes three types of investments. The types depend on whether the appliance to be fabricated is fixed or removable.

Classification

Type-I Investment

These are employed for the casting of inlays or crowns, when the alloy casting shrinkage compensation is accomplished principally by thermal expansion of the investment.

Type-II Investment

These are used for casting of inlays or crowns, but the major mode of compensation is by the hygroscopic expansion of the investment.

Type-III Investment

These are used for construction of partial dentures with gold alloys.

Composition

Essential ingredients of the dental inlay investment employed with the conventional gold casting alloys are α-hemihydrate and a form of silica. The detailed composition of gypsum bonded investments was given in Table 13.1.

Setting Reaction

The most recognized theory of the mechanism of setting is the crystalline theory given by **Henry Loui's in 1887**. The crystalline theory of $CaSO_4$ α-hemihydrate has been discussed in Gypsum Products chapter of this book.

Table 13.1 Composition of gypsum bonded investment

Ingredient	Wt %	Functions
Calcium sulfate α-hemihydrate	25–45	• Acts as a binder. • Improves strength.
Silica	55–75	• Refractory material and can withstand high temperatures. • Regulates the thermal expansion.
Modifiers E.g. Boric acid, NaCl, etc.	Trace	• Regulates the setting expansion and setting time. • Also prevents most of the shrinkage of gypsum, when it is heated above 300°C.
Reducing agents E.g. Carbon, powdered graphite or powdered copper	Trace	• To provide a nonoxidizing atmosphere in the mold when the gold alloy is cast.
Coloring agents	Trace	Provides characteristic color.

Setting Time

It is the time from the beginning of mixing until material hardens. According to ADA specificationn number 2, it ranges between 5–25 minutes.

Factors Influencing Setting Time

Theoretically, there are at least three methods by which such control can be achieved.
1. The solubility of hemihydrate can be increased or decreased by addition of potassium sulfate (accelerator) or Borax (Retarder).
2. The number of nuclei of crystallization can be increased or decreased, i.e. the greater the nuclei of crystallization, the faster the gypsum crystals form and the sooner the hardening of mass will occur.
3. If the rate of crystal growth can be increased or decreased by addition of accelerator or retarder, the setting time can be accelerated or retarded.

Factors Controlled by Manufacturer

Effect of Varying the Composition

More amount of silica in the investment powder increases the manipulation time, initial setting time, because the particles of refractory filler interfere with the interlocking of growing gypsum crystals and making this less effective in developing a solid structure.

Fineness

The finer the particle size of the hemihydrate, the faster the mix hardens. (More number of gypsum nuclei hence more rapid rate of crystals).

Impurities

If the calcination is not complete so that gypsum particles remain, or if the manufacturer adds gypsum, the setting time will be shortened because of increase in potential nuclei of crystallization.

Factors Controlled by Operator

In practice, these methods have been incorporated into the commercial products available. The operator can vary the setting time by altering w/p ratio and mixing speed.

W/P Ratio

The more the water that is used for mixing, the fewer nuclei are there per unit volume, i.e. setting time is prolonged.

Mixing

Within the practical limits, the longer and the more rapidly the mixing is done, the shorter is the setting time, i.e. some gypsum crystals form immediately as it is brought into contact with water. As the mixing begins, the formation of these crystals increases and at the same time the crystals are broken up by the mixing spatula and are distributed throughout the mixture which results in formation of more nuclei of crystallization, thus setting time is decreased.

Effect of Temperature

The temperature of the water used for mixing as well as room temperature affects setting time.
- Increased water temperature acts as an accelerator. But temperature above 50°C has a reverse effect.
- A change in temperature results in variation in the solubility of $CaSO_4$ hemihydrate and dihydrate, which may change the rate of chemical reaction.

Normal Setting Expansion (NSE)

The volumetric or linear increase in physical dimensions of an investment caused by chemical reactions that occur during hardening to a rigid structure is called normal setting expansion.

Regardless of the type of gypsum product used, an expansion of the mass can be detected during the change from the hemihydrate to the dihydrate.

As the amount of gypsum increases during setting period, the mass thickens because of the formation of needle-like crystals. The crystallization procedure is an outgrowth of crystals from nuclei of crystallization. Crystals growing from the nuclei can intermesh with and obstruct the growth of adjacent crystals. If this process is repeated by thousands of the crystals during growth, an outward thrust or stress develops that produces an expansion of the entire mass. Thus a setting expansion takes place, this crystal impingement and movement results in the production of micropores. The structure immediately after setting is composed of interlocking crystals, between which are micropores and pores containing the excess water required for mixing. On drying, the excess water is lost and the void space is increased.

- A mixture of silica and hemihydrate results in setting expansion greater than that of the gypsum product when it is used alone. The silica particles interfere with the intermeshing and interlocking of the crystals as they form. Thus, the thrust of crystals is outward during growth and they increase expansion.
- The ADA specification no. 2 for type-I investments permits a maximum setting expansion 'in air' of only 0.6%. But the setting expansion of modern investments is approximately 0.4%.
- The purpose of the setting expansion is to aid in enlarging of the mold to compensate partially for the casting shrinkage of the mold.

Hygroscopic Setting Expansion (HSE)

If the setting process is allowed to occur under water, the setting expansion may be more than double in magnitude. The reason for the increase expansion when the hemihydrate is allowed to react under water is related to the additional crystal growth permitted.

The hygroscopic setting expansion differs from the normal setting expansion in that it occurs when the gypsum product is allowed to set under or in contact with water and that it is greater in magnitude than normal setting expansion. The hygroscopic setting expansion may be 6 or more times the NSE of a dental investment. The HSE is one of the methods for expanding the casting mold to compensate for the casting shrinkage of the gold alloy.

ADA specification no. 2 for such type-II investments requires a minimum setting expansion in water of 1.2%, the maximum expansion permitted is 2.2%.

Factors Controlling the Hygroscopic Expansion

Effect of composition: The magnitude of the hygroscopic setting expansion of a dental investment is generally proportional to the silica content of the investment. The finer the particle size of silica the greater is the expansion.

Effect of w/p ratio: The higher the w/p ratio of the investment the lesser is the expansion.

Effect of spatulation: With most investments, as the mixing time is reduced, the hygroscopic expansion is decreased.

Shelf-life of investment: The older the investment, the lower the hygroscopic expansion.

Effect of confinement: The confining effect on the hygroscopic expansion is much more pronounced than the similar effect on the normal setting expansion. Both the expansions are confined by opposing forces, such as the walls of the container in which the investment is placed or the walls of the wax pattern. Therefore, the effective hygroscopic expansion is likely to be less in proportion to the expected expansion than is the normal expansion.

Effect of the amount of added water: The magnitude of the hygroscopic expansion is in direct proportion to the amount of water added during the setting period until a maximum expansion occurs. No further expansion is evident regardless of any amount of water added.

The walls of the ring restrict both the expansions. Hygroscopic setting expansion is particularly sensitive to any kind of restraining effect. To counteract the effect of restraining action of the ring, disposable paper rings are used for investing wax pattern to facilitate free expansion.

Thermal Expansion

Thermal expansion is the increase in dimension of a set investment due to temperature increase during burnout.

The expansion of a gypsum-bonded investment is directly related to the amount of silica present and to the type of silica employed. A considerable amount of quartz is necessary to counterbalance the contraction of the gypsum during heating. The contraction is entirely balanced when the quartz content is increased to 75%.

The thermal expansion of quartz investment is influenced by—
• The particle size of the quartz.
• Type of gypsum binder
• W/p ratio.

According to ADA specification no.2 for type-I investment, which rely principally on the thermal expansion for compensation, the thermal expansion must be 1–1.6%.

For type-II investment, which relies on hygroscopic expansion for compensation of the contraction of the gold alloy, the thermal expansion is 0%–0.6% at 500°C.

An inlay investment undergoes maximum thermal expansion at a temperature not higher than 700°C. Hence when a thermal expansion technique is employed, the maximum mold temperature for the casting of gold alloy should be less than 700°C because gold alloy can become contaminated at a mold temperature higher than this.

Factors Affecting Thermal Expansion

W/P ratio: The more the water used in mixing the investment, the less is thermal expansion achieved during heating.

Effect of chemical modifiers: The addition of small amount of Na, K, or lithium chloride to the investment eliminates the contraction caused by the gypsum and the expansion without the presence of an excessive amount of silica. Boric acid also has similar effect.

Thermal Contraction

On cooling from 700°C an investment can undergo contraction, which is less than its original dimension. This contraction results in contraction of gypsum and not related to the amount and any property of silica. On reheating it may expand, thermally to the same dimensions when it was first heated. But reheating of investment is not advisable as it develops internal cracks.

Strength

The strength of an investment increased rapidly as the material hardens after initial setting time. However, the free water content of the set product definitely affects its strength. Hence two strengths of a gypsum product are recognized.

1. *Wet or green strength:* Strength obtained when the water in excess of that required for the hydration of the hemihydrate is left in the test specimen.
2. *Dry strength:* When the specimen has been dried of the excess water, the strength obtained is dry strength. The dry strength is 2 or more times the wet strength.

The strength of an investment must be adequate to prevent or chipping of the mold during heating and casting of the gold alloy. The strength of an investment is measured in terms of compressive strength.

- The compressive strength is increased according to the type and amount of gypsum binder present.
- The use of chemical modifies also helps in increasing the strength because more of the binder can be used without a marked reduction in thermal expansion.

According to ADA specification no. 2, the compressive strength for the inlay investment should not be less than 2.4 MPa (350 psi) when tested 2 hrs after setting.

Factors Affecting Strength

W/P ratio: The greater the w/p ratio, the greater will be porosity. The more the water is employed in mixing; the lower is the compressive strength because the greater is the porosity, fewer crystals are available per unit volume for a given weight of hemihydrate.

Temperature: Heating the investment to 700°C may increase or decrease the strength as much as 65%, depending on the composition, i.e. greatest reduction with NaCl containing investment.

1. After the investment has cooled to room temperature its strength decreases considerably mainly because of fine cracks that form during cooling.
2. The addition of an accelerator or retarder lowers both the wet and dry strength.

Manipulation

Selection of Materials

Clean rubber bowl, plaster spatula, required amount of investment material and distilled water.

Proportioning

The water and powder should be measured by using an accurate graduated cylinder for the water volume (i.e. by use of scoop), as it does not pack uniformly. It may vary from product to product. If the container is shaken, the volume will increase as a result of entrapment of air. Preweighed envelopes are better as they promote accuracy, reduce waste and save time.

Mixing

Hand mixing: A measured amount of water is placed in the bowl and the weighed powder is shifted in and the mixture is then vigorously stirred with the periodic wiping of the inside of the bowl with the spatula to ensure the wetting of all of the powder and breaking up any agglomerates or lumps. Entrapment of air in the mix must be avoided to avoid porosity leading to weak spots and surface inaccuracies. The use of an automatic vibrator of high frequency and of low amplitude can reduce the air entrapment. The mixing should continue until a smooth mix is obtained usually, within a minute.

Mechanical mixing: The preferred method of mixing is to add the measured water first, followed by gradual addition of the preweighed powder. The powder is incorporated during approximate –15 seconds of mixing with a hand spatula, followed by 20–30 seconds of mechanical mixing under vacuum by a mixture. The strength and hardness achieved by such mechanical mixing exceeds that obtained by one minute of hand mixing.

PHOSPHATE BONDED INVESTMENTS

The rapid growth of the use of metal ceramic restorations and the increased use of higher melting alloys has resulted in an increased used of phosphate bonded investments.

Classification

Type I—For crowns, inlays and other fixed restoration.

Type II—For partial denture and other cast removable restorations.

In case of silver-palladium or base metal alloys, it is believed that carbon embrittles the alloys, even though the investment is heated to temperature that burns out the carbon. But latest evidences indicate that palladium reacts with carbon at temperature above 1504°C. Thus if the casting temperature of a high palladium alloy exceeds this critical point, a phosphate investment without carbon should be used. Also, a carbon crucible should not be employed for melting the alloy.

Composition

Powder composition is given in Table 13.2.

Liquid

Colloidal silica liquid suspensions: Colloidal silica suspensions are used with the phosphate investments in place of water as it requires greater expansion. Some phosphate investments are made to be used with water for the casting of many alloys. For predominantly base metal alloys, a 33% dilution of the colloidal silica is required.

Setting Reactions

The setting reaction for the binder system that causes the investment to set and harden is generally written as follows:

$$NH_4H_2PO_4 + MgO + 5H_2O \rightarrow NH_4MgPO_4.6H_2O$$

The final product of the reaction is mono-ammonium diacid phosphate or magnesium ammonium phosphate.

Working and Setting Time

- Phosphate investments are affected by temperature. The warmer the mix, the faster it sets. The setting reaction itself is exothermic, and this further accelerates the rate of setting.
- Increased mixing time and mixing efficiency, results in a faster set and a greater rise in temperature.
- In general, the more efficient the mixing, the better the casting in terms of smoothness and accuracy.
- Mechanical mixing under vacuum is preferred.

Setting and Thermal Expansion

In practice, setting reaction shows slight expansion, and this expansion can be increased by the use of a colloidal silica solution instead of water.

When phosphate investments are mixed with water they exhibit shrinkage between the temperatures of 200°–400°C. This contraction is practically eliminated by replacing the water with colloidal silica solution.

For phosphate bonded material combined setting and thermal expansion of around 2% is normal, provided the special silica liquid is used with the investment.

Manipulation

Required amount of powder and liquid are dispensed in vacuum mixer bowl and hand

Table 13.2 Composition of phosphate bonded investment

Ingredient	Wt %	Functions
Powder		
Binder	20	Increases strength, setting and thermal expansions.
E.g. Mixture of basic MgO and acidic ($NH_4H_2PO_4$)		
Refractory materials	80	• Withstand higher temperatures.
E.g. Quartz or cristobalite or mixture of both		• Give large setting expansions.
Carbon	Trace	Acts as reducing agent.

spatulated for 30 seconds until the powder is wetted by the liquid. Then the mixing bowl is attached to the vacuum mixer and mechanically spatulated according to manufacturer's recommended mixing time. Then it is placed in a mechanical vibrator to remove air bubbles. Then the mix is poured in the casting ring.

Advantages

- They have the ability to withstand high temperatures.
- They have sufficient green and fired strength.
- They can withstand the impact forces and pressure of centrifugally cast molten alloy.
- They provide setting and thermal expansion high enough to compensate for the thermal contraction of cast metal prosthesis or porcelain veneers during cooling.

Disadvantages

- Using the casting temperature greater than 1375°C, results in mold breakdown and rougher surfaces of the castings.
- The high strength of these investments makes removal of the casting from the investment a difficult and tedious task.

The higher strength of phosphate bonded materials means that these products can be used for casting all types of alloys, i.e. precious, semiprecious and base metal. The wax burn out temperature is varied to suit the type of alloy being cast. Typical burn out temperatures are as follows:

Gold alloys: 700–750°C
Palladium-silver alloy: 730–815°C
Base metal alloy: 815–900°C.

ETHYL SILICATE BONDED INVESTMENTS

The ethyl silicate bonded investments require more complicated and time-consuming procedures. It is used in the construction of the high fusing base metal partial denture alloys.

It is supplied as a powder that requires mixing with a liquid to bind the mixed mass via setting reaction at room temperature.

- The powder consists of refractory particles of silica and glasses in various forms along with MgO and some other oxides in minor amount.
- The liquid that is used for the setting reaction may be supplied as a stabilized alcohol solution of silica gel or it may form from two liquids that are supplied.

When the system uses two liquids then one is ethyl silicate and the other may be an acidified solution of denatured ethyl alcohol.

Handling Technique

The powder is added to the hydrolyzed ethyl silicate liquid, mixed quickly and vibrated into a mold that has an extra collar to increase the height. The mold is placed on a vibrator to settle heavier particles quickly while the excess liquid and some of the fine particles rise to the top. In about 30 minutes, the accelerator in the powder hardens the settled part and the top excess is poured off. Thus the liquid: powder ratio in the settled part is greatly reduced, and the setting shrinkage is decreased to 0.1%.

This type of investment can be heated from 1090°C– 1180°C (2000°F–2150°F) and is compatible with higher fusing alloys. Its low setting expansion minimizes distortion. The expansion of the investment is mainly due to thermal expansion. Thus distortion of the pattern is minimized. These investments are more suited for large precise castings.

Properties

The green strength of these investments is low, and refractory models are best handled by reinforcing them with a resin dip.

Compressive strength: 1.5 MPa.
Setting contraction: 0 – 0.4%.
Thermal expansion: About 1.5%–1.8% can be attained between room temperature and 1000°C–1177°C (1800°F – 2150°F).

Advantages

- These investments offer the ability to cast high temperature Co – Cr and Ni – Cr alloys.

- Good surface finish.
- Low distortion and high thermal expansion.
- They are less dense (i.e. more permeable) than phosphate bonded investments and thin sections with fine detail can be reproduced.
- The low-fired strength makes removal of casting from investment easier than with phosphate bonded investment.

Disadvantages

- Added processing attention and extra precaution needed in handling the low strength fired molds.
- The low strength and high thermal expansion requires a more precise burn out process and firing schedule to avoid cracking.

The silica-bonded investments undergo slight contraction during setting and the early stages of heating. This is due to the nature of the setting reaction and subsequent loss of water and alcohol from the material.

Of the three main types of investment—the phosphate bonded products are becoming popular. Silica bonded materials are rarely used nowadays due to the fact that they are less convenient to use than the other products and that ethanol produced in the liquid can spontaneously ignite or explode at elevated temperature.

DIE STONE INVESTMENT COMBINATION

In this method the die material and the investing medium have a comparable composition. A commercial gypsum bonded material, called *'Divestment'* is mixed with colloidal silica liquid. The die is made from this mix and the wax pattern is constructed on it. Then the entire assembly (die and pattern) is invested in a mixture of divestment and water, thereby eliminating the possibility of distortion of the pattern on removal from the die or during the setting of the investment.

The setting expansion of the material is 0.9% and thermal expansion is 0.6%, when it is heated to 677°C. Because divestment is a gypsum bonded material, it is not recommended for high fusing alloys, as used in metal ceramic restoration. It is a highly accurate technique for use with conventional gold alloys.

Divestment phosphate is a phosphate bonded investment that is used in the same manner as divestment and is suitable for use with high fusing alloys.

SUGGESTED READING

1. Curtis RV. The suitability of dental investment materials as dies for superplastic forming of medical and dental prostheses. Mater Sci and Eng Tech (Superplastic Forming). 2008;39(4-5):322-6.
2. Canay S, Hersek N, Çiftçi Y, Akça K. Comparison of diametral tensile strength of microvave and oven-dried investment materials. J Prosthet Dent. 1999;82(3):286-90.
3. Eliopoulos D, Zinelis S, Papadopoulos T. The effect of investment material type on the contamination zone and mechanical properties of commercially pure titanium castings. J Prosthet Dent. 2005;94(6):539-48.
4. Ito M, Yamagishi T, Oshida Y, Munoz CA. Effect of selected physical properties of waxes on investments and casting shrinkage. J Prosthet Dent. 1996;75(2):211-6.
5. Low D, Swain MV. Mechanical properties of dental investment materials. J Mater Sci: Mater in Medicine. 2000;11(7):399-405, DOI: 10.1023/A:1008942223938.
6. Nilner K, Owall B. Reproduction of details using dental stones and investment material in impressions of elastomers and waxes. Swed Dent J. 1982;6(6):249-55.
7. Okabe T, Ohkubo C, Watanabe I, Okuno O, Takada Y. The present status of dental titanium casting. J Minerals, Metals and Materials Soc. 1998;50(9):24-9, DOI: 10.1007/s11837-998-0410-7
8. Papadopoulos T, Axelsson M. Influence of heating rate in thermal expansion of dental phosphate-bonded investment material. Eur J Oral Sci. 1990;98(1):60-5.
9. Papadopoulos T, Zinelis S, Vardavoulias M. A metallurgical study of the contamination zone at the surface of dental Ti castings, due to the phosphate-bonded investment material: the protection efficacy of a ceramic coating. J Mater Sci. 1999;34(15):3639-46, DOI: 10.1023/A:1004639002688.
10. Wang RR, Welsch GE, Castro-Cedeno M. Interfacial reactions of cast titanium with mold materials. Int J Prosthodont. 1998; 11(1):33-43.

Dental Casting Alloys (Casting Gold and Base Metal Alloys)

14

HISTORY OF DENTAL CASTING ALLOYS

- Taggart was the first to describe the "lost wax technique" in 1907. The existing jewelry alloys were adapted for dental casting purposes. These alloys can be strengthened by the addition of Cu, Ag and Pt.
- By 1948, their composition had become diverse, palladium began to substitute platinum.
- In the 1950's, metal-ceramic alloys were introduced.
- Base metal removable partial denture alloys were introduced in 1930's. Due to their many advantages over conventional gold alloys, they have become increasingly more popular. (Advantages of base metal alloys are their lighter weight and increased mechanical properties).

TERMINOLOGY

Noble Metals

Gold, platinum, palladium, rhodium, ruthenium, iridium, osmium, and silver are the eight noble metals. They are less reactive in the oral cavity and have high resistance to tarnish and corrosion.

- However, in the oral cavity, silver is more reactive and therefore is not considered as a noble metal.
- The noble metals have been the basis of inlays, crowns and bridges because of their resistance to corrosion in the oral cavity.

Precious Metals

The term precious indicates the "intrinsic value" of the metal.

- All noble metals are precious but all precious metals are not noble metals.
- Of the eight noble metals, four of major importance in dental casting alloys, they are gold, platinum, palladium and silver.
- All four have FCC crystal structure and all are white in color except gold.

Semiprecious Metals

There is no accepted composition, which differentiates precious from semiprecious. The term semiprecious should be avoided.

Base Metals

These are non-noble metals. They are invaluable components of dental casting alloys because of their influence on physical properties, control of the amount and type of oxidation or their strengthening effect. Such metals are reactive with their environment, and are referred to as "base metals".

Some of the base metals can be used to protect an alloy from corrosion by property known as "Passivation". Although they are frequently referred as nonprecious. But the preferred term is base metal, e.g.: chromium, cobalt, nickel, iron, copper, manganese, etc.

IDEAL PROPERTIES OF CASTING ALLOYS

- Biological requirement: They should be biocompatible, that means, they should be nonallergic, nontoxic and noncarcinogenic either during usage or fabrication.
- Chemical requirement: They should be chemically inert, that means, they should have a good tarnish and corrosion resistance.
- Physical/mechanical requirements–
  — They should have high strength and wear resistance to resist the forces in the oral cavity.
  — They should be sufficiently ductile and resilient (otherwise it may fracture during burnishing).
  — They should have sufficient hardness for grinding and finishing of the alloy.
  — The solidification shrinkage should be minimum or zero.
  — They should have high fatigue strength.
- Alloys should be inexpensive both in terms of metal and laboratory expenses.
- They should have good fluidity when molten and ease of melting and are easier to cast.
- They should have high sag resistance (metal – ceramic alloys).
- Ease of soldering.
- They should fit accurately into the prepared cavity or onto the prepared tooth structure.
- They should be amenable to heat treatment so that the physical properties cannot be altered.

CLASSIFICATION OF DENTAL CASTING ALLOYS

According to ADA Specification No. 5

The ADA specification no.5 classified these alloys as type-I, type-II, type-III, and type-IV, with the content of gold and platinum group metals ranging from 83–75% respectively.

Based on their Hardness

I. *Soft (type – I):* For restoration subject to very slight stress such as inlays (VHN = 50–90)

II. *Medium (type – II):* For restoration subject to moderate stress such as onlays.

III. *Hard (type – III):* For high stress situations, including onlays, crowns, thick Veneer crowns and short span fixed partial dentures.

IV. *Extra hard (type – IV):* For extremely high stress states, such as endodontic posts and cores, thin veneers crowns, long-span fixed partial dentures and removable partial dentures.

Based on their New ADA Specification or on their Nobility

I. *High noble:* With a noble metal content of greater than or equal to 60 wt% and gold content of greater than or equal to 40%.

II. *Noble:* With a noble metal content of greater than or equal to 25 wt%.

III. *Predominantly base metals:* With a noble metal content of less than 25 wt%.

Based on their Function

- In 1927, Bureau of Standards classified gold casting alloys function as type I, II, III and IV. Hardness increases from type I–V.
- Later in 1960, metal-ceramic alloys were introduced and added to the classification. Removable partial denture alloys were also included, e.g. For metal-ceramic hard and extra hard: For veneering with dental porcelain copings, hard type, for short span bridges, and extra hard for long span bridges.
  Removable partial denture alloys for RPD frames and denture bases.

Based on their Description

I. Crown and bridge alloys:
   a. Noble metal alloys
      E.g. Gold-based – type – III and type – IV and low gold alloys, nongold-based silver, platinum alloys.
   b. Base metal alloys:
      E.g. Ni-based and cobalt-based.

II. Metal-ceramic alloys:
   a. Noble metal alloy for porcelain bonding
      E.g. Gold, Pt and Pd

Gold, Pd and Ag
Gold and Pd
Pd and Ag
High palladium.
b. Base metal alloys for porcelain bonding
E.g. Ni – Cr and
Co – Cr.
III. Removable partial denture (RPD) alloys
a. Gold alloy – only type – IV is used
(**Note**: Majority of the RPD frameworks
is made from base metal alloys)
b. Base metal alloys:
E.g. Co – Cr, Ni – Cr, Co – Cr – Ni.

Based on the Color of the Alloy

I. Yellow gold alloys
Those with more than 60% gold and those
with low gold or economy gold with 42–55%
gold has yellow color.
E.g. Noble, high noble, predominantly
base metals and Japanese gold (also called
technic alloy).
II. White gold alloys
Those with gold more than 50% but
palladium give white color.
E.g. Ag – Pd with or without gold but of
mainly Ag gives white color.
Pd – Ag with mainly Pd gives white color.

DENTAL CASTING GOLD NOBLE METAL ALLOYS

Pure gold is a soft and ductile metal and so
is not used for casting dental restoration and
appliances. Dental casting golds are alloyed
commonly with copper, silver, platinum,
palladium, nickel, and zinc. Alloying gold with
these metals not only improves its physical and
mechanical properties but also reduces its cost.

Applications

* Inlays and onlays
* Crowns and bridges
* Metal-ceramic bridges
* Resin bonded bridges

* Endodontic post
* Removable partial denture frameworks.

Composition and Functions of Each Ingredient

Gold

* It is the principal ingredient of gold colored
alloys.
* It increases tarnish resistance of the final alloy.
* Provides ductility.
* Increases specific gravity and plays an
important role in its heat treatment process.

General composition of gold alloys	
Ingredients	Weight %
Gold	50–90
Platinum	0–20
Palladium	0–12
Copper	0–17
Silver	0–20
Zinc	0–2
Indium, Iridium, Osmium, and Ruthenium	0–0.5

Traditionally, the gold content of a dental
alloy has been specified in terms karat and
fineness.
* "Karat" refers to the parts of pure gold in 24
parts of an alloy. For an example, 24 – karat
gold is pure gold; where- as 22 – karat gold
is an alloy containing 22 parts pure gold and
2 parts of other metal.
* "Fineness" describes gold alloys by the
number of parts per 1000 of gold. For
example, pure gold has a fineness of 1000,
and 650 fine alloy has a gold content of 65%
thus, the fineness rating is 10 times the gold
percentage in an alloy.
The terms karat and fineness are rarely used
to describe the gold content of current alloys.

Copper

* Very active and red in color.
* Copper and gold dissolves in all proportion
to form solid solutions. It reduces the melting
point of the alloy.

- Improves hardness and strength.
- It does not reduce the malleability and ductility of gold but produces an alloy that can be cold worked.
- It plays an important role in heat treatment.
- It imparts reddish color to the gold.

Silver

- Active element and white in color
- Improves strength and hardness slightly by solution hardening.
- It neutralizes the reddish color of copper (a small addition Ag makes the gold paler or whitens).
- It reduces the malleability and ductility very slightly and lowers the melting point.
- It reduces tarnish and corrosion resistance, as it tarnishes readily in the presence of sulfides.

Platinum

- It forms solid solutions with gold.
- It increases the melting temperature and also raises the recrystallization temperature.
- It is a noble metal, increases the corrosion resistance.
- It is better hardener and strengthener than copper.
- It whitens the color of alloy.

Palladium

- It is similar to platinum in its effect.
- It hardens as well as whitens the alloy.
- It also raises the melting temperature to a certain extent by sharply than by platinum.
- Increases the resistance to tarnish and corrosion.
- It is less expensive than platinum, thus reducing the cost of an alloy.

Zinc

- It acts as scavenger for oxygen. Without zinc the silver in the alloy causes absorption of oxygen during melting. Later during solidification, the oxygen is released producing gas porosities in the casting.
- It lowers the melting point.

- It decreases surface tension and increases fluidity of the alloy.

Other Metals (Indium, Osmium, and Ruthenium)

- They refine grain size, when present only in small quantities.
- They lower the melting point.
- They reduce tarnish resistance but better than zinc.
- Indium acts as deoxidizer, decreases surface tension and increases fluidity of the alloy.

Properties of Gold Alloy

Biological Property

Gold alloys are relatively biocompatible.

Chemical Properties

Gold alloys have excellent tarnish and corrosion resistance in oral cavity, due to their high noble metal content.

Physical and Mechanical Properties

Density: Density of gold alloy is higher than base metal alloys. The density of casting gold alloys is around 15.2 gm/cm^3 and base metal alloys contains around 8.5 gm/cm^3. The high density of alloys has both advantages and disadvantages:
- *Advantages:* Alloys with a higher density have a better castability than alloy with a lower density.
- *Disadvantages*
  - High density improves gravitational forces. So, the problem arises when these alloys are used for upper removable partial dentures.
  - Due to high density, it requires more amount of material for casting.

Melting range:
- The melting range sets basis for the casting temperature and the type of investment material.
- Ideally type I–IV gold alloys should have a lower fusion temperature if they are to be cast

Table 14.1 Melting range of casting gold alloys

Type	Melting range (°C)
Type I	943–960
Type II	924–960
Type III	843–916
Type IV	921–943
Metal-ceramic	1270–1304

with conventional equipment and if gypsum investment is to be used. Melting range of all types of casting gold alloys is given in Table 14.1.

- Gypsum investments can withstand the temperature up to 1000°C. So, the gold alloys can cast with gypsum investments. Beyond 1000°C gypsum bonded investments undergo degradation.

Modulus of elasticity: The gold alloys have less MOE, and they are more flexible than base metal alloys. The average value is approximately 90 × 10^3 MPa.

Elongation: Elongation of the metal indicates ductility. A reasonable amount is required specially if the alloy is to be deformed during clinical use.

For example:
- Clasp adjustment for removable partial dentures, margin adjustment and burnishing of crowns and onlays.

- Percentage elongation decreases from type I–IV alloys.
- Type-I alloys can be easily deformed even under a low stress and they possess sufficient ductility.
- Type-II alloys have a percentage elongation, which is equal to that of type-I alloys indicating good ductility.

Yield strength: Yield strength increases from type I–IV alloys.

Hardness: Hardness also increases from type I–IV alloys so that they show high wear resistance from type I–IV alloys.

The values of percent elongation, yield strength and hardness of the gold alloy were given in Table 14.2.

Casting shrinkage or dimensional changes: Most metals and alloys, including gold and the noble metal alloys have the tendency to shrink or contract when they change from the liquid state to the solid state. The shrinkage occurs in three stages.

I. The thermal contraction of the liquid metal between the temperature to which it is heated and the liquidus temperature.

II. The contraction of the metal inherent in its change from the liquid to solid state.

III. The thermal contraction of the solid metal that occurs down to room temperatures.

- The values of the casting shrinkage differ for the various alloys presumably

Table 14.2 Mechanical properties of casting gold alloys

Type	Yield strength (MPa)	Ultimate tensile strength (MPa)	Elongation (%)	Hardness (VHN)
Type-I (High noble)	103	200	25-30	60-80
Type-II (High noble)	186	345	38	101
Type-III High noble Noble	207 H 275 241	365	39 H 19 30	121 H 182 138
Type-IV High noble Noble	275 H 493 434	445	35 H7 10	149 H264 180

Where H – Age hardened conditions, other values are for the quenched (softened condition)

Table 14.3 Casting shrinkage (%) of casting gold base metal alloys

Alloy	Casting shrinkage (%)
Type I, gold based	1.56
Type II, gold based	1.37
Type III, gold based	1.42
Base metal alloys	
Ni – Cr – Mo – Be	2.3
Co – Cr – Mo	2.3

because of differences in their composition (Table 14.3).

- Platinum, palladium and copper are effective in reducing the casting shrinkage of an alloy. This is one of the reasons that the gold alloys show less casting shrinkage than base metal alloys (Table 14.4).
- The value for the casting shrinkage of pure gold closely approaches that of its maximal linear thermal contraction.

Compensation for Solidification Shrinkage

Either one or both of the following two methods may obtain the compensation for the shrinkages inherent in the dental casting procedure.
1. Setting or hygroscopic expansion of the investment.
2. Thermal expansion of the investment.

Both techniques are currently in use and are commonly termed the "hygroscopic expansion (low-heat)" and the "Thermal expansion (high-heat)"methods. The high-heat method requires thermal expansion of the investment to increase from room temperature to a high temperature (650°C–700°C for gypsum-bonded investments and up to 871°C for phosphate bonded investments).

Casting shrinkage and method of compensation can be summarized as shown in Table 14.4.

Despite these stated differences, the overall procedures involved in investing and casting are quite similar and, therefore, are described simultaneously. For better results, the manufacturer's recommendations for the specific alloy used should be followed.

Ringless Casting System

To provide maximum expansion of investment, a ringless system is available, commercially is called as "power cast ringless system", consists of three sizes of rings and formers, preformed wax sprues and shapes, investment powder, and a special investment liquid.

The tapered plastic rings allow for removal of the investment mold after the material has set. This system is suited for the casting of alloys that require greater mold expansion than traditional gold-based alloys.

Heat Treatment of High Noble and Noble Metal Alloys

Gold alloys can be significantly hardened if the alloy contains a sufficient amount of copper. Type-I and–II alloys usually do not harden or they harden to a lesser degree than do the type-III and type-IV alloys. The actual mechanism of hardening is probably the result of several different solid-state transformations. The purpose of heat treatment may be:
a. To soften the alloy—so that having the alloy in a softened state may facilitate shaping and working of the appliance in the laboratory. This is called "softening heat treatment".

Table 14.4 Casting shrinkage and methods of compensation

Wax shrinkage	+	Alloy shrinkage	= Total shrinkage =	Setting expansion	+	Thermal expansion	
(0.3%)		(1.4%)	(1.7%)	NSE 0.4%		1.3%	For high heat technique
				NSE 1.0%		0.7%	For low heat technique

b. To harden the alloy—so that the mechanical properties are improved to withstand the constant oral stresses to a greater degree, when the appliance is finally fitted to the mouth. This is called "hardening heat treatment".

Softening Heat Treatment

It is also called as "solution heat treatment". This is done before an appliance is grinded, adjusted, or in any other way could work outside the mouth.

Mechanism: The casting is placed in an electric furnace for 10 minutes at a temperature of 700°C and then it is quenched in water. During this period, all intermediate phases are changed to a disordered solid solution, and the rapid quenching prevents ordering that occurs during cooling. This results in reduction of tensile strength, proportional limit and hardness, but the ductility is increased.

The appliance in the soft condition can easily be adjusted and grinded in the laboratory. But it cannot be fitted into the mouth having such reduced physical properties. Therefore, the appliance or cast is now subjected to "hardening" or "age hardening heat treatment".

Hardening Heat Treatment

It is also known as "age hardening". This is done after the try in stage of the cast, during which adjustments are made, while the appliance is soft. The arrangement of atoms in space lattices is disordered after softening heat treatment. Cast is strain hardened or cold worked due to adjustments, grindings, etc. Ideally all the effects of strain hardening must be removed by softening heat treatment. Therefore, the cast is once again subjected to softening heat treatment, to cause ordered arrangements of atom in space lattice before age hardening.

Mechanism: The casting is "soaked" or "aged" at a specific temperature for about 15–30 minutes, before it is water quenched. The aging tempera-

ture depends upon the alloy composition but is generally between 200°C to 450°C. Manufacturer specifies the proper time and temperature.

This hardening heat treatment makes an alloy strong and hard. But reduces ductility. This type of hardening is done to metallic partial dentures and bridges but not to inlays. Such age hardened appliance will not deform in the mouth easily but, if at all deformed, will break easily because of its reduced ductility.

Alloys for Metal-ceramic Restorations

Because of the poor tensile and shear strength, all porcelain restorations are weak and brittle and so break easily. But porcelain is necessary for esthetics. This problem can be solved by making the restoration in metal and applying porcelain to labial or buccal areas of the appliance or cast in thin layer (veneer) for esthetics. Thus both strength and appearance are met in restoration.

Alloys used for metal ceramics can be classified as:
1. High noble alloys—with high gold
2. Noble alloys—with low gold or gold free
3. Base metal alloys (discussed in the Base Metal Casting Alloys topic).

Ideal Requirements of Alloys for Metal Ceramics

1. Should be rigid and strong.
2. The coefficient of thermal expansion should be similar to that of porcelain.
3. Should have high proportional limit.
4. Should have high MOE.
5. Should be resistant to tarnish and corrosion.
6. Should have high melting temperature to withstand the high temperature of porcelain firing procedure.
7. Should have sag-resistance to prevent sagging under its own weight because of high temperature involved in porcelain baking.
8. Should be hard.
9. Should have capacity to bond to dental porcelain.

High Noble Alloys

Composition

Ingredient	Wt %	Functions
Gold	82	Main ingredient
Platinum	12	Increases the melting temperatures
Palladium	4	Reduces COTE
Silver	2	Strengthens the alloy
Indium	1	
Iridium	0.3	Refines the grain structure
Zinc	1	
Tin	0.2	Produces thin oxide film on the surface of the alloy.
Copper	2	

Other Combinations of High Noble Alloys

1. Au – 87, Pd – 6, Pt – 5, Ag – 1
2. Au – 77, Pd – 10, Pt – 3, Ag – 9
3. Au – 52, Pd – 39, Ga – 2.

Noble Alloys

These are gold-free alloys and are mainly palladium-based alloys. These alloys stand between high noble and base metals alloys with respect to price and they are more popular than high gold alloys.

Composition
1. Palladium-silver alloys: Pd – 60%, Ag – 28%
   Disadvantage: Discoloration of porcelain due to Ag, i.e. green-yellow in color and therefore was described as "greening effect".
2. Palladium-copper alloys: Pd – 74%, Cu – 15%, Ga – 9%

3. Palladium-cobalt alloys: Pd – 78%, Co – 10%
4. Palladium-gallium-silver-gold: Pd – 75%, Ga – 6%, Ag – 6%, and Au – 6%.

All these combinations, contain a small percentage of tin and indium as bond forming elements between metal and porcelain.

BASE METAL ALLOYS

Alloys, which contain little or no noble metals are known as base metal alloys (contains <25 weight percent of noble metals. These metal alloys are introduced to overcome the drawbacks of noble metal alloys such as higher density, low modulus of elasticity and expensive.

These base metal alloys can be used as casting metal alloys or as wrought alloys for orthodontic treatment and dental instruments.

The first base metal alloys were cobalt-chromium alloys primarily used for removable partial denture framework. The latest base metal alloys are titanium alloys. Commonly used base metal alloys are Ni-Cr-Mo, Ni-Cr-Be, Ni-Ti, Co-Cr-W, pure titanium and Ti-Al-V.

Classification of Base Metal Alloys
1. Based on composition:
   i. Cobalt-based alloys:
      For example, Co-Cr-W, Co-Ni-Cr, and Co-Cr-Mo
   ii. Nickel-based alloys:
      For example, Ni-Cr-Mo, Ni-Ti, and Ni-Cr-Be.
   iii. Titanium-based alloys:
      For example, pure titanium, Ti-Al-V, and Ni-Ti.
   iv. Aluminum bronzes.
2. Based on applications (Fig. 14.1).

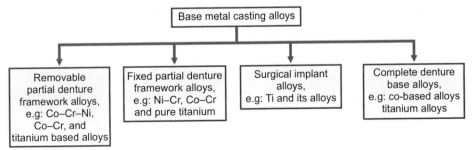

Fig. 14.1 Application of base metal alloys

Properties of Alloying Elements

Cobalt

- Melting point: 1495°C.
- Density: 8.9 gm/cc.
- Imparts hardness, strength, and rigidity to the alloy.
- Decreases tarnish and corrosion.
- Decreases ductility and malleability.

Chromium

- Melting point: 1875°C
- Density: 7.6 gm/cc.
- Very good corrosion resistance by forming Cr_2O_3 film.
- It helps in attaining maximum mechanical properties.
- More amount of chromium causes brittleness to the alloy.

Nickel

- Melting point: 1453°C.
- Density: 8.9 gm/cc.
- Decreases strength, hardness, and modulus of elasticity.
- Decreases fusion temperature.
- Increases ductility.
- Nickel vapor inhalation causes lung cancer.

Molybdenum or Tungsten (Mo or W)

- Increases mechanical properties specially hardness.
- It is used for grain refinement.

Iron, Copper, Beryllium (Fe, Cu, Be)

- Used as hardeners.
- Reduces fusion temperature and grain size.
- Beryllium dust causes health hazards – dermatitis.

Manganese, Silicon, Zinc (Mn, Si, Zn)

- Used as oxide scavengers to prevent oxidation of other elements during melting.
- Also used as hardeners.

Iridium, Ruthenium

- Grain refiner and hardeners.

Carbon

- It increases strength, hardness, and ductility when added in small amounts.
- Excess carbon increases brittleness.

Boron

- Acts as a deoxidizer.
- Also used as hardener.
- It reduces ductility.

Nickel-Based Alloys

According to ADA specification no. 14, base metal alloys should contain more than 85% by weight major elements (Co, Ni, Cr). Nickel-based alloys mainly used in metal-ceramic fabrications.
E.g. Ni-Cr-Mo: Commercial name – Neptune
Ni-Cr: Commercial name – Ticonium.
Ni-Cr-Mo-Be: Commercial name: Rexillium.

General Composition of Nickel-Based Alloys

Ingredients	Weight %
Ni	61–81
Cr	11–27
Mo	2–9
Be	0.5–2
Al	0.2–4.2
Fe	0.1–0.5
Cu	0.1–1.6
Mn	0.1–3.0
Sn	1.25

Nickel-based alloys are the cheapest of all alloys.

Properties

Biological properties: Nickel may produce allergic reaction and also inhalation of toxic vapor or dust causes lung cancer. Beryllium may cause dermatitis and inhalation of dust causes berylliosis (flue-like symptoms and granulomata of the lungs).

Precautions: The work area should be well-ventilated and good exhaust system should be installed to remove the fumes and dust during melting.

Chemical properties: Decreases tarnish and corrosion because of the passivating effect.

Passivation: It is the formation of an impervious layer (Cr_2O_3) on the surface, when the base metal alloys containing Cr, Ti, or Al are exposed to atmospheric oxygen. This layer protects alloy from tarnish and corrosion.

Thermal properties
- **Melting range:** 1155–1304°C.
- **COTE** nearly mismatches with ceramics.

Physical properties
Density: 7.8–8.4 gm/cc.
- *Hardness:* High hardness, 175–360 VHN, makes them very difficult to cut, grind and polish.
- **Yield strength:** 310–828 MPa.
- **Modulus of elasticity:** 150–210 GPa. These are very stiff materials thus thickness of copings can be reduced to 0.3 mm.
- *Sag resistance:* Higher sag resistance. So these alloys are more stable at porcelain firing temperature.
- *Casting shrinkage:* Since melting point of these alloys is high, it undergoes more casting shrinkage. So greater mold expansion is needed to compensate this.
- *Porcelain bonding:* These alloys form an adequate oxide layer because of the presence of passivating elements, such as Cr, Ti, and Al, which is essential for successful porcelain bonding. The bonding mechanisms between metal and ceramic have been discussed in the Dental Ceramic chapter of this book.

Advantages

- Less expensive.
- Resistance to tarnish and corrosion.
- Low density (lighter in weight).
- Greater ductility and percent elongation.
- Less brittle than Co-Cr alloys.

Disadvantages

- Nickel vapor inhalation causes lung cancer.
- Beryllium vapor inhalation causes berylliosis.
- High fusion temperature.
- High hardness.

Uses

- Used mainly for metal-ceramic crowns and bridges.

Cobalt Based Alloys

Cobalt based alloys have bright lustrous, hard, strong, and non-corrosion and tarnishing qualities.
E.g. Co-Cr: Commercial name – Vitallium.
Co-Cr-Ni: Commercial name – Ultra 100 (Unitec)
Co-Cr-Ru: Commercial name – Genesis II
Co-Cr-W-Ru: Commercial name – Novarex.

Composition

Ingredients	Weight %
Co	35 – 65
Cr	23 – 30
Ni	0 – 20
Mo	0 – 70
Fe	0 – 5
C	0.4
Mn, Bi, Pt	Trace

Properties

Biological properties: These are highly biocompatible, non-toxic and nonirritant alloys.

Chemical properties: High tarnish and corrosion resistance when compared to nickel-based alloys because of the presence of chromium as basic element.

Mechanical properties
- **Density:** 8–9 gm/cc.
- **Fusion temperature:** 1250°C–1480°C.

- **Yield strength:** 700–800 MPa.
- **Modulus of elasticity:** 200–250 GPa.
- **Hardness:** 300–432 VHN. Hardness is very high so cutting, grinding and polishing is difficult.
- *Casting shrinkage:* Due to high fusion temperature casting shrinkage is high so more mold expansion is needed to compensate this.

Advantages

- Lighter in weight.
- Good mechanical properties.
- Good tarnish and corrosion resistance.
- Good biocompatibility.
- Less expensive.

Disadvantages

- More casting shrinkage.
- High hardness.
- Low ductile and malleability and more brittle in nature.
- High fusion temperature.

Uses
- Mainly used for cast removable partial denture frameworks.
- Denture bases.
- Crown and bridges.
- Bar connectors.

Titanium Alloys

Titanium and its alloys have been adopted in dentistry because of its light weight, good strength and ability to passivated (Fig. 14.2).
They are mainly used in:
- Metal-ceramic restorations.
- Partial denture frameworks.
- Crown and bridges.
- Implants.

Pure Titanium or C$_p$Ti (Commercially Pure Titanium)

Composition
Pure titanium: 100 Wt%.
Trace amounts of oxygen (0.18%) and iron (0.20–0.05).

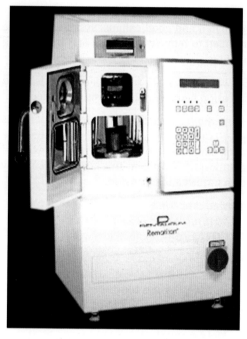

Fig. 14.2 Casting machine for titanium alloys

Allotropic forms: Titanium undergoes allotropic changes from HCP (α–Titanium) martensitic form to BCC (β–Titanium) austenitic form when heated above 883°C.

Properties
- Excellent biocompatibility.
- Good tarnish and corrosion resistance because of the presence of passivating elements.
- Melting point: 1668°C.
- Density: 4.1 gm/cc.
- Yield strength: 340 MPa.
- Ultimate tensile strength: 345 MPa.
- Hardness: 210 VHN
- COTE: 8.4×10^{-6} /°C.

Advantages
- Excellent biocompatibility.
- Good resistance to tarnish and corrosion.
- Good mechanical properties.

Disadvantages
- High melting point.
- Highly active at higher temperatures.
- Poor fit.

Titanium Alloys

Alloying other metals with titanium enables attainment of the benefits of lower melting point and casting temperature and also it provides a means to stabilize or expand either the α–phase or β–phase.

E.g. Ti-30Pd, Ti-20Cu, Ti-15V, Ti-6Al-4V.

More frequently used alloy is Ti-6Al-4V, which has α + β structure and has better mechanical properties for casting purpose.

Composition

Ti-30Pd	Ti-6Al-4V
Ti – 70%	Ti – 90%
Pd – 30%	Al – 6%
Trace elements	V – 4%
	Trace elements

Properties
- Excellent biocompatibility.
- Good tarnish and corrosion resistance because of the presence of passivating metal.
- The reaction of the tissues that contacts titanium and its alloys are extremely mild and direct in bone growth or osseointegration does occur.
- Yield strength: 870 MPa.
- Ultimate tensile strength: 925 MPa.
- Hardness: 320 VHN.
- Modulus of elasticity: 117 GPa.
- Melting temperature: 1440°C.
- Very low density: 4.5 gm/cc.

Casting procedure: Because of very high melting point and oxygen sensitivity, phosphate bonded investment with Al_2O_3, ZrO_2, and MgO refractory material is needed for the investment.

Electric tungsten arc or induction melting in vacuum, or inert argon gas atmosphere is required because of high fusion temperature. Modified casting machines with added compression as well as vacuum suction techniques are required.

Advantages
- Low density.
- Excellent biocompatibility.
- Good tarnish and corrosion resistance.
- Good mechanical properties.

Disadvantages
- Expensive.
- Oxygen sensitivity (special investment is required).
- High fusion temperature (tungsten arc or induction melting is needed).

Uses
- Metal-ceramic restorations.
- Dental implants.
- Partial denture framework.
- Complete denture base.
- Bar connectors.

Aluminum Bronze (Cu-Zn-Al)

Common name is Japanese gold and these alloys are copper rich alloys.

Composition

Copper: 54 wt%
Zinc: 34 wt%
Aluminum: 12 wt%.

Properties
- Low tarnish and corrosion resistance (formation of copper sulfide gives the dark color).
- Low density: 8–8.2 gm/cc.
- Low fusion temperature: 750–850°C. Gypsum-bonded investment material and ordinary gas torch flame is needed for melting of an alloy.
- Mechanical properties are similar to type-II and type-III dental casting gold alloys.
- Gold-like appearance hence the name "Japanese gold".

Advantages
- Less expensive
- Low density
- Low fusion temperature.

Disadvantages
- Low tarnish and corrosion resistance.
- Mechanical properties are inferior to other base metal alloys.

Table 14.5 Comparison of selected indirect restorative dental materials

Factors	Ceramic	Metal-Ceramic	Cast-Gold (High Noble) Alloys	Base metal alloys (Non-Noble)
General description	Porcelain, ceramic or glass-like fillings and crowns.	Ceramic is fused to an underlying metal structure to provide strength to a filling, crown or bridge.	Alloy of gold, copper and other metals resulting in a strong, effective filling, crown or bridge.	Alloys of non-noble metals with silver appearance resulting in high-strength crowns and bridges.
Principal uses	Inlays, onlays, crowns and esthetic veneers.	Crowns and fixed bridges.	Inlays, onlays, crowns and fixed bridges.	Crowns, fixed bridges and partial dentures.
Leakage and recurrent decay	Sealing ability depends on materials, underlying tooth structure and procedure used for placement.	The commonly used methods used for placement provide a good seal against leakage. The incidence of recurrent decays is similar to other restorative procedures.		
Durability	Brittle material, may fracture under heavy biting loads. Strength depends greatly on quality of bond to underlying tooth structure.	Very strong and durable.	High corrosion resistance prevents tarnishing; high strength and toughness resist fracture and wear.	
Cavity preparation considerations	Because strength depends on adequate ceramic thickness, it requires more aggressive tooth reduction during preparation.	Including both ceramic and metal creates a stronger restoration than ceramic alone; moderately aggressive tooth reduction is required.	The relative high strength of metals in this section requires the least amount of healthy tooth structure removal.	
Clinical considerations	These are multiple-step procedures requiring highly accurate clinical and laboratory processing. Most restorations require multiple appointments and laboratory fabrication.			
Resistance to wear	Highly resistant to wear, but ceramic can rapidly wear opposing teeth if its surface becomes rough.	Highly resistant to wear, but ceramic can rapidly wear opposing teeth if its surface becomes rough.	Resistant to wear and gentle to opposing teeth.	
Resistance to fracture	Prone to fracture when placed under tension or on impact.	Ceramic is prone to impact fracture; the metal has high strength.	Highly resistant to fracture.	

Contd…

Contd...

Factors	Ceramic	Metal-Ceramic	Cast-Gold (High Noble) Alloys	Base metal alloys (Non-Noble)
Biocompatibility	Well-tolerated.	Well-tolerated, but some patients may show allergenic sensitivity to base metals.	Well-tolerated.	Well tolerated, but some patients may show allergenic sensitivity to base metals.
Post-placement sensitivity	Sensitivity, if present, is usually not material-specific.			
	Low thermal conductivity reduces the likelihood of discomfort from hot and cold.	High thermal conductivity may result in early post-placement discomfort from hot and cold.		
Esthetics	Color and translucency mimic natural tooth appearance.	Ceramic can mimic natural tooth appearance, but metal limits translucency.	Metal colors do not mimic natural teeth.	
Relative cost to patient	Higher; requires at least two office visits and laboratory services.	Higher; requires at least two office visits and laboratory services.		
Average number of visits to complete	Minimum of two; matching esthetics of teeth may require more visits.	Minimum of two; matching esthetics of teeth may require more visits.	Minimum of two.	

Uses

- Crown and bridges.
  Comparison of selected indirect restorations was given in Table 14.5.

SUGGESTED READING

1. Baran GR. The metallurgy of Ni-Cr alloys for fixed prosthodontics. J Prosthet Dent. 1983;50:639.
2. Clark GCF, Williams DF. The effects of proteins on metallic corrosion. J Biomed Mater Res. 1982;16:125.
3. Geis-Gerstofer J, Passler K. Studies of the influence of the content on corrosion behaviour and mechanical properties of Ni25Cr10Mo alloys. Dent Mater. 1993; 9: 177.
4. German RM, Wright DC, Gallant RF. *In vitro* tarnish measurements on fixed prosthodontics alloys. J Prosthet Dent. 1982;47: 399.
5. Gülþen Can, Gül Akpýnar, Ahmet Aydýn. The release of elements from dental casting alloy into cell-culture medium and artificial saliva. Eur J Dent. 2007;1:86-90.
6. Iijima M, Yuasa T, Endo K, Muguruma T, Ohno H, Mizoguchi I. Corrosion behavior of ion implanted nickel-titanium orthodontic wire in fluoride mouth rinse solutions. Dent Mater J. 2010;29(1): 53-8.
7. Kikuchi M. Dental alloy sorting by the thermoelectric method. Eur J Dent. 2010;4:66-70.
8. Leinfelder KF. An evaluation of casting alloys used for restorative procedures. J Am Dent Assoc. 1997;128:37.
9. Lucas LC, Lemons JE. Biodegradation of restorative metal systems. Adv Dent Res. 1992;65: 32.
10. Malhotra ML. Dental gold casting alloys: a review. Trends Tech Contemp Dent Lab. 1991;8:73.

11. Malhotra ML. New generation of palladium-indium-silver dental cast alloys: a review. Trends Tech Contemp Dent Lab. 1992;9: 65.
12. Pekkan G, Pekkan K, Hatipoglu MG, Tuna SH. Comparative radiopacity of ceramics and metals with human and bovine dental tissues. J Prosthet Dent. 2011;106:109-17.
13. Vallittu PK, Kokkonen M. Deflection fatigue of cobalt-chromium, titanium and gold alloy cast denture clasps. J Prosthet Dent. 1995; 74:412.
14. Wostmann B, Blober T, Gouentenoudis M, Balkenhol M, Ferger P. Influence of margin design on the fit of high-precious alloy restorations in patients. J Dent. 2005;33:611-8.
15. Wostmann B, Blober T, Gouentenoudis M, Markus Balkenhol. Paul Ferger. Influence of margin design on the fit of high-precious alloy restorations in patients. J Dent. 2005;33:611-8.
16. Yong T, De Long B, Goodkind RJ, et al. Leaching of Ni, Cr and Be ions from base metal alloys in an artificial environment. J Prosthet Dent. 1992;68:692.

Casting Procedure for Dental Alloys

15

Many dental restorations such as inlays, crowns, RPD frameworks. etc. are made by casting. Casting can be defined as the act of forming an object in a mold. The fundamental principles are same, regardless of the size of the casting; the techniques differ only in sprue design, type of investment method of melting the alloy.

CLINICAL EVALUATION OF CASTING FIT

The objective of the casting procedure is to provide a metallic duplication of missing tooth structure with as much accuracy as possible. Casting fit mainly depends on the solubility and disintegration of the dental cement or luting agent used for cementation. If the luting agent is highly soluble in oral fluids that reduces the quality of fit of casting and also leads to the marginal leakage and secondary caries. The marginal adaptation also depends on the differences in COTE of tooth and the casting.

CASTING TECHNIQUE

The objective of casting procedure is to provide a metallic duplication of missing tooth structure with as much accuracy as possible. The lost wax casting process, through one of the oldest existing technologies, is still the preferred and most commonly used method for casting dental restorations.

The following are the steps involved in the casting procedure:

1. Preparation of tooth or teeth to receive a cast restoration.
2. Make an impression of the prepared tooth.
3. Preparation of die.
4. Preparation of a wax pattern.
5. Sprue the wax pattern.
6. Invest the wax pattern.
7. Burn out procedure.
8. Casting.
9. Recovery.
10. Finishing and polishing.
11. Cementation on the prepared tooth.

Tooth Preparation

The operation field should be isolated using a rubber dam. A cavity is then prepared on the tooth or teeth without any under cuts. Diamond burs are used to cut the enamel on occlusal surface. A proper finish line should be there in the preparation to which the pattern preparation will be done.

Impression Making

An impression of the prepared tooth or teeth is recorded with a suitable impression material followed by cast pouring.

Preparation of Master Die

After recording the impression of patients prepared teeth, a positive replica of that is prepared on which the subsequent procedures will be done. This is called as die.

To pour a die, a set of materials are available which are different from normal materials are used for the preparation of casts. The various die materials have been discussed in die materials chapter of this book.

In conclusion, there are varieties of die materials that can be used. Although they may be harder and stronger than die stone but it is difficult to prepare such dies. So usually die stone will be prepared in the laboratory.

Waxing

Wax is applied over dies that will be replaced by molten metal in lost wax technique. For the casting of noble metal alloys the choice of material is inlay wax, which is of two types according to ADA specification no. 4, type–I medium for direct technique and type–II for indirect technique (soft). Both the types have a flow of 70–90% above 45°C. With 20°C rise the wax will expand as much as 0.7% and contraction will be about 0.35%.

During adding stresses may incorporate which may distort the pattern later. It is poor conductor of heat so time is required for uniform softening and cooling of the wax. To avoid distortion it is advised to invest the pattern as early as possible.

The requirements and selection criteria of inlay casting wax to prepare the wax patterns have been discussed in Dental Waxes chapter of this book.

Technique of Waxing

The first step is to use a sharp black or red pencil and precisely survey all margins. This is valuable when trying to locate them after the wax has been applied.

Next a die lubricant must be applied to the die. This is light oil like film (μ - film, a colloidal suspension of wax), otherwise it becomes impossible to remove the wax pattern from the die as a single unit. The lubricant must be very thin to avoid any discrepancy between the pattern and die. It must be necessary to apply largely more than one coat as the stone usually largely absorbs the first coat. Two types of waxing techniques can be used.

1. *Direct technique:* In this type–I wax is softened and forced into the prepared tooth cavity and is directly carved in the mouth.

2. *Indirect technique:* Pattern is prepared on the die, which is positive replica of prepared tooth, outside the mouth.

Wax Addition Procedure

Wax is uniformly softened and melted. The melted wax may be added in layers with spatula or a waxing instrument or it may be painted with a brush. The prepared cavity is over-filled and the wax is then carved to the proper contour. When margins are being carved, extreme care should be taken to avoid abrading any surface of stone die. A silk cloth may be used for a final polishing pattern rubbing towards the margins. Prepared pattern should be invested as early as possible.

Spruing

Purpose of Spruing

- To form and mount for the wax pattern and fix the pattern in sprue so that a mold can be made.
- To create a channel for elimination of wax during burn out procedure.
- To form a channel for the ingress of molten alloy during casting.
- To compensate for alloy shrinkage during solidification.

Sprue Size and Design

The sprue must be large enough so that it remains open until the casting solidifies, and short enough to allow rapid filling of the mold cavity. Large and small inlays require a sprue that is one μ-gauge (4–5 mm long) and 16 gauge (3–4 mm long) respectively. Long and small crowns require 10 and 12 gauges respectively with an average sprue length of 4–5 mm.

Point of Attachment

The bulkiest part of the pattern is the best location for attaching the sprue. This will usually be on the mesial or distal part of the pattern. When the pattern has more than one surface the sprue will be angled at near 45° to horizontal plane, to facilitate metal flow. If two bulky positions are separated by a thin cross-section a y-shaped sprue must be added. Various types of sprues and their attachment to the wax pattern are shown in Figure 15.1A.

Sprue Selection

The wax sprue is the most commonly used. A hallow metal pin is preferable to a solid metal pin because of its stronger attachment. Sticky wax must be used to fill the hallow sprue cone before use. Plastic sprues (Fig. 15.1B) are not recommended because of their higher flow temperatures and thermal expansion characteristics, which make it difficult to eliminate the sprue.

Patterns may be sprued either directly or indirectly. The sprue former provides a direct connection between the pattern area and the sprue base or crucible former area in the former, whereas in latter a connector or reservoir bar is positioned between the pattern and crucible former. For multiple single units in fixed partial dentures it is common to use indirect spruing.

A reservoir should be added to a spruing network to prevent localized shrinkage porosity when the molten alloy fills the heated casting ring; the pattern area should solidify first and the reservoir last. Because of its large mass of alloy and position in the heat center of the ring, the reservoir remains molten to furnish liquid alloy into the mold as it solidifies.

The space between the wax pattern and the end of casting ring should be 6 mm as shown in Figures 15.3A and B.

If the pattern is less than 6 mm from the end of the casting ring, there will not be enough thickness of investment to keep the molten alloy from breaking through. If there is more than 6 mm of space, the alloy will solidify before the entrapped air can escape resulting in back pressure porosity.

Wax Pattern Removal

The sprue former should be attached to the wax pattern. The pattern can be removed directly in

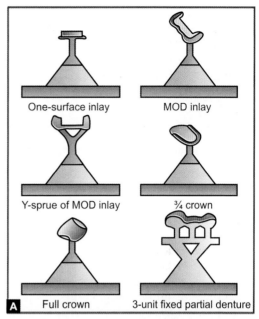

One-surface inlay   MOD inlay

Y-sprue of MOD inlay   ¾ crown

A   Full crown   3-unit fixed partial denture

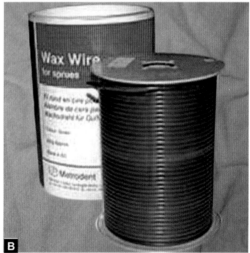

B

Figs 15.1A and B (A) Different types of sprues and their attachments (B) Plastic sprues

the line with its path of withdrawal from the die. Teasing wax pattern should be avoided during removal.

Casting Ring Liners

The most casting techniques the investment mold sets and is heated in a casting ring made

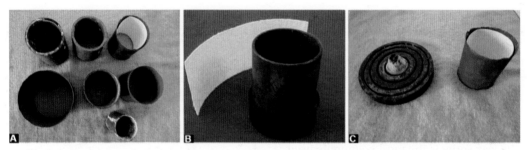

Figs 15.2A to C (A) Metal casting ring (B) Casting ring and liner (C) Sprue base and casting ring with liner

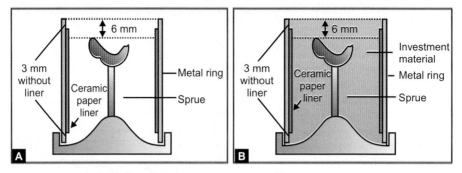

Figs 15.3A and B (A) Wax pattern in casting ring prior to investing
(B) Wax pattern in casting ring after investing

of heat resisting alloy. Souder, who advocated the use of asbestos tape to provide the necessary cushioning, first recognized the need for a soft ring liner to eliminate or at least reduce restraint to investment expansion by the ring. Since asbestos readily absorbs water, the liner was prewetted to prevent its absorbing water from the unset investment mix.

The technique of lining a casting ring with asbestos was first described by "Taylor and coworkers" and from the use of wet asbestos was a standard procedure. This makes additional water available to the setting investment and causes an increased setting expansion.

To ensure uniform expansion, the liner is cut to fit the inside diameter of the casting ring with no overlap as shown in Figures 15.2A to C. The dry liner is tacked in position with sticky wax and then is used either dry or wet. With a water liner technique, the lined ring is immersed in water for some time, and then the excess water shaken away. Squeezing the liner should be avoided because this leads to variable amounts of water removal and uneven expansion.

Recently attention has been drawn to the danger that asbestos fibers in casting ring liners could cause asbestosis. It is claimed that acceptable threshold limit for asbestos fibers in air can be considerable exceeded when casting are removed from asbestos lined castings. For this reason, because of the increasing unavailability asbestos products, two alternate materials such as ceramic and cellulose liners have replaced asbestos as a ring liner.

1. Ceramic materials based on the aluminosilicate fibers, which at atmospheric pressure will not absorb water and are normally used dry. The aluminosilicate ceramic materials are highly heat resistant. Although ceramic liners do not absorb water under atmospheric conditions they readily absorb large amount of water when vacuum investing techniques are used. This markedly lowers the water/powder ratio of

the investment mix, reducing its working time and more importantly increasing both the setting and thermal expansion to an uncontrolled extent.

2. Cellulose, which readily absorbs water and like asbestos must be prewetted. Cellulose liners, being paper products, are burned away during the burn out procedure. So a technique must be found to secure the investment in the ring.

The designed length of the liner remains a matter of controversy. If the length of the liner is shorter than the ring itself the investment is confined at one or both ends of the ring. The expansion of the investment is always greater the unrestricted longitudinal direction than in the lateral direction, i.e. towards the ring itself. Therefore, it is desirable to reduce the expansion in the longitudinal direction. The ring liner should be placed some short (3.25 mm) of ends of the casting ring as shown in Figures 15.3A and B; to produce more uniform expansion; thus, there is less chance for distortion of the wax pattern and mold.

Investing

After the wax pattern has been prepared and sprued, a surface tension reducing agent is applied; it then should be invested promptly. To invest the prepared wax pattern three types of investment materials are available such as gypsum bonded, phosphate bonded and silica bonded investments. Former one is used for gold casting alloys and later two are used for high fusing alloys. Usually these materials are supplied as powder and liquid. They contain, in general, a binder, refractory and modifiers.

Refractory materials are used to withstand high temperature and to provide thermal expansions to compensate for the solidification shrinkage of alloys.

Gypsum bonded investments cannot be used for high fusing alloys because at temperatures above 1100°C decomposition of investment occurs, that will spoil the casting. But it is ideally suited for gold casting, which melts at around 700°C.

Phosphate and silica bonded investments are used for high fusing alloys and a good fit restorations can be obtained. These materials can also be used for gold casting alloys but usually gypsum bonded is preferred for gold alloys.

Investing Procedure

The proper and correct water/powder ratios of the investment mix, a required number of spatulation turns and a proper investing technique are essential to obtain acceptable casting results. There are two different methods of investing the wax pattern:
1. Hand investing
2. Vacuum investing.

Hand investing: The correct amount of water or special liquid is measured and placed in a rubber-mixing bowl and the investment powder is added to the water or special liquid in the bowl. The powder and liquid are mixed briefly with a plaster spatula until all the powder is wetted and then the mix is spatulated. During spatulation, one should follow the manufacturer's recommendations carefully; because setting expansion is critically depending on the number of spatulation turns.

After the spatulation, the mixing bowl is placed on vibrator to remove air bubbles and also to collect the mix from the sides of the bowl. Then paint the wax pattern with investment mix by using a camel hairbrush. During this, the sprue base should be held firmly in a hand to prevent distortion of wax pattern. Use vibratory forces to prevent air entrapment. Then inlay ring is placed over the sprue base and filled. The ring is filled by holding it with slight angle so that the investment will flow slowly down its side to fill the bottom to the top. The filled ring is then set aside for the investment to set completely, which usually requires 45–60 minutes.

Vacuum investing procedure: The powder and water or special liquid are mixed in a specially designed vacuum investing equipment (Fig. 15.4) under vacuum and the mixed investment is permitted to flow into the ring around the

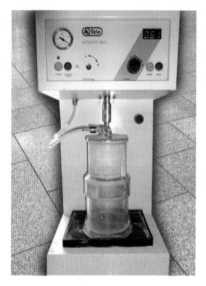

Fig. 15.4 Vacuum investing machine

wax pattern with the vacuum present. Although vacuum does not remove all the air from the investment and the inlay ring, the incorporation of air usually is reduced to such a degree that a smooth adoption of the investment to the pattern can be obtained in this manner. Vacuum investing often yields casting with improved surfaces when compared to castings produced from patterns that are hand invested. The degree of difference between the two procedures depends to a great extent on the care used in hand investing.

Whether hand or vacuum investing procedures employed in filling the casting ring, the investment should be allowed to harden in air if the thermal expansion technique is to be used, on the other hand, if the hygroscopic water immersion technique is to be employed. The casting ring containing the investment should be placed immediately in a water bath at 37°C and the investment is allowed to harden under water.

Divestment Technique

An optional modality to casting fabrication is the divestment technique. Briefly it involves investing of the die and pattern together. The die,

therefore, becomes an actual part of the mold cavity. The basic nature of divestment material is not unlike that of silica and gypsum products except in the liquid, which is an aqueous mixture of 30% ethyl silicate. It differs from conventional investment in setting and thermal expansion. It has a large setting expansion with a small thermal expansion.

Wax Elimination or Burn Out

Once the investment is set for an appropriate period approximately 1 hour for most gypsum and phosphate bonded investments, it is ready for burn out. The procedures for two types of investments are similar. The crucible former and any metal sprue former are carefully removed. Any debris from the in gate area is cleaned with a camel hair brush. If the burn out procedure does not immediately follow the investing, the investing ring is placed in a humidor at 100% humidity. If at all possible, the investment should not be permitted to dry out. Rehydration of set investment that has been stored for an extended period may not replenish all of the lost water.

The invested rings are placed in a room temperature furnace and heated to a prescribed maximum temperature. For gypsum bonded investments that temperature can be either 468°C for the hygroscopic or 650°C for the thermal expansion technique and for phosphate bonded investments, the maximum temperature setting may range from 700°C–870°C depending on the type of alloy selected. See the Figures from 15.5A to D for steps involved in burnout process.

During burn out, the ingredients of inlay wax is composed of C, H and N will decompose and form CO_2, water and NO, all of which are in gaseous form and can be easily eliminated. The formation of these gases however depends on the pressure of a sufficient supply of oxygen, the relatively high temperature of oven and adequate time of heating of the ring.

During burn out, some of the melted wax is absorbed by the investment and residual carbon produced by ignition of the liquid wax becomes trapped in the porous investment. It is advisable to begin the burn out procedure while the mold is still wet. Water trapped in pores of the

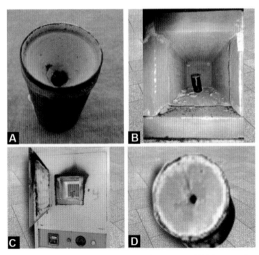

Figs 15.5A to D (A) Before wax burnout, (B) Placing the casting ring in burnout furnace, (C) During burn out and (D) After wax elimination

investments reduces the absorption of wax from the mold. This process is facilitated by placing the ring with the sprue hole down over slot in a ceramic tray in the burn out furnace.

Ringless Casting

To save more time, the use of a ring and a liner is eliminated, the metal ring being replaced with a plastic ring that is tapered so that once the investment has set it can be pushed out of the ring, held for a specified time to complete setting and then placed directly into the hot furnace. Obviously, the expansion on setting is different (more) when a lined ring is used so that the changes in overall fit must be considered. The required expansion may be adjusted by varying the liquid concentration. The system is called the power cast ringless system, consists of three sizes of rings and a special investment liquid. This system is suited for the casting of alloys that require greater mold expansion than traditional gold-based alloys.

Casting Crucibles

Generally, three types of casting crucibles are available such as clay, carbon and quartz (including zircon-alumina) (Fig. 15.6).

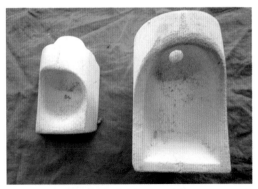

Fig. 15.6 Casting crucibles

Clay crucibles are appropriate for many of crown and bridge alloys such as high noble and noble types.

Carbon crucibles can be used not only for high noble crown and bridge alloys but also for the higher fusing gold based metal ceramic alloys.

Quartz crucibles are recommended for high fusing alloys of any type. They are specially suited for alloys that have a high melting range and are sensitive to carbon contamination. For example, nickel based, cobalt based and Pd-Ag alloy.

Methods of Melting Alloys

Torch Melting

The most common method of heating gold alloys for full cast metal restorations have been by the use of a gas-air blow torch. The main objective of melting procedure is to develop the most efficient gas-air flame that will quickly yet clearly melt the metal. The relative proportions of gas and air influence the temperature of the flame.

The properly adjusted flame contains well-defined component parts as shown in Figure 15.7. The most part of the flame can be identified by the conical areas. (1) The inner-most, conical portion of the gas flame has no heat content and is only gas and air (or oxygen) mixture. (2) Next outer green colored cone is the combustion zone, can not be used. (3) Next outer, pale blue colored zone, is the reducing flame, which is the hottest part and should be used for alloy melting. (4) The outer most yellow colored oxidising zone also should never be used.

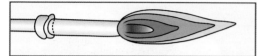

Fig. 15.7 Different zones of flame

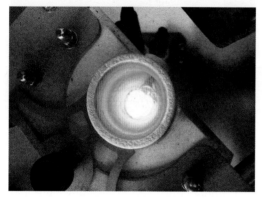

Fig. 15.8 Molten alloy in the crucible

Air/acetylene and oxygen/acetylene generate much higher temperatures with later providing the hottest flame. Though the air or oxygen/acetylene flame have the advantage of melting alloys faster than the gas/air or oxygen modes.

The alloy first appears spongy and then small globules of fused metal appear, following which the bulk of the alloy assumes an spheroidal shape and begin to slide down to the bottom of the crucible (Fig. 15.8). If this is to be cast by a centrifugal machine, bring the casting ring out the burn out oven and place it securely in the casting cradle as the metal begins to liquefy.

Electrical Melting

Electrical mode of melting includes electric resistance melting, which is suitable for all gold alloys, as well as induction melting and electric arch melting, which are capable of melting the Co-Cr and titanium alloys. Gold and palladium alloys require a reducing atmosphere as supplied by the use of the middle cone of the torch, with flux being added to the melt. A greater convenience is approached by the electrical furnace, which uses a carbon (rather than ceramic) crucible thus providing a reducing environment throughout the melting regime.

Casting

Time Allowable for Casting

The burn out oven and the casting machine must be convenient to each other to avoid any time loss during the actual casting process. To prevent any noticeable contraction in the investment as the temperature drops, the casting should be made within one minute upon removal from the furnace.

A cool or cold mold is not indicated for any casting technique. Although mold temperatures in the low heat technique is low, an accurate casting will result when the mold temperature is maintained and metal solidification will not be premature.

Casting Machines

These are the devices, which force the molten alloy into the investment mold required for casting.

Alloys are melted in one of three following ways, depending on the available types of casting machines.

1. The alloy is melted in a separate crucible by a torch flame and the metal is cast into the mold by centrifugal force.
2. The alloy is melted electrically by a resistance or induction furnace, then the casting into the mold centrifugally by motor or spring action.
3. The alloy is melted as in the first two ways, but it is cast by air pressure, a vacuum or both.

Centrifugal Casting Machine

The metal is melted by a torch flame in a glazed ceramic crucible and attach the crucible to the broken arm of the casting machine (Fig. 15.9A). The broken arm feature accelerates the initial rotational speed of this crucible and casting ring. Thus increasing the linear speed of the liquid casting alloy as it moves into and through the mold. Once the metal has reached the casting temperature and the heated casting ring is in position, the machine is released and the spring triggers the rotational motion (Fig. 15.9B).

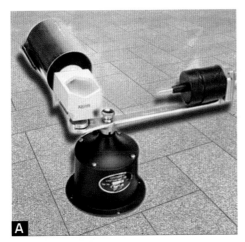

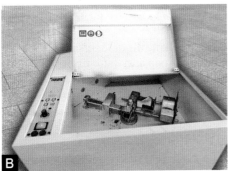

Figs 15.9A and B (A) Spring driven centrifugal casting machine (B) Motor driven centrifugal casting machine

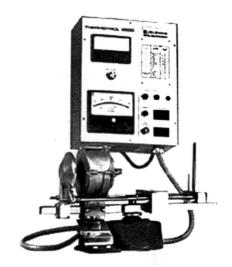

Fig. 15.10 Electrical resistance casting machine

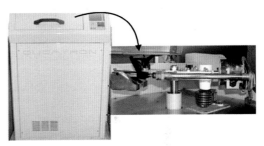

Fig. 15.11 Induction casting machine

Electrical Resistance-Heated Casting Machine

In this instance there is an automatic melting of the metal in a graphite crucible within a furnace rather than by use of a torch flame (Fig. 15.10).

Advantages
- Solidification can be delayed, since sprue former contains molten alloy.
- Proper adjustment of temperature of the alloy.

Induction Casting Machine

With this unit, an induction field that develops within a crucible surrounded by water-cooled metal tubing melts the metal. Once the metal reaches the casting temperature, it is forced into the mold by air pressure, vacuum or both, at the other end of the ring (Fig. 15.11). The device has become popular for base metal alloys and noble alloy castings.

Recovery and Cleaning the Cast

After the casting is completed, the molten alloy appears like a red button in the investment as shown in Figure 15.12A. Then the ring is removed and quenched in water. The Figure 15.12B shows the casting after cooling to room temperature. Advantages of quenching:
1. The noble metal alloy is left in an annealed condition for burnishing and polishing and similar procedures.
2. When the water contacts the hot investment, the investment becomes soft and granular and the casting is more easily cleaned.

After quenching, the casting is retrieved by careful breaking the investment. Some

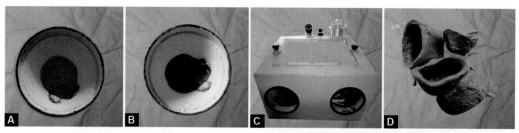

Figs 15.12A to D (A) Immediately after casting—molten metal can be seen in the casting investment (B) Cooling to room temperature (C) Sand blaster (D) Metal casting after recovery

investment may be sticking to the casting and that can be removed by a process called sand blasting. Sand blasting apparatus can be seen in Figure 15.12C and the casting after sand blasting is done as shown in Figure 15.12D.

The dark surface of the alloy due to oxidation and tarnish can be removed by a process known as "pickling", which consists of heating the discolored casting in an acid. Commonly used acids for picking are 50% HCl 'or' H_2SO_4. In pickling, costing is placed in a test tube or dish and acid is poured and heated to 50°C–70°C. Boiling should be avoided as it releases fumes, they may corrode laboratory furnishings.

Pickling removes oxide layer and also residual investment.

Ultrasonic devices are also available for cleaning the casting as one commercial pickling solution made of acid salts.

Finishing

After the casting has been pickled and thoroughly washed, it must be carefully examined to determine if any imperfections are present. These include incomplete margins or small nodules on the casting. The nodules are removed by using inverted cone bur.

If the casting is satisfactory, it is separated from the sprue and button by using carborundum disk.

When the proximal contours and occlusal contacts are satisfactory the final finishing should be done prior to cementation.

After occlusal adjustment in the casting it may be smoothened to final contours using small round finishing burs, small peter disks,

small rubber wheels. Additional polishing may also be done by use of a wheel brush with a polishing agent such as "Tripoli", lightly over the metal surfaces but be careful that the polishing material is not lodged in the internal portion of the casting.

After blocking the drain in the sink scrub the casting with soap and water using a toothbrush and then place the casting in the ultrasonic cleaner, following which it should be ready for cementation (Figs 15.12A to D).

Cementation

The final link to a successful cast restoration is dependent upon the care taken during cementation. The process requires hard intermediate cementing materials placed between the casting and the tooth for the purpose of immobilizing the restoration.

The purpose of the cement is to fill the irregularities on the preparation and those on the casting surface to provide a rigid core mechanically lodged in the surface irregularities, resulting in a secure restoration.

Usually for final cementation Zn phosphate, polycarboxylate and GIC are used.

DEFECTS IN CASTING

The precision casting should have an exact shape, size and fitting. If suitable precautions are not taken during casting procedure, there may be chance of casting defects in various steps.

The various casting defects can be classified as follows:

    i. Distortion.

Table 15.1 Causes and remedies for distortion of casting

Causes	Remedies
Careless removal of the wax pattern from the die	Apply lubricant and remove the wax pattern carefully from the die
Release of stresses during manipulation	• Manipulation of wax pattern at high temperature • Invest the wax pattern within one hour • Apply uniform pressure during manipulation
Casting too large— excessive expansion. Casting too small—less expansion	• Controlled setting and thermal expansion • 3 mm gap, free of ring liner at the end restricts the expansion

   ii. Surface roughness and irregularities.
  iii. Porosity.
  iv. Incomplete or missing details.

DISTORTION

Distortion results in the misfit of the prosthesis. Dimensional errors also result in the distortion of the prosthesis. Various causes for distortion in casting and remedies to prevent the distortion were discussed in Table 15.1.

ROUGH SURFACE AND SURFACE IRREGULARITIES

Surface of the dental casting should be an accurate reproduction of the surface of the wax pattern from which it is made. Rough surfaces can be removed by additional finishing and polishing otherwise it affects the esthetic qualities and also leads to corrosion. Irregularities prevent a proper seating of the casting or prosthesis. Various causes for surface irregularities in casting

Table 15.2 Causes and remedies for surface roughness and irregularities of casting

Causes for surface roughness and surface irregularities	Remedies
Rough wax pattern	Wax pattern should be polished well to remove any irregularities
High W/P ratio and large particle size of the investment	Using correct W/P ratio and select investment of correct particle size
Improper mixing of the investment	Homogeneous mixing of investment
Insufficient wetting of the wax pattern	Apply surfactants and vacuum mixing of investment
Air bubbles collection on the wax pattern	Apply surfactants and vacuum mixing of investment
Thin water film on the surface of the wax pattern	Apply surfactants and vacuum mixing of investment
Incomplete dewaxing	Should not be left any wax residue in the mold cavity
Impact of the molten alloy—molten alloy should not strike a weak portion of the mold surface. Molten alloy may fracture or abrade mold surface results in rough surface	Proper spruing can eliminate this problem
Temperature of the alloy too high—attacks the surface of the mold and results in rough surface	Use gas air torch
Too high pressure during casting results in rough surface	A gauge pressure of 0.10–0.14 MPa in an air pressure casting machine

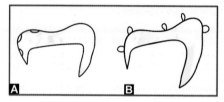

Figs 15.13A and B (A) Rough surface (B) Nodules

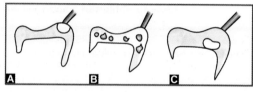

Figs 15.14A to C (A) Localized shrinkage porosity; (B) Micro-porosity; (C) Hot-spot/suck back porosity

and remedies to prevent them were discussed in Table 15.2.

Rough surface can be defined as finely spaced surface imperfections, characterize the total surface area. Irregularities refer to isolated imperfections such as nodules that do not characterize the total surface area (Figs 15.13A and B).

POROSITY

Porosity may occur both within the interior region of the casting and on the external surface. External surface porosities lead to rough surface. Internal porosities will lead to weakening of the casting and also sometimes it may lead to secondary caries (Tables 15.3 and 15.4).

Classification of Porosity

a. *Solidification defects*
   i. Localized shrinkage porosity.
   ii. Microporosity.
   iii. Hot spot or suck back porosity.

b. *Trapped gases*
   i. Pin hole porosity.
   ii. Gas inclusions.
   iii. Subsurface porosities.
   iv. Back pressure porosity.

Solidification Defects

During solidification, almost all metal alloys contract and result in some amount of defects and these defects will be irregular in shape.

Table 15.3 Causes and remedies for solidification defects (porosity) of casting

Types of defect	Causes	Remedies
Localized shrinkage porosity These are the large irregular voids and formed close to the sprue attachment at the bulkiest portion (Fig. 15.14A)	Incomplete feeding of the molten metal during solidification	• Using sprue of correct thickness • Attach sprue to the thickest portion of the wax pattern • Placing the reservoir close to the wax pattern
Microporosity These are fine small irregular voids, formed throughout the casting (Fig. 15.14B)	Rapid solidification or when the mold or casting temperature is too low	Temperature of the casting liquid should be higher
Hot spot or suck back porosity This occurs at the occlusal line angle that is not well-rounded (Fig. 15.14C)	Molten metal alloy impinging on the mold wall near the sprue, the hot spot cause in this region and freezes last. Since the sprue has already solidified, no more molten alloy available and the resulting shrinkage causes suck back porosity	• Flaring of te point of sprue attachment • By reducing the temperature difference between the mold and the molten alloy

Table 15.4 Types of causes and remedies for trapped gas porosity in casting

Type of defect	Causes	Remedies
Pinhole porosity These are small spherical pinhole like porosities occur throughout the casting (Fig. 15.15A)	Entrapment of gas during solidification, e.g. Cu and Ag dissolve oxygen in the liquid state, on solidification absorbed gas expelled and porosity results	• Molten metal should not be kept for longer time and temperature should not be low • Investment should be porous
Gas inclusion porosity These are larger spherical voids (Fig. 15.15B)	• Entrapment of the gas that is mechanically trapped by the molten metal in the mold or that is incorporated during casting procedure • Using the oxidizing zone of the flame instead of reducing zone	• Investment should be porous • Proper adjusting and positioning of the torch flame
Subsurface porosity These are regular small air bubble voids (Fig. 15.15C)	Simultaneous nucleation of solid grains and gas bubbles below the surface of casting	Temperature of the molten metal should be high
Back pressure porosity These are seen at the inner surface of the casting (Fig. 15.15D)	Inability of the air trapped in the mold to escape through the pores in the investment (insufficient venting), which exerts the back-pressure preventing the liquid alloy to occupy the entire mold surface	• Casting and mold temperature should not be low • Proper burn out • Proper W/P ratio of the investment • Thickness of the investment between the tip of the pattern and the end of the ring should not be greater than 6 mm • The extra vent sprue former to the wax pattern

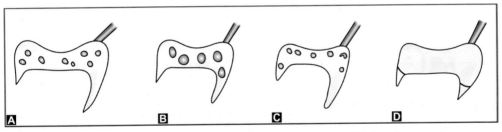

Figs 15.15A to D (A) Pinhole porosity (B) Gas inclusion porosity (C) Subsurface porosity (D) Back pressure porosity

Trapped Gas Porosities

Air and gases like H_2, N, etc. get absorbed during casting procedure are released during solidification result in voids. These defects will be regular in shape.

INCOMPLETE CASTING

Molten alloy is prevented in some manner from complete filling of the mold results in incomplete casting (Fig. 15.16) (Table 15.5).

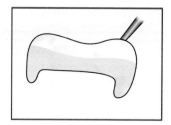

Fig. 15.16 Incomplete casting

Table 15.5 Causes and remedies for incomplete casting

Causes	Remedies
Insufficient venting of the mold	Investment should be porous. Additional venting sprues should be provided.
High viscosity of the molten metal	Temperature of the molten alloy should be high so that viscosity and surface tension lowered, prevents premature solidification.
Incomplete dewaxing that blocks the sprue	Complete dewaxing.

OTHER DEFECTS

FINS

These are the feathers like extensions on the casting surface (Fig. 15.17) (Table 15.6).

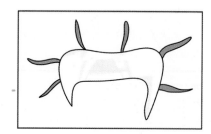

Fig. 15.17 Fins

Table 15.6 Causes and remedies for fins in casting

Causes	Remedies
Produced by the molten alloy enters the cracks formed in the fractured investment that may produce by the overheating of the investment.	• Use proper W/P ratio of investment • Take precautions during wax burn out • Use proper heating technique.

Black Casting

This is the discoloration of the casting (Table 15.7).

Table 15.7 Causes and remedies for discoloration in casting

Causes	Remedies
Overheating of the investment results in decomposition of material releases sulfur dioxide. This combines with the alloy and discoloration occurs	Pickling removes this discoloration
Carbonized wax residue sticks to the surface of the casting leads to discoloration	It can be removed by heating over the flame

SUGGESTED READING

1. Anusavice KJ. Philips' Science of dental materials, ed 11, St Louis, Saunders, 2003.
2. Dootz ER. Technology of casting and soldering alloys for metal-ceramic applications. Ceramic Eng Sci Proc. 1985;6:84.
3. Ito M, Yamagishi T, Oshida Y. Effect of selected physical properties of waxes on investments and casting shrinkage. J Prosthet Dent. 1999;75:211.
4. Mackert JR. An expert system for analysis of casting failures. Int J Prosthodont. 1988;1:268.
5. Powers JM, Sakaguchi RL. Craig's restorative dental materials. ed 12, St Louis, Elsevier, 2006.

Dental Ceramics

16

The word 'ceramic' is derived from the Greek word "Keramikos", which literally means 'burnt stuff', but which has come to mean more specifically a material produced by burning or firing. Ceramic is a compound of metallic and non-metallic elements. Metals are aluminum, calcium, lithium, magnesium, potassium, sodium, tin, titanium and zirconium. Nonmetals are silicon, boron fluorine, and oxygen.

Ceramics are characterized by their refractory nature, hardness, and chemical inertness and susceptible to brittle fracture. Ceramics are used for pottery, porcelain glasses, refractory and abrasives.

Porcelain is defined as a white translucent ceramic that is fired to glazed state. All porcelains and glass ceramics are ceramics but not all ceramics are porcelains or glass ceramics.

CLASSIFICATION OF DENTAL CERAMICS

1. Based on fusion temperature:
   a. High fusing porcelain—1300–1400°C
   b. Medium fusing porcelain—1100–1300°C
   c. Low fusing porcelain—850–1100°C
   d. Ultra-low fusing porcelain—less than 850°C.
2. Based on its use:
   Used for–
   a. Artificial or denture teeth – mainly made from high fusing porcelain
   b. Jacket crowns, bridges, inlays – medium fusing porcelain
   c. Veneers over cast metal crowns (metal ceramics) – low fusing ceramics.
   d. Used for titanium and titanium alloys – ultralow fusing.

3. Based on processing methods:
   a. Condensation and sintering
   b. Pressure molding and sintering
   c. Casting and ceramming
   d. Slip casting
   e. Sintering and glass infiltration
   f. Machining (milling by computer control) – CAD-CAM ceramics.
4. By type:
   a. Feldspathic porcelain
   b. Leucite reinforced
   c. Aluminous porcelain
   d. Alumina
   e. Glass infiltrated porcelain
   f. Glass infiltrated alumina porcelain
   g. Glass ceramic
   h. CAD – CAM ceramics
5. By substructure or core material:
   a. Cast metal
   b. Swaged metal
   c. Glass ceramic
   d. CAD – CAM ceramic
   e. Sintered ceramic core.

CLASSIFICATION OF PORCELAIN CROWN

According to composition the porcelain crown is divided into all-ceramic crowns and porcelain fused to metal (PFM).

All-ceramic crowns
- Feldspar ceramic
- Cast glass ceramics
- Core reinforced
  — Aluminous
  — Injection – molded
  — Magnesia high expansion.

Porcelain Fused Metal (PFM)
- Cast alloy
- Wrought alloy.

DISPENSION

Ceramics are supplied in powder form, which is mixed with water.

Composition

The detailed composition of dental ceramics is discussed in Table 16.1.

Stains

These are supplied in kits and are made in the same way as the concentrated color frits. Stains are often made from low porcelain glasses that they can be applied at temperature below the maturing temperature of the restoration.

These stains are employed as surface colorants or to replicate the enamel check lines, hypo-calcification areas or other defects in the body of porcelain.

MANUFACTURING OF PORCELAIN POWDER

Manufactured by mixing the components, fusing them in a furnace and quenching the fused mass into water. Quenching results in internal stresses that produce considerable cracking and fracturing throughout the glass, this process is known as 'fritting' and the product is called 'frit'. The resultant brittle structure can then be grounded to fine powder to use.

During the prefusing of porcelain, the flux reacts with the outer layer of grains of silica, kaolin (pyrochemical reaction) and partly combines them together.

During subsequent firing in the dental lab, the powder is fused to form the restoration.

Color Frits

Color frits are produced by fusing metallic oxides together with fine glass and feldspar and then regrinding to a powder. These various powders are blended with-pigmented powder frit to produce the proper use and shade.

STRUCTURE OF PORCELAIN

The various components of the porcelain blended together by the manufacturers, results in two principal phases:
1. Vitreous (glass) phase.
2. Crystalline (mineral) phase.

Vitreous (Glass) Phase

Glass is considered to be a noncrystalline solid. The ordered arrangement of glass is more or less localized with a considerable number of disordered units between them. Since such an arrangement may be considered typical of liquid structure and such solids are sometimes called as 'super cooled liquids'. Such a structure is called "vitreous" and the process of formation is known as 'vitrification'.

In ceramic term, vitrification is the development of the liquid phase by the reaction or melting, which on cooling, produces the glass phase. The glass phase formed during the firing process has properties typical of glass such as brittleness, nondirectional fracture pattern, flow under stress and high surface tension in the fluid state. Devitrification is nothing but crystallization of glass. It is not good for glass.

Crystalline (Mineral) Phase

The crystalline phase includes silica and metal oxides as coloring agents or opacifiers. Dental porcelain uses SiO_4 network as the glass-forming matrix.

PROPERTIES

- Excellent biocompatibility.
- Chemically inert in oral cavity.
- Esthetics of porcelain are excellent.

The structure of porcelain restoration is probably most important mechanical property. The structure of porcelain depends upon its composition, surface integrity and presence of voids. The strength is also reduced by the presence of surface ingredients.

Table 16.1 Composition of dental ceramics

	Component	%	Functions
1.	Feldspar (naturally occurring minerals composed of potash [K_2O], soda [Na_2O], alumina and silica). Mixture of K_2O. $Al_2O_3.6\ SiO_2\ Na_2O\ Al_2O_3.6\ SiO_2$	75–85	It is the lowest fusing component, which melts first and flows during firing, initiating these components into a solid mass.
2.	Silica (Quartz)	12–22	1. Strengthens the fired porcelain restoration 2. Remains unchanged at the temperature normally used in firing porcelain and thus contribute stability to the mass during heating by providing framework for the other ingredients.
3.	Kaolin ($Al_2O_3.\ 2SiO_2.\ 2H_2O$) (Hydrated aluminosilicates)	4	1. Used as a binder 2. Increases moldability of the unfired porcelain 3. Imparts opacity to the finished porcelain product
4.	Glass modifiers, e.g. K, Na, or Ca oxides or basic oxides	Minute	They interrupt the integrity of silica network and act as flux. 1. Added to provide porcelain at different firing temperatures. 2. Responsible for lowering the softening temperature of glass and increase fluidity.
5.	Color pigments or frits, e.g. Fe/Ni oxide–brown, Cu oxide–green, MgO - lavender, TiO_2–yellowish brown, Co oxide – blue.	Trace	To obtain the delicate shade necessary to simulate the natural teeth.
6.	Zr/Ce/Sn oxides	Trace	To develop the appropriate opacity.
7.	Uranium oxide	Trace	Acts as opacifier.

- Compressive strength – 330 MPa.
- Diametral tensile strength – 34 MPa – low because of surface defects.
- Transverse strength – 62 to 90 MPa.
- Shear strength – 110 MPa – low due to brittle nature or lack of ductility.
- MOE – 69 GPa
- Surface hardness – 460 KHN – high abrasion resistance.
- Specific gravity – 2.2–2.3 gm/cm^3
- Good insulator.
  - Thermal conductivity – 0.0030.
  - Thermal diffusivity – 0.64 mm^2/sec.
- COTE – 12 × 10^{-6}/°C.
- **Dimensional changes (shrinkage on firing):** During firing any residual water is lost from the material accompanied by loss of any binders that results in volume shrinkage of about 30–40%, due to elimination of voids during sintering. Therefore, a precise control of the condensation and firing technique is required to compensate for such shrinkage value during the construction of porcelain restoration.

METHODS OF STRENGTHENING CERAMICS

The major drawbacks of ceramics are brittleness, low fracture toughness and low tensile strength.

Methods used to overcome the deficiencies of ceramics fall into two categories (Flow chart 16.1).

1. Methods of strengthening brittle materials— occurs through one or both of the two mechanisms.
   a. Development of residual compressive stress within the surface of the material.
      i. Chemical binding
      ii. Thermal tempering
      iii. Thermal compatibility
   b. Interruption of crack propagation through the material.
      i. Dispersion of crystalline phases
      ii. Transformation toughening
2. Methods of designing components to minimize stress concentration and tensile stress.

Methods of Strengthening Brittle Materials (Flow Chart 16.1)

Development of Residual Compressive Stresses within the Surface of the Material

In this method, residual compressive stresses are introduced within the surface of glass and ceramic objects. Strengthening is gained by virtue of the fact that developing of tensile stresses before any net tensile stress develops must first negate these residual stresses.

Flow chart 16.1 Strengthening methods of ceramics

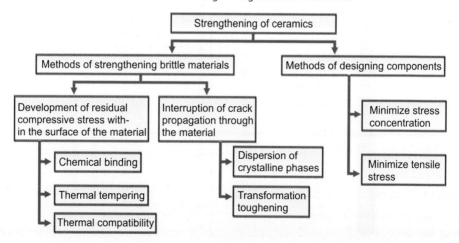

i. *Chemical tempering or ion exchange:* It is one of the most effective methods of introducing residual compressive stresses into the ceramic. In this process the larger K^+ ions exchange the smaller Na^+ ions (a common constituent of variety of glasses). When dental porcelain possessing sufficient soda (Na_2O) is immersed in a KNO_3 salt bath at 400°C for 4 hours, K^+ ions will replace or exchange some of the Na^+ ions located close to the surface layers. The K^+ ions are 35% larger than the Na^+ ions, create larger residual compressive stresses (700 MPa) in the surface of the glass subjected to this treatment. This surface compression results in increased strength of porcelain.

ii. *Thermal tempering:* On rapid cooling the surface of the object from the molten state can introduce residual compressive stresses. The rapid cooling produces skin of glass surrounding soft (molten) core. During solidification, the molten core tends to shrink, but the outer skin remains rigid. This shrinkage in molten core creates the residual tensile stress in core and residual compressive stresses within the outer surface.

iii. *Thermal compatibility:* This method applies to porcelain fused metals. The metal and porcelain should be created with slight mismatch in their thermal contraction coefficient. Typically porcelains have COTE 13.0–14.0 × 10^{-6}/°C and metals have between 13.5–14.5 × 10^{-6}/°C. The difference of 0.5 × 10^{-6}/°C in thermal expansion between metals and porcelain causes the metal to contract slightly more than does the ceramic during cooling after firing the porcelain. This condition puts the ceramic under slight residual compression, which makes it less sensitive to tensile stresses. These are known as thermally compatible system.

Interruption of Crack Propagation through the Material

A dispersed phase, which is capable of obstructing the crack propagation through the material, is reinforced into the glasses or ceramics to strengthen them. Two different types of dispersions are used to interrupt crack propagation.

i. *Dispersion of crystalline phase (Alumina–Al_2O_3) or Aluminous porcelain:* Al_2O_3 is added to glasses as a dispersed phase to strengthen them. Al_2O_3 is a tough crystalline material, which can prevent the crack propagation through them and strengthen the glass. The technique has found application in dentistry in the development of aluminous porcelain for PJC.

ii. *Transformation toughening:* A crystalline material such as 'Partially Stabilized Zirconia' (PSZ) is incorporated into glasses or ceramics. PSZ is capable of undergoing change in crystal structure when placed under stress and can improve the strength. As the refractive index of PSZ is much higher than that of surrounding glass matrix results in scattering of light as it passes through the bulk of porcelain, and this scattering produces an opacifying effect that may not be esthetic in most restorations.

Design of Dental Restoration involving Ceramics

a. *Minimizing tensile stresses:* The design of ceramic should avoid exposure of the ceramic to high tensile stress.

b. *Reducing stress raisers:* The design should also avoid stress concentrations at sharp angles or marked changes in thickness.

MANIPULATION

Fabrication Porcelain Jacket Crown (PJC) or all Ceramic Restorations

General techniques for the construction of porcelain jacket crown are as follows:

1. Tooth preparation
2. An impression is taken with an elastomeric impression material
3. Preparation of die
4. Adaptation of thin sheet of platinum foil

5. Condensation
6. Firing
7. Cooling
8. Staining
9. Glazing
10. Removal of platinum foil
11. Cementation.

After tooth preparation, an impression of prepared tooth is made with an elastomeric impression material and a die is formed by a suitable die material. Now the portions of the die is carefully covered with the thin layer of platinum foil approximately 0.025 mm thick. The platinum matrix retains the porcelain mix in the shape during firing and determines to a greater extent the fit of the restoration.

A proper shade of powder is mixed with water to a consistency and then applied to the platinum foil matrix in several increments.

Condensation

Condensation is the process of particle packing together and of removing the water.

Objectives

- To adapt the material to the requisite shape.
- To remove as much water as possible. The more water is removed, the less is the contraction.
- To produce desired strong porcelain.

Methods of Condensation

Condensation can be achieved by several methods:

Vibration: It consists of applying the wet porcelain to the platinum matrix and then vibrating the die in which the matrix rests. As the particles condense, the water rises to the surface. The excess water is then blotted with a clean tissue paper or an absorbent medium.

Spatulation: The wet porcelain is applied with a spatula and then the surface is smoothened with instrument. This will distribute the particle and cause them to become more closely packed. The water rises to the surface and it is removed with a lined cloth or blotting paper.

Brush technique or capillary action: It consists of adding paste to the matrix and dry powder is sprinkled onto the wet surfaces. The dry powder removes the excess water by capillary action from the mixture already applied. The particles move close together as the water is withdrawn.

Whipping: After the paste has been applied to the matrix, it may be whipped with brush. The water is thus brought to the surface and it is removed.

Factors Affecting Condensation

The success of condensation depends on skills of operator and the range of size of the particles.
- If the particles are of same size, 45% of a given volume will consist of voids.
- If a number of particles are blended with larger ones, void or space is considerably reduced.
- If three or more particle sizes are used that will achieve an even greater degree of compaction. Powder consisting of mixtures of particle sizes compact more easily than those with particles of one size.

A well-compacted crown reduces firing shrinkage and show regular contraction over the entire surface. Thus maintaining the original form on a slightly reduced space.

Firing

Firing is the process of heating closely packed particle to achieve interparticular bonding and sufficient diffusion to decrease the surface area or increase the density of the structure.

Purpose of firing is to sinter the particle of powder together properly to form restoration.

Procedure

After the condensation has completed, the condensed mass is placed in front or below the muffle of a preheated furnace (approximately 650°C). A porcelain furnace (Fig. 16.1) consists of an electrically heated muffle with a pyrometer, which indicates the temperature in the part of the muffle where condensed mass is placed. Most modern porcelain furnaces allow firing under

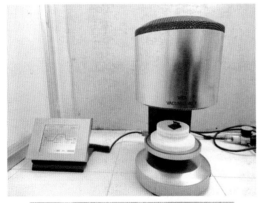

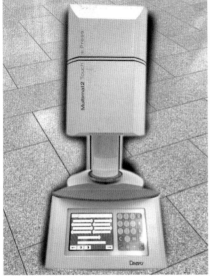

Fig. 16.1 Ceramic firing furnace

vacuum. Another method of firing apart from vacuum firing is firing under highly diffusible gas and pressure cooling process.

During firing porcelain undergoes many changes, they are as follows:

a. The first change involves the loss of water, which was added to the powder to form a workable mass.

b. The second change occurs as the temperature is raised and the particles of porcelain fuse together by sintering. Sintering is a process responsible for the fusion of the particles to form a condensed or dense mass. As a result of sintering porcelain shrinks.

c. The glazing stage is reached in the last firing and is held only through a glossy surface to form.

Stages of Firing

Low bisque: As the temperature increases, particles soften and started to flow between particles. Fired articles exhibit rigidity. There is no contraction or volume shrinkage and no cohesion between the particles.

Medium bisque: Powder particles exhibit complete cohesion. There is slight contraction or shrinkage.

High bisque: Shrinkage is complete and mass exhibits smoother surface. A very slight amount of porosity may be visible, but the body does not exhibit a glazed appearance.

Firing of Porcelain Jacket Crown

In the first firing, the dentin portion which is formed approximately 30% oversized is fired. The temperature is approximately 56°C below the fusion temperature of porcelain. After cooling, the enamel portion is added is also oversized when the second firing is made. After the firing process, the structure is cooled slowly. At this stage the matrix may not be distributed properly. Then if it is necessary stains are applied, it is returned to the furnace for initial firing. As it is held at correct firing temperature, complete fusion takes place and a thin glaze is formed onto the surface. After being annealed by careful slow cooling, the platinum matrix removed and the completed restoration is prepared for cementation.

Precautions of Firing

• The condensed porcelain should be placed on a fine clay tray and not be permitted to come into contact with the floor or wall of furnace. The initial rate of heating should be slow otherwise water will be converted to strain so rapidly that unfired porcelain may be crumbled. So it is better to place it in a preheated tray for the elimination of water.

- Uniform heating is desirable to give sufficient time for the interior of the porcelain to heat up.
- Initially the furnace door should be left open for the steam to escape.

Cooling

The proper cooling of porcelain forms its firing temperature to room temperature is the subject of considerable controversy. Cooling should be done slowly and uniform after firing. Rapid cooling results in brittle fracture.

Glazing

Porcelain for PJC's may be characterized with stains and glazes to provide a more life-like appearance.

Purpose of Glazing

The surface of the crown should be smooth when the restoration is placed in the mouth, otherwise food and other debris may cling to it. The rough surfaces can be removed by glazing the body using glazes (Fig. 16.2).

Glazes

A glaze is a ceramic veneer, which may be added to the porcelain restoration after it has been fired.

A glaze for the dental purpose is generally a transparent glass with a fusing temperature lower than that of the porcelain body.

A glaze is applied as a paste and the crown is again fired to the fusion temperature of the glaze. The resulting glossy or semiglossy surface is completely nonporous.

The most important requirement of glaze is its COTE should be equal to that of porcelain body to which it is applied. High COTE results in crazing (tension) and low COTE results in compressive stress may develop cracks in the glazing known as 'peeling'.

Types of Glazing

1. Self-glazing or autoglazing
2. Add-on glazing.

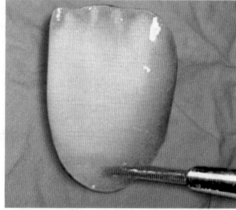
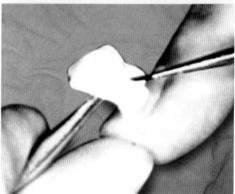

Fig. 16.2 Glazing of ceramic crown

Self-glazing: The finished article is kept in the muffle chamber of the furnace and temperature is lowered very quickly to melt the surface particle. A thin layer of glossy material is formed during this self-glazing firing procedure at a temperature and time that causes localized softening of the glass phase and setting of crystalline particles within the surface region. This self-glaze ensures adequate chemical durability.

Add-on glazing: A glaze porcelain mix having a low fusion temperature is applied as a thin coating and then fired carefully.

Precaution during Glazing

Over-glazing should be avoided since it gives the restoration as an unnatural glossy appearance and may cause slumping or loss of contour as well as weakens the mass.

Advantages of Glazed Porcelain

- High strength
- Better esthetic
- Better hygienic
- Reduces crack propagation
- Reduces the abrasion caused due to opposing teeth or restoration.

Stains

A mixture of one or more pigmented metal oxides and usually a low fusing glass that when dispersed in aqueous slurry applied to the surface of porcelain and dried or fired, will modify the shade of the ceramics-based restoration.

Uses of Stains

- Slight marking or defects are placed in porcelain restoration in imitation of a similar dental condition.
- Stains are used in incisal area to imitate enamel rods and hypocalcified structures.

Removal of Platinum Foil

After firing, platinum foil is removed and ready for cementation.

Cementation

Cementation can be done using glass ionomer cement or zinc polycarboxylate cement. Mostly preferable luting media for PJC's is resin cement.

FABRICATION DEFECTS

Volume Shrinkage

The cause of shrinkage during firing of dental porcelain is the loss of water and densification through sintering. Volume shrinkage is of the order of 30–40%, particularly due to elimination of voids during sintering.

Remedy

a. Manufacturers should use variation of particle size to minimize space between the particles.
b. The external shape of the crown should be 1–1½ mm longer in all directions in order to compensate for the shrinkage.

Internal Porosity

It is due to inclusion of air during firing. This can be seen in bulk of the material and reduces its translucency and these voids rarely appear on the surface of ceramic tooth or crown, because the entrapped gases can be released.

Remedy

a. Vacuum firing in which the air is removed before it is entrapped during vitrification process (formation of glass-like structure). It is most normally used method for producing dental porcelain.
b. Diffusible gases such as noble gases are substituted for the ordinary furnace atmosphere. The air is then driven out of the interstices during firing and the diffusible gas is substituted. During fusion, such entrapped gases diffuse outwards through the porcelain.
c. Cooling the porcelain under pressure, which causes compression of the gas, thereby reducing the size so that their effect is negligible.

Advantages of PJC as Restorative Material

- Esthetically porcelain is most perfect material for the replacement of the missing tooth substance. It is available in a range of shades and various levels of translucency such that a most life-like appearance can be obtained.
- It is hard and resists wear extremely well.
- Extremely compatible with soft tissues.
- Correctly formulated porcelain is very resistant to chemical attack being unaffected by the wide variations of pH, which may be encountered in mouth.
- Good insulating properties because the metal atoms transfer their outermost atoms to the

nonmetallic atoms and thereby stabilize highly mobile electron. This fact is important when the gross amount of enamel and dentin are to be replaced and the residual layer of dentin.

Disadvantages

- Susceptibility to brittle fracture particularly when flow and tensile stress exist in the same region of the ceramic restoration.
- Low fracture toughness and tensile strength. The relatively poor mechanical properties can be improved by using alumina or metal supporting structure.
- High degree of shrinkage upon firing.
- Excessive hardness may be a disadvantage when it contacts the opposite natural teeth, which may result in excessive wear of the teeth in opposing arch.
- Problems in matching in the exact color and texture of the natural teeth.

METAL CERAMIC RESTORATION OR PORCELAIN FUSED TO METAL

All ceramic anterior restorations can appear very natural. Unfortunately, the ceramics used in these restorations are brittle and subject to fracture from high tensile stress. All metal restorations are strong and tough but from esthetic point of view they are acceptable for posterior restorations. Fortunately, the esthetic qualities of porcelain can be combined with strength and toughness of metal to produce restorations that have both a natural tooth-like appearance and very good mechanical properties. Therefore, if a strong bond is affected between the porcelain veneer and such proper design and physical properties of porcelain and metal, the porcelain is reinforced. So that brittle fracture can be avoided or at least minimized. This is often referred to metal restorations or more popularly called metal ceramic restorations.

Requirements for Alloys for PFM Bonding

1. Good corrosion resistance.

2. The alloys used for metal-ceramic restorations should be capable of withstanding porcelain-firing temperature without melting. Hence alloy must have high fusion temperature.
3. Must resist deformation at temperature encountered during the firing of ceramic (sag resistance).
4. Alloys should have high MOE (to minimize elastic deformation) and high-yield strength (no permanent deformation) to avoid excess stress in the porcelain, which is brittle.
5. Should have a value of COTE similar to that of porcelain, which it is bonded.
6. Should be capable of forming a bond with porcelain veneer that the porcelain does not become detached.
7. Alloys must allow good wetting to porcelain and must form surface oxides for chemical bonding to occur.
8. Components of the alloy must not discolor the porcelain (discoloration can occur due to presence of copper in some alloys).

Requirements of Ceramics for PFM Bonding

1. Must simulate the appearance of natural teeth.
2. Must fuse to metal at relatively low temperature so that the metal does not melt.
3. Must have COTE compatible with the alloys used.
4. Must withstand oral environment.
5. Porcelain during firing must wet and flow over the metal surface (low contact angles indicate good wetting).

Composition of PFM Alloys

- High gold alloys
- Low gold alloys
- Au–Pd alloys
- Ni–Cr alloys
- Co-Cr alloys
- Ni-Ti alloys.

The composition of alloys used for metal-ceramic restorations have been discussed in the Dental Casting Alloys chapter of this book.

Composition of Ceramics For PFM Restorations

The composition of the ceramic generally corresponds to that of the glasses except for an increased alkaline content. The addition of greater quantities of soda and potash (glass modifiers) in order to increase the thermal expansion to a level compatible with metal coping and to reduce fusion temperature. The addition of glass/metal modifier (K_2O) results in the formation of high expansion leucite crystals.

Leucite ($K Al_2 Si_2O_6$) is potassium aluminum silicate with a large COTE increases the thermal expansion of porcelain, so that it could match that of dental alloys. Color pigments and opacifiers control the color and translucency of the restoration.

Bonding between Ceramic and Metal

The primary requirement for the success of metal ceramic restoration is the development of durable wall between the porcelain and the alloy. The nature of the bonding can divide into three types:

- Mechanical bonding
- Compressive (thermal) bonding
- Chemical bonding.

Mechanical Bonding

If the fused porcelain is able to wet the metal rough surface efficiently, it will flow into surface irregularities on the surface resulting in mechanical interlocking. Sand blasting is often used to roughen the surface of the metal coating to improve the bonding with the ceramic.

Precautions

- Excessive roughening resulting in stress concentration at the metal ceramic interface.
- Excessive rough surface can also reduce adhesion if the ceramic does not penetrate into the surface and voids are present at the interface. This may happen with improperly fined metals that are poorly wetted by porcelain.

Compressive (Thermal) Bonding

A critical requirement for the adhesion is thermal expansion compatibility between the ceramic and the metal. Ceramo-metallic systems are designed with a very small degree of mismatch in order to leave the porcelain in a state of compression.

$$\alpha_{Porcelain} - 13 \text{ to } 14 \times 10^{-6}/°C$$
$$\alpha_{Metal} - 13.5 \text{ to } 14.5 \times 10^{-6}/°C$$

The difference of $0.5 \times 10^{-6}/°C$ causes the metal to contract slightly more than the porcelain on cooling from firing temperature. This mismatch leaves porcelain in residual compression and makes it less sensitive to apply tensile forces (increase bond strength).

Chemical Bonding

The principal mode of porcelain metal binding is by a direct electron transfer that occurs between oxides of glass and oxidisable metal in the coping alloy, this is a chemical bonding.

Alloys of purely noble metals do not bind chemically. Addition of oxidisable elements such as Indium (In), Tin (Sn) such an alloy establishes the potential for the oxidation of the alloy and component adhesion to the glass.

Ceramic bonding to the metal in certain cases requires the electrodeposition of metal coatings and heating to form suitable metal oxides.

Clinical Failure

The major problems associated with metal ceramic restoration is the failure of porcelain veneer, crazing, cracking and separation of the porcelain from the underlying substrate (Figs 16.3A to C), may be caused by several conditions. When the porcelain veneers crack away from the casting, the failure develops in one or several conditions.

Technical Considerations of Metal–Ceramic Restoration

Because of the high melting temperature of the alloy, gypsum bonded investment material

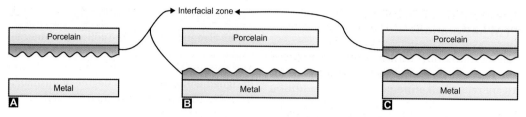

Figs 16.3A to C Bond failure (A) between interfacial zone and metal (B) between porcelain and interfacial zone (C) in interfacial zone itself

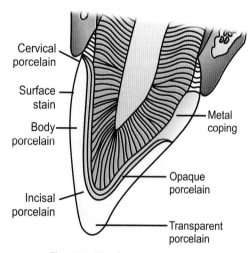

Fig. 16.4 Metal-ceramic restoration

cannot be used, thus phosphate or silica bonded investment material must be used. A gas-oxygen flame or induction is generally employed for melting the alloy (Fig. 16.4).

Surface treatment of metal casting before porcelain application is important for good bonding. This treatment is used to toughen the casting and form surface oxides. The surface may be roughened by sand blasting with a fine alumina abrasive. In most cases, the metal casting is heat treated either in air or under partial vacuum to produce surface oxide to improve bonding. The opaque porcelain is condensed with a thickness of approximately 0.1–0.2 mm. It is then fired, the translucent enamel is applied and tooth form built. The unit is again fired. A final glaze is then obtained as with the PJC.

Advantages

- The properly made ceramic crown is stronger and more durable than PJC.
- Permanent esthetic quality of the porcelain properly designed reinforced ceramic unit.
- Bridgework is possible and excellent fit.

Drawbacks

- More tooth structure may be needed to be removed to provide a proper bulk of the crown with all porcelain restoration.
- Appearance of metal margins.
- Discoloration of metal (green color by silver).
- Appearance of translucency is difficult to produce.
- Possible disadvantage of the alloy used.

Porcelain Bonded to Platinum Foil

Porcelain with the metal bonded ceramic restoration is that a considerable thickness of tooth substance removed to allow space for the metal casting and porcelain veneer. An alternative approach is to make a porcelain crown, which is bonded to platinum foil.

The objective of this technique is to improve the esthetics by the replacement of the thicker metal casting with a thin platinum foil, thus allowing more room for porcelain.

This technique involves laying down two platinum foils in the working die as a boost to the normal single foil. The exposed surface of the outer foil is then tin-plated and the porcelain crown is constructed and fired on the top of the tin plated surface. Porcelain bonded to the layer of tin oxide on the tin plated surface. The liner platinum foil is removed prior to cementation of the crown while the outer platinum face remains bonded to the inner surface of the crown. These foils help to prevent the crack formation on the inner surface.

Metal-ceramic Based on Swaged Foil Coping

These are the products designed to fabricate the metal coatings of metal-ceramic crown with the use of a melting and casting process. Swaged (work hardened) foil porcelain crowns consist of porcelain fused to a coping of wrought (swaged) palladium-gold alloy.

ALL CERAMIC RESTORATIONS

To overcome the drawbacks of metal-ceramics, all-ceramic systems for dental restorations have been developed with the help of novel processing techniques introduced to dentistry, such as heat-pressing, slip-casting, Computer Aided Design-Computer Aided Machining (CAD-CAM), etc. All-ceramic materials have been developed to match dental requirements, offering increasingly greater performance from a mechanical standpoint.

All-ceramics contain a significantly greater amount of crystalline phase (from about 35 to about 99 volume %). This higher level of crystallinity is responsible for an improvement in mechanical properties through the following mechanisms.
- Dispersion strengthening.
- Transformation toughening.
- Thermal incompatibility between glass matrix and crystalline phase.

Unfortunately, higher crystallinity is also associated with higher opacity, which is not always desirable for dental ceramics.

However, crystallinity is only one of many intrinsic factors contributing to materials performance. Other factors such as crystal size and geometry, modulus of elasticity, phase transformation and thermal expansion mismatch between crystal and glassy phase play a crucial role in determining the final mechanical properties of the ceramic.

CLASSIFICATION OF ALL-CERAMIC RESTORATIONS

Based on Processing Methods

1. Sintered porcelains
   - Leucite-reinforced feldspathic porcelain. E.g.: Optec HSP.
   - Alimina based porcelains.
   - Magnesia based porcelains.
   - Zirconia based porcelains. E.g.: Mirage II.
2. Ceramming and sintering such as glass-ceramics
   - Mica based porcelains E.g.: Dicor
   - Hydroxyapatite based porcelains E.g.: Cerapearl
   - Lithia based porcelains E.g.: High strength ceramics.
3. Machinable ceramics
   - Machinable ceramic E.g.: Vitabloc MK II, Dicor MGC (Machinable Glass Ceramic), Clay In-Ceram
   - CAD-CAM Ceramics E.g.: CEREC system (Siemens), Procera system (Nobelbiocare)
   - Copy milling ceramics E.g.: Clay system (Mikrona Tech)
4. Slip-cast ceramics
   - Inceram alumina.
   - Inceram spinell.
   - Inceram zirconia.
5. Heat-Pressed and Injection Molded Ceramics.
   - Leucite based E.g.: IPS Empress.
   - Spinell Based E.g.: Magnesia spinell: Alceram.

Based on Microstructure

1. Glass based systems E.g.: Silica type.
2. Glass based systems with crystalline fillers E.g.: Leucite crystals, Lithium disilicate crystals, etc.
3. Crystalline based systems with glass fillers. E.g.: Alumina, etc.

4. Polycrystalline solids.
   E.g.: Alumina and Zirconia.

Based on Strengthening

1. Based on dispersion strengthening
   E.g.: Aluminous porcelains.
2. Based on transformation toughening.
   E.g.: Leucite-reinforced feldspathic porcelain, zirconia based
   Porcelains, mica based porcelains, hydroxy-apatite based
   porcelains, lithia based porcelains, etc.
3. Based on thermal incompatibility
   E.g.: Leucite-reinforced feldspathic porcelain (Optec HSP), etc.

Aluminous Porcelain

The major disadvantage of the porcelain is brittleness and this is the factor, which limits its use. Several methods are available, which are aimed at preventing the formation and propagation of cracks on the surface of the porcelain restoration. One approach is to use a core of pure alumina on which the porcelain crown is constructed.

Alumina is a very hard, opaque material, which is less susceptible to crack propagation than porcelain. Porcelain, which contains alumina is referred to as aluminous porcelain and alumina extent is normally around 40% by volume.

Functions of Alumina

Powdered alumina may be added to porcelain in order to achieve a significant strengthening. The mechanism of strengthening is that the alumina particles act as crack stoppers preventing the propagating crack throughout the body of the porcelain.

The improvement of properties not only as a result of good mechanical properties of alumina with porcelain, the two materials having closely matching values of COTE and MOE. In addition, alumina is slightly soluble in low fusing porcelain allowing for a continuity of atomic bonding through the ceramic. This ensures that the interface region between the alumina particles and the porcelain in virtually stress-free and not likely to encourage crack propagation around the alumina particles.

For example, Transverse strength – 125 MPa
Shear strength – 145 MPa.

Fabrication

The crown is formed on a platinum matrix with a core of aluminous porcelain. A veneer of usually glass type is then fired over the crown for esthetics. Less tooth structure needs to be removed since the aluminous porcelain core requires a thinner veneer for good esthetics than a metal crown. Aluminous porcelain has also application in denture teeth in which brittleness has been a problem.

Disadvantages

Alumina is opaque and therefore can only be used to construct the inner core region of the porcelain crown. This is generally acceptable since it is the inner region from which the crack propagates and this is therefore they are in need of reinforcement.

Glass Ceramic/Castable Glass Ceramic

A glass ceramic is a material fabricated in a vitreous or noncrystalline state and then converted to crystalline state by heat treatment. The strength and toughness of glass ceramics can be increased by the formation of the crystalline plates, particles or needles during the cerammin process. These crystalline structures increase strength by interrupting the crack propagation through them under masticatory forces.

Composition

The first commercially available castable ceramic material for dental use is 'Dicor', which was developed by Dentsply international and supplied as silicon glass plate ingots containing MgF_2.

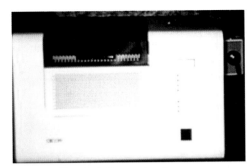

Fig. 16.5 Ceramming furnace

Manipulation

The restoration is waxed on a die and then wax pattern of the crown is invested by phosphate bonded investment material and ingot of ceramic material is placed in a spherical crucible and melted and cast with a motor driven centrifugal machine at 1380°C (Fig. 16.5).

After removal of sprue, the glass is invested again and heat-treated at 1075°C for 6 hours to produce crystallization of glass to form a mica-ceramic. This crystal nucleation and crystal growth process is called 'ceramming'.

The final shape is achieved by applying a thin layer of porcelain veneer of the required shape and fire.

Advantages

- Fracture toughness is improved by devitri-fication.
- Little shrinkage as a result of processing.
- Good esthetics because of the 'chameleon effect' where part of color of restoration is picked up from the adjacent teeth as well as treated cement used for restoration.

Uses

- Used for inlays, full crown restoration by a lost wax casting process.

Leucite Reinforced

Manufacturers have introduced high strength ceramic using leucite (potassium aluminium silicate) crystals dispersed in glass matrix.

- IPS Empress

- IPS Empress 2
- Optec HSP.

PRESSIBLE CERAMICS

IPS Empress

IPS-Empress introduced as an injection molding system that uses leucite (4%–50%) reinforced feldspathic porcelain. The leucite crystals may improve the strength and fracture resistance of the feldspathic glass matrix in a manner similar to that which occurs in glass-ceramics like Dicor or in dispersion strengthened aluminous porcelains.

IPS empress all ceramic permits light to be reflected, scattered, and absorbed throughout the entire crown and the underlying tooth structure. Opalescent properties of an empress crown in-vitro viewed by transmitted white light.

IPS empress is a heat-pressed glass-ceramic that has superior mechanical properties for several reasons. The high shrinkage of leucite crystals creates compressive stress in the vitreous phase, which prevents the development of surface cracks. The randomly oriented leucite crystals are tightly packed in the vitreous phase and stop the propagation of microcracks. The combination of heat pressing, initial firing, and stain and glaze of the veneers creates an additional 50% increase in strength. This higher cohesive strength and fracture toughness allows for thicker areas of porcelain with a lesser risk of fracture.

Chemical Composition of IPS Empress

$$
\begin{array}{lcl}
SiO_2 & : & 59.0\text{--}63.0 \\
Al_2O_3 & : & 19.0\text{--}23.5 \\
H_2O & : & 10.0\text{--}14.0 \\
Na_2O & : & 3.5\text{--}6.5 \\
CeO_2 & : & 0\text{--}1.0 \\
CaO & : & 0.5\text{--}3.0 \\
BaO & : & 0\text{--}1.5 \\
TiO_2 & : & 0\text{--}0.5
\end{array}
$$

Manufacturing of IPS Empress Glass Ceramic

The powder to which the stabilizers, additives, fluorescent agents and pigments have been added, then pressed to form ingot. Once the ingot has been sintered to about 1200°C it is ready for sale on the market for processing in EP500 press furnace.

Fabrication of IPS Empress Restoration

The fabrication of a dental crown according to layering technique, for example is characterized by wax up of a reduced model that is invested in a special investing material, after a muffle has been preheated the wax is burnt out, it is placed in an EP500 press furnace.

Subsequently, a glass-ceramic ingot for layering technique is pressed into the mold of the reduced crown at 1180°C according to the viscous flow process. The crown framework is exposed to this temperature for 35 minutes. It is then cooled, divested and finished. Then the ceramic incisal materials for layering technique for short "layering ceramic" and glazes are applied. These materials are sintered at about 910 to 870°C respectively. Glass-ceramic ingots for sintering technique is preferred for fabrication of the various restorations like inlay, onlays, veneers, etc. The ingot is pressed at 1050°C for staining technique. This provides IPS Empress glass-ceramic with its ultimate strength and esthetic properties.

IPS Empress 2

IPS empress 2 is a successor of the original IPS empress. It is manufactured the same way as IPS empress, but consists of completely different components. Whereas IPS empress is a leucite-reinforced glass ceramic, IPS empress 2 consists of a lithium disilicate glass-ceramic core that is layered with a sintered glass-ceramic, and the chemical basis for the material is the SiO_2-Li_2O system. The first lithium disilicate glass-ceramic was developed in as early as 1950's.

This development was the work of STOOKEY. Following his fundamental discovery, lithium disilicate glass-ceramic became the subject of considerable amount of research. The nucleation mechanism and kinetics of crystallization of the main lithium disilicate phase received the

most attention. The disadvantage of the lithium disilicate glass-ceramic was their poor chemical resistance.

Chemical Composition of IPS Empress 2

SiO_2	:	57 to 80
Al_2O_3	:	0 to 5
La_2O_3	:	0.1 to 6
K_2O	:	0 to 13
MgO	:	0 to 5.0
ZnO	:	0 to 8.0
Li_2O	:	11 to 19
P_2O_5	:	0 to 11
Other additives up to 8.		

Manufacturing of IPS Empress 2 Glass Ceramic

Melting a glass, which is powdered and crystallized in a sintering and heat-press process using a heat-press furnace, produces the glass-ceramic.

The base glass is melted at a temperature of 1400°C to 1600°C. Raw materials like oxides, carbonates and phosphates are used. The molten material is poured into water and afterwards grounded to fine powder. Then the sieved powder is pressed in a uniaxial press to form cylinders measuring 13 mm in diameter and 12 to 24 mm in height.

These cylinders are then sintered at 850°C to 900°C under vacuum. During this process the cylinders are also crystallized. Thus an intermediate product in the form of a glass-ceramic ingot is produced in this manner. The ingots are cooled to room temperature after sintering process.

Fabrication of IPS Empress 2 Restoration

The fabrication of a dental crown using IPS Empress 2 is characterized by wax up of a reduced model that is invested in a special investing material, after a muffle has been preheated the wax is burnt out, IPS Empress 2 glass-ceramic ingot is placed in an EP500 press furnace.

Subsequently, a glass-ceramic ingot is pressed into the mold of the reduced crown at 920°C. The crown framework is exposed to this temperature for 20 minutes. The effective pressure applied through the plunger is 20 bar. The pressing process is conducted under a partial vacuum of 20 to 50 mbar in the furnace chamber. Under these conditions, the glass-ceramic becomes viscous and consistently flows into the mold. The typical pressing time varies from 5–20 minutes depending on the volume and complexity of the mold. It is then cooled to room temperature. During the heat-press process and the cooling phase the final microstructure of the glass-ceramic is formed. Then the pressed part is divested and finished.

The heat pressed IPS empress 2 glass-ceramic should be glazed or layered with additional glass-ceramic to obtain dental restoration such as crowns for the anterior and posterior region or FPD's for the anterior region. The layering material is sintered on the heat-pressed frame using a sintering furnace at a temperature of 800°C (Table 16.2).

This sintered glass-ceramic contains fluorapatite crystals similar to the needle-like fluorapatite crystals found in fluoride-enriched natural tooth structure. This process mimics natural tooth structure, not only in composition through the use of fluorapatite, but through the layering process of providing a strong dentinal framework overlaid with a translucent enamel-like layer. The sintered glass-ceramic also has inherent fluorescence, opalescence, and an enamel-like translucency.

Indications

3-unit FPD's in the anterior and the premolar region (up to the second premolar as the abutment).

Single crowns in the anterior and the posterior regions.

Advantages

- Specially developed lithium disilicate framework ceramics.
- Newly developed fluorapatite layering ceramics.
- Improved fracture resistance.

Table 16.2 Comparison of heat-pressed ceramics

Property	IPS Empress	IPS Empress 2
Flexural Strength (MPa)	112 ± 10	400 ± 40
COTE (ppm/—°C)	15 ± 0.25	10.6 ± 0.25
Pressing Temperature (°C)	1150–1180	890–920
Veneering Temperature (°C)	910	800

- Very high chemical resistance of both framework and layering ceramics.
- High translucency.
- Outstanding light optical properties due to apatite (also a component of natural teeth).
- Wear behavior similar to that of natural enamel.
- Ingots available in the most popular chromoscope shades.
- Excellent esthetic appearance.

Injection Molded Core Ceramic/Shrink-Free Ceramics/ Cerestore (Alceram)

These materials were reported in 1983 for the production of all ceramic, single anterior or posterior crowns. The method involved in the production of crown cores by injection molding, partially eliminating the need for use of a platinum foil and improving adoption of the crown. The nonshrink property is achieved by incorporating significant qualities of MgO into the ceramic frit. These react with the alumina during firing to form a mixed metal oxide called spinel ($MgAl_2O_6$). The spinel is less dense than the original mix of oxides of its formation results in an expansion, which compensates for firing shrinkage.

Composition

A mixture of an alumina, MgO, aluminosilicate glass frit, wax, and silicon-resin plasticizers.

Manipulation

The technique for fabricating ceramic coping from this type of material involves the formation of a wax pattern on epoxy resin die. The lost wax process obtains the volume intended for forming the coping. A plastic composition containing alumina, magnesia, wax glass and silicon resin is heated to 180°C and injection molded and the injection pressure in the mold to form new coping. Firing is then carried on a special furnace using controlled temperature up to 1300°C, during this formation of spinel occurs. Veneer porcelains are packed into the surface of the coping to produce finished crown. The drawback of this manipulation is complexity and high cost of process.

OPTEC HSP (High Strength Porcelain)/ OPTEC VP (Veneer Porcelain)

Many porcelain systems cause wear to the opposing dentition during function, which usually necessitates nightguard use. New low-wear ceramics may remove the need for a nightguard in the future. With the advent of low-fusing, low-wear ceramics built over a pressable ceramic (Optimal Pressable Ceramic [OPC]), has excellent esthetics, translucent margins and many of the new colors are designed to match bleached teeth.

It is a leucite-reinforced all-ceramic material (leucite is 45–50%). IPS Empress and OPC basically are the same; however, OPC's leucite crystal (filler) is smaller, resulting in higher compressive strength (187 to 320 psi) and a flexural strength of over 23,000 psi. The process of heat pressing the ceramic rather than stacking the material differentiates OPC from IPS Empress.

It has 50% leucite in a glass matrix therefore stronger than conventional feldspathic porcelain. These leucite crystals are dispersed in a glassy matrix by controlling their nucleation during production. No core is required like Dicor. VP is higher in chroma than HSP. OPC is the second-generation product of IPS empress.

Indications

- Anterior single units.
- Posterior single units.
- Veneers.

Contraindications

- Clenching and bruxism.
- Short clinical crowns.
- Large or immature pulp chambers.
- Abnormal occlusal relationships.
- Existing periodontal disease.

INFILTRATED CERAMICS

In-ceram

In-ceram was developed in 1985, by Sadoun. It makes use of aluminous cores that are infiltrated with a glass to achieve high strength substructures that can support crowns and bridges.

In-ceram belongs to a class of materials known as interpenetrating-phase composites. These materials consist of at least two phases that are inter-wined and extend continuously from the internal to the external surface. These materials may possess improved mechanical and physical properties compared with the individual components. They may have improved strength and fracture resistance due to the fact that a crack must pass through alternative layers of both components no matter what direction the crack takes.

Slip Casting

An all-ceramic restorative system, in-ceram, is based on the slip casting of an alumina core with its subsequent glass infusion. An impression of the master cast preparations is made with elastomeric impression materials. Special gypsum supplied with in-ceram is poured to produce the die onto which the in-ceram alumina is applied.

Alumina powder (38 g) is mixed with 5 ml of deionized water supplied in a premeasured container. One drop of a dispersing agent is added to help create a homogeneous mixture of alumina in the water. One half of the alumina is added to a beaker containing the water/dispersant and then sonicated for 3 minutes in a Vitasonic. This initiates the dispersion process. A second quantity of powder equal to one half of the remaining amount is added to the beaker and sonicated for 7 minutes; during the last minute, a vacuum is applied to eliminate air bubbles.

This solution of alumina is referred to as 'slip', which is then 'painted' onto the gypsum die with a brush. The alumina is built up to form the underlying core for the ceramic tooth. The water is removed via capillary action of the porous gypsum, which packs the particles into a rigid network.

The alumina core is then placed in the in-cerament furnace and sintered. The cycle involves a slow heating of approximately 2°C per minute to 120°C to remove water and the binding agent. A rapid temperature rise would boil of remaining water and binder, producing cracks in the framework. The second stage of sintering involves a temperature rise of approximately 20°C/min to 1120°C for 2 hours to produce approximation of the particles with minimal compaction and minimal shrinkage of alumina. Shrinkage is only about 0.2% thus an interconnected porous network is created, connecting pores on the outer surface with those on the inner surface.

A lanthanum aluminosilicate glass is used to fill the pores in the alumina. The glass is mixed with water and placed on a platinum-gold alloy sheet. The external surface of the core is placed on the glass. The core is then heated in the Inceramat to 1100°C for 4–6 hours. The glass becomes molten and allows flowing into the pores by capillary diffusion. A 4-hour infusion time is used for bridges. The excess glass is removed by sand blasting with alumina particles. The last step in the fabrication of the restoration involves the application of aluminous porcelain core to produce the final form of the restoration. The in-ceram core material is apparently the strongest material available for restorative procedures. Flexural strength values for the core range up to 600 MPa, but may decline as the veneer porcelain is added or the core thickness decreases.

In-Ceram Spinell

A second-generation material, in-ceram spinell is based on the in-ceram technique, has recently been introduced. The technique of fabrication is essentially the same as the original system.

The primary difference is a change in composition to produce a more translucent core. The porous core is fabricated from a magnesium-alumina powder to form the porous core after sintering instead of alumina powder as in in-ceram alumina. This type of material has a specific crystalline structure referred to as "Spinell".

The porous spinell is secondarily infiltrated with a low viscosity, lanthanum aluminosilicate glass, which produces a more translucent substructure upon which Vitadur Alpha is veneered to form the final restoration. The glass infiltration of in-ceram spinell should be done in a vacuum environment.

In-ceram spinell is twice as translucent as in-ceram alumina because the refractive index of its crystalline phase is closer to that of glass and the vacuum infiltration leaves less porosity. The translucency of in-ceram spinell closely matches that of dentin.

Indications

- Anterior crowns
- In clinical situations where maximum translucency is needed.

Contraindications

- Posterior restorations.
- Anterior and posterior FPDs.

In-Ceram Zirconia

In-ceram zirconia is also a second-generation material based on in-ceram fabrication technique. The difference is being a change in composition to produce a material that has improved flexural strength and fracture toughness.

The porous core fabricated with in-ceram zirconia has a tetragonal form of crystal. The porous core is secondarily infiltrated with a low viscosity, lanthanum aluminosilicate glass, which produces a stronger substructure.

Zirconia has a physical property called transformation toughening (strengthening)

Table 16.3 Comparison of glass-infiltrated ceramics

Property	In-ceram alumina	In-ceram spinell	In-ceram zirconia
Composition	Al_2O_3 and lanthanum glass	$MgO - Al_2O_3$	$Al_2O_3 - ZrO_2$
Flexural strength (MPa)	500	350	700
Translucency	Translucent	Highly translucent	Opaque
Strength	Better	Good	Best
Indications	Anterior and posterior crowns, anterior 3-unit bridge	Anterior crown inlays and onlays	Posterior crown and bridges

when an external energy source is applied to the material it goes through a phase transformation to a monoclinic form of zirconia. The monoclinic form of crystal is 3%–5% larger, thus in places of microcracks this process of crystallization can seal the cracks.

Properties of three types of glass infiltrated ceramics are compared in Table 16.3.

MACHINABLE CERAMICS

CAD-CAM Ceramics

CAD—Computer Aided Designing

CAM—Computer Aided Manufacturing/ Machining/Milling

A system has been available for dental use, which consists of miniature 3D–video camera, monitor, keyboard, image processing module and a milling machine (to cut the ceramic). The camera produces a stereographic image of cavity preparation and digital data are used to control cutting of the filling surface of ceramic inlays. These ceramics are supplied as small blocks that can be grounded into inlays and veneers in a computer driven CAD-CAM system.

Advantages

- Freedom of making an impression.
- The need for only single appointment.
- Negligible porosity in CAD – CAM ceramic material.
- Good patient appearance.

Drawbacks

- Need of costly equipments.
- The lack of computer controlled support for occlusal adjustment.
- The technique sensitive nature of surface imaging is required for prepared tooth.

Zirconia Ceramics

One of the most difficult areas in dentistry today is the restoration of dental structures with biocompatible materials that are strong enough to withstand the forces of chewing (500–1000 lbs pressure on molar teeth). Patients now have a choice of a material that is esthetic, strong, pure, biocompatible and capable of being used for single and long span dental bridgework. That material is called zirconium oxide.

Properties

- Excellent biological compatibility: absolutely bioinert.
- Tasteless.
- Hardness: 1200 VHN
- Compressive strength: 2000 MPa
- Bending strength: 1000 MPa
- Modulus of elasticity: 210 GPa
- Tensile strength: 7 MPa
- Zirconium oxide is manufactured and optimized industrially so that the material qualities remain unchanged through the complete production chain.
- Radiopaque.

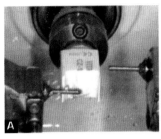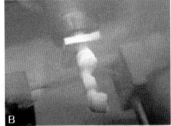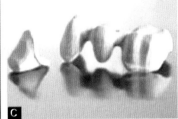

Figs 16.6A to C Milling of (A) Ceramic block; (B) Ceramic bridge designed on a ceramic block; (C) Milled ceramic crown and bridge copings

- No pulp irritation because there is no need to use adhesive cements and minimal invasive preparation by dentist.

Zirconium oxide forms the core of each crown and provides the cross-link that bridges the gap of missing teeth (Figs 16.6A to C). The precision fit of the zirconium core is derived from computer-guided lathes that cut the form out of a solid zirconium oxide block. Once formed, new synthetic porcelain (99.9% pure) is baked onto the zirconium core and then shaped like a tooth. Because of the extreme accuracy of the crown fit, the crowns can be cemented with biocompatible dental luting material.

Advantages

- Posterior bridges can be fabricated since it has high tensile strength.
- High resistance to corrosion.
- Stability to hydrolysis.
- High biocompatibility in comparison with other ceramics (Table 16.4).

In medicine, zirconium oxide is being used more and more as the material of choice specially for hip prosthesis. For years, there have existed substantial clinical tests and examinations, which confirm the high quality of zirconium oxide.

Comparison of selected indirect restorations are discussed in Dental Casting Alloys chapter of this book in Table 14.5.

Porcelain Teeth

They are used for both complete and partial denture. The anterior teeth have one or two gold covered pins to provide retention to denture base. The porcelain teeth in general have undercuts 'dentoric holes' located centrally in the underside of the teeth. The differences between porcelain teeth and acrylic teeth have been discussed in the Denture Base Resins chapter of this book.

Advantages

- Excellent esthetics.
- Excellent biocompatibility.
- Highly resistant to wear and distortion.

Table 16.4 Comparison of all-ceramic restorations

Property	Castable	Pressable	Infiltrated	Machinable
Margin quality	Good	Excellent	Good	Good
Translucency	Good	Slightly	Opaque	Slight
Strength	Weak	Moderate	High	Moderate
Acid etchable	Etchable	Etchable	Not indicated	Etchable
Abrasiveness	Minimum	Moderate	High	High
Treatment time	Two visits	Two visits	Two visits	One visit

Disadvantages

- Brittle.
- Do not bind to acrylic denture base and require mechanical retention.
- Cannot be easily polished after grinding.
- High density, increased weight of tooth.
- Produce clicking sound on contact.
- Mismatch of COTE produces stresses in acrylic denture base.

SUGGESTED READING

1. Anusavice KJ. Recent developments in restorative dental ceramics. J Am Dent Assoc. 1993;124:72-84.
2. Augstin-Panadero R, Fons-Font A, Roman-Rodriguez JL, Granell-Ruiz M, Del Rio-Highsmith J, Sola-Ruiz MF. Zirconia versus metal: a preliminary comparative analysis of ceramic veneer behaviour. Int J Prosthodont. 2012;25(3):294-300.
3. Blatz MB, Dent DR, Sadan A, Arch GH, Lang BR. In vitro evaluation of long term bonding of Procera. All-ceram alumina restorations with a modified resin luting agent. J Prosthet Dent. 2003;89:381-7.
4. Chong KH, Chai J, Takahashi Y, Wozniak W. Flexural strength of in-ceram alumina and in-ceram zirconia core materials. Int J Prosthodont. 2002;15:183-8.
5. Cornell D, Winter R. Manipulating light with the refractive index of an all-ceramic material. Prac. Proced. Aesthet. Dent. 1999; 11(8):913-7.
6. Davis BR, Aquilino SA, Lund PS Diaz-Arnold AM, Denehy GE. Colorimetric evaluation of the effect of porcelain opacity on the resultant color of porcelain veneers. Int J Prosthodont. 1992; 5:130-6.
7. Denry I, Holloway JA. Ceramics for Dental Applications: A Review, Materials. 2010;3:351-68; doi:10.3390/ma3010351.
8. Denry IL. Recent Advances in Ceramics for Dentistry, Crit Rev Oral Biol Med. 1996;7(2):134-43.
9. Dong JK, Luthy H, Wohlwend A, Scharer P. Heat Pressed ceramics: Technology and strength. Int J Prosthodont. 1992;5:9-16.
10. Duret F, Blouin JL, Duret B. CAD-CAM in dentistry. J Am Dent Assoc. 1988;117:715-20.
11. Fairhurst CW. Dental ceramics: the state of the science. Adv Dent Res. 1992;6:78-81.
12. Faull TW, Hesby RA, Pelleu Jr. GB, Eastwood GW. Marginal opening of single and twin platinum foil-bonded aluminous porcelain crowns. J Prosthet Dent. 1985;53:29-33.
13. Giordano R, Cima M, Pober R. Effect of surface finish on the flexural strength of feldspathic and aluminous dental ceramics. Int J Prosthodont. 1995;8:311-9.
14. Griggs JA. Recent advances in materials for all-ceramic restorations. Dent Clin North Am. 2007;51(3):713-viii. doi:10.1016/j.cden.2007.04.006.
15. Guazzato M, Albakry M, Swain MV, Ironside J. Mechanical properties of in-ceram alumina and in-ceram zirconia. Int J Prosthodont. 2002;15:339-46.
16. Hasleton DR, Diaz-Arnold AM, Hillis SL. Clinical assessment of high strength all-ceramic crowns. J Prosthet Dent. 2000;83: 396-401.
17. Holand W. Materials science fundamentals of the IPS Empress 2 glass-ceramic. Ivoclar Vivadent Rep. 1998;12:3-10.
18. Holloway JA, Denry I, Rosenstiel SF. Surface layer characterization after dual ion exchange of a leucite reinforced dental porcelain. Int J Prosthodont. 1997;1:136-41.
19. Iseri U, Ozkurt Z, Yalnýz A, Kazazoðlu E. Comparison of different grinding procedures on the flexural strength of zirconia. J Prosthet Dent. 2012;107(5):309-15.
20. Jones WD. Development of dental ceramics: an historical preview. Dent Clin North Am. 1985;20:4:621-66.
21. Josephson BA, Schulman A, Dunn ZA, Hurwitz W. A compressive strength study of an all-ceramic crown. J Prosthet Dent. 1988; 59:12-6.
22. Kelly JR, Nishimura I, Campell SD. Ceramics in dentistry: Historical roots and current perspective. J Prosthet Dent. 1996; 75:18-32.
23. Kern M, Thompson VP. Sandblasting and silica coating of a glass infiltration alumina ceramic: Volume loss, morphology and changes in surface composition. J Prosthet Dent. 1994;71:453-61.
24. Koh N, Hino T, Miyauchi S. Clinical use of a new glass ceramic material. Int J Prosthodont. 1991;4:138-46.
25. Leinfelder KF. Porcelain esthetics for the 21st century. J Am Dent Assoc. 2000;131:47-51.
26. Lund PS, Davis PW. Shear bond strength of textured opaque porcelain. Int J Prosthodont. 1992;5:503-9.
27. Lund PS, Piotrowski TJ. Colour changes of porcelain surface colorant resulting from firing. Int J Proshtodont. 1992;5:22-7.

28. Luthardt RG, Holzhuter MS, Rudolph H, Herold V, Walter MH. CAD/CAM machining effects on Y- TZP Zirconia. Dent Mater. 2004;20:655-62.

29. Mainjot A, Schajer GS, Vanheusden AJ, Sadoun MJ. Influence of zirconia framework thickness on residual stress profile in veneering ceramic: Measurement by hole-drilling. Dent Mater 2012;28:378-84.

30. Mante FK, Brantley WA, Dhuru VB, Ziebert GJ. Fracture toughness of high alumina core dental ceramic: The effect of water and artificial saliva. Int J Prosthodont. 1993;6:546-52.

31. Miyazaki T, Hotta Y, Kunii J, Kuriyama S, Tamaki Y. A review of dental CAD/CAM: current status and future perspectives from 20 years of experience. Dent Mater J. 2009;28(1):44.

32. Nilgün Öztürk A, Ýnan O, Ýnan E, Öztürk B. Microtensile Bond Strength of CAD-CAM and Pressed-Ceramic Inlays to Dentin. Eur J Dent. 2007;1:91-6.

33. Oh S, Dong J, Luthy H, Scharer P. Strength and microstructure of IPS Empress 2 Glass Ceramic after different heat treatments. Int J Prosthodont. 2000;13:468-72.

34. Özkurt Z, Iþeri U, Kazazoðlu E. Zirconia ceramic post systems: a literature review and a case report. Dent Mater J. 2010;29(3): 233-45.

35. Piddock V, Qualtrough AJE. Dental ceramics: an update. J Dent. 1990;18:227-35.

36. Probster L. Compressive strength of two modern all-ceramic crowns. Int J Prosthodont. 1992;5:409-14.

37. Raigrodski AJ. Contemporary materials and techniques for all ceramic fixed partial dentures: A review of the literature. J Prosthet Dent. 2004;92:557-62.

38. Rekow EF. Dental CAD-CAM systems: What is the state of art? J Am Dent Assoc. 1991;122:42-8.

39. Rosenblum MA, Schulman. A review of all ceramic restorations. J Am Dent Assoc. 1997;128:297-307.

40. Seghi RR, Denry I, Brajevic F. Effects of ion exchange on hardness and fracture toughness on dental ceramics. Int J Prosthodont. 1992;5:309-14.

41. Seghi RR, Denry IL, Rosenstiel SF. Relative fracture toughness and hardness of new dental ceramics. J Prosthet Dent. 1995;74:145-50.

42. Sivakumar A, Valiathan A. Dental ceramics and ormocer technology—navigating the future!, trends. Biomater Artif Organs. 2006;20(1):40-3.

43. Sobrinho LC, Cattell MJ, Glover RH, Knowles JC. Investigation of the dry and wet fatigue properties of three all-ceramic crown systems. Int J Prosthodont. 1998;11:255-62.

44. Stephen J Chu. Use of a synthetic low-fusing Quartz Glass-ceramic material for the fabrication of metal-ceramic restorations. Pract Proced Aesthet Dent. 2001;13(5):375-80.

45. Suchanek WL, Riman RE. Hydrothermal Synthesis of Advanced Ceramic Powders, Advances in Sci and Tech. 2006;45:184-93.

46. Sukumaran VG, Bharadwaj N. Ceramics in dental applications, trends biomater. Artif Organs. 2006;20(1):7-11.

47. Sulaiman F, Chai J, Jameson LM, Worzniak WT. A comparison of the marginal fit of in-ceram, IPS Empress, and Procera Crowns. Int J Prosthodont. 1997;10:478-84.

48. Thamaraiselvi TV, Rajeswari S. Biological evaluation of bioceramic materials—a review, trends biomater. Artif Organs. 2004;18(1):9-17.

49. Thompson JY, Bayne SC, Heymann HO. Mechanical properties of new mica based machinable glass ceramic for CAD/CAM restoration. J Prosthet Dent. 1996;76:619-23.

50. van der Zal JM, Vlaar S, Ruiter J, Davidson C. The Cicero system for CAD/ CAM fabrication of full ceramic crowns. J Prosthet Dent. 2001;85:261-7.

51. Willi Paul, Chandra P Sharma. Nanoceramic matrices: biomedical applications. Am J Biochem and Biotech. 2006;2(2):41-8.

Mechanics of Cutting with Dental Burs

17

Before any dental restoration can be placed in the mouth, the teeth or other tissues must be prepared to receive the restoration. Usually such a process requires the cutting of the tooth structure (tooth preparation). Cutting is generally understood to mean the removal of a part of a structure or surface by means of shearing action. In a cutting tool the blade cuts through the work at a predetermined rate, which is controlled by many factors.

DENTAL BURS

Dental burs are essentially miniature milling cutters as used in industry. Many shapes and sizes of dental burs are available for various purposes in the preparation and finishing of cavities and restorations.

Design of Dental Burs

A dental bur has three parts such as head, shank and shaft (Fig. 17.1).

Head: Portion carrying the cutting blades.

Shank: Portion connecting the head to the shaft.

Shaft: Portion, which will be engaged within the handpiece.

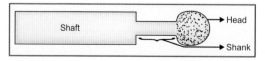

Fig. 17.1 Dental bur

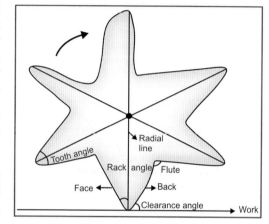

Fig. 17.2 Cross-section of dental bur

Face

The side of the tooth ahead of the cutting edge in the direction of rotation is known as the tooth face (Fig. 17.2).

Back or Flank

It is the side of the tooth on the trailing edge (Fig. 17.2).

Rake Angle

It is the angle between the face of the bur, tooth and the radial line from the center of the bur to the blade or cutting edge. It can be either positive, negative or zero.

Negative rake angle: If the face is beyond or leading the radial line in reference to the

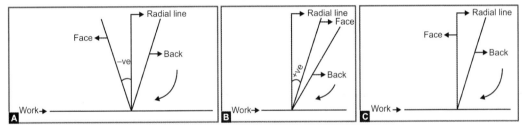

Figs 17.3A to C (A) Negative rake angle (B) Positive rake angle (C) Zero rake angle

direction of rotation the rake angle is said to be negative rake angle (Fig. 17.3A).

Burs made with negative rake angle are frequently used in dentistry.

Advantages of negative rake angle:
- Easy to design
- Less temperature rise during use
- Longer service
- Less clogging.

Positive rake angle: If the radial line leads the face so that the rake angle is on the inside of the radial line the rake angle is said to be positive (Fig. 17.3B).

Zero or radial rake angle: Rake angle can be zero if the radial line coincides with face of the bur tooth (Fig. 17.3C).

Zero rake angled bur has lower efficiency.

Land

The plane of surface immediately following the cutting edge is called land (Fig. 17.4A).

Clearance Angle

The angle between the back of the tooth and the work is known as the clearance angle. The angle between the land and the work is called as the primary clearance angle. The angle between the back and the work is called secondary clearance angle (Fig. 17.4A). If the back of the tooth is curved the clearance is said to be radial (Fig. 17.4B).

Tooth Angle

It is measured between the face and the back or if a land is present between the face and the land (Figs 17.5A and B).

Flute or Chip Space

The space between the successive teeth is known as flute or chip space (Fig. 17.6).

Factors Affecting the Cutting Efficiency of Burs

1. Rake angle

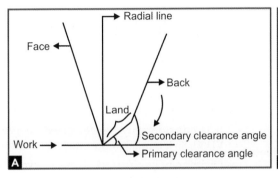

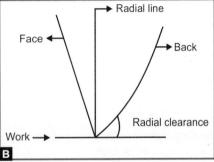

Figs 17.4A and B (A) Clearance angle (B) Radial clearance angle

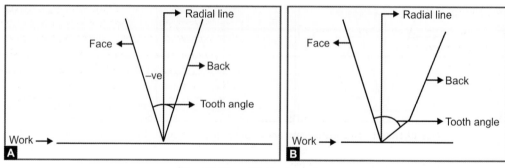

Figs 17.5A and B Tooth angle

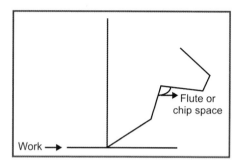

Fig. 17.6 Flute or chip space

2. Clearance angle
3. Number of teeth in the bur
4. Concentricity and run-out
5. Influence of load
6. Influence of speed
7. Coolants.

CLASSIFICATION OF DENTAL BURS

According to their composition
   a. Steel burs
   b. Tungsten carbide burs
   c. Diamond burs.

According to their mode of attachment to the handpiece
   a. Latch type
   b. Friction type.

According to the handpiece they designed for
   a. Contra-angle burs
   b. Straight handpiece bur.

According to the length of the head
   a. Long
   b. Short
   c. Regular.

According to their shape
   a. Round burs
   b. Wheel burs
   c. Inverted cone burs
   d. Plane cylindrical fissure bur and cross cut cylindrical fissure bur
   e. Plane taper and cross cut taper fissure bur
   f. Pear-shaped bur
   g. End cutting burs.

Steel Burs

Steel burs are made from hypereutectic alloy; they usually contain manganese and molybdenum as hardening agents in small amounts. The steel bur is usually from blank stock by a rotating cutter that cuts parallel to the axis of the bur.

Tungsten Carbide Bur

It was introduced in 1947. They have largely replaced the steel burs for cavity preparation.

Advantages

- It is considerably harder (1650 to 1700 VHN). So it is much more efficient in cutting enamel.
- It is very rigid with the high MOE.

Disadvantages

- It is not as resilient or tough as steel.
- Being more brittle cannot be used in thin sections.

Diamond Burs

Diamond is the hardest material known. It is called as super abrasive. Burs and abrasive wheels are made with diamond chips (either natural or synthetic) bonded to the surface of the metallic shaft. Since the diamond chips are very hard there is no need for the exposure of new abrasive particles during grinding. So the binders are manufactured specially to resist abrasive particle loss rather than to degrade at a certain point and release particles. They are used in the preparation of crowns. Finishing diamonds are used for resin bonded composites they contain diamond particles of 40 μm or less in diameter. The main disadvantage of these burs is diamond grits are very expensive.

Abrasion and Polishing

18

Before any dental restoration or appliance is placed permanently in the mouth, it is important that all these restorations or appliances should be highly polished and therefore should have a smooth surface.

Rough surfaces occur unavoidably during the construction of an appliance. For example, in spite of all the care, an acrylic denture base may have minor surface roughness.

A rough surface is:
- Uncomfortable to the patient.
- Poor oral hygiene: Food and other debris cling to it. It is difficult to remove these deposits from the rough surface.
- Tarnish and corrosion: Apart from unhygiene, these deposits will produce suitable conditions for corrosion or tarnishing of any metallic materials.
- Poor esthetics.

Therefore minor surface roughness should be removed from the denture before polishing is done.

ABRASION

Surface roughness is removed by a process known as abrasion. It is the smoothening of rough surface before preparing it for polishing. The term "abrasion" in the strict sense of the word denotes "a wearing of one surface against another by friction."

Abrasion is the process of wear on the surface of one material by another material by scratching, gouging, chiseling, tumbling or other mechanical means.

The material that causes the wear is called an "abrasive", and the material being abraded is called "substrate". An abrasive removes the rough areas on the surface by removing chips or shavings from the material.

In an abrasive tool (e.g. Diamond rotary instrument) containing thousands of abrasive points, which are not arranged in an ordered pattern. Each point acts as an individual blade and removes a chip or shaving from the material, producing innumerable scratches on the surface.

Abrasive particles remove some material from the surface in a manner similar to the action of a chisel in carving a piece of wood.

In the abrading of metals, the crystalline surface of the metal is disturbed, sometimes to a depth of 10 µm. The grains become disoriented and strain hardening may occur. More the abrasion greater is the disorientation. Strain hardening accompanies the disorientation and the superficial hardness of the surface is increased.

The surface effect varies with different metals for example, in a ductile metal like gold; less amount of the surface may be removed by the abrasive than in a brittle metal.

The surface disturbance of a resin, as in a denture base, undoubtedly includes the introduction of surface stresses, which may cause distortion if the abrasion is too vigorous. The generation of heat during the abrasion partially relieves such stresses, but if it is too great, it may relieve processing stresses, so that a general warpage results, as well as an actual melting of the surface of the resin.

Factors Affecting Rate of Abrasion

The rate of abrasion of a given material by a given abrasive is determined primarily by factors as follows:

Difference in Hardness

An abrasive must be harder than the material, which it abrades. This relationship is appreciable even at high temperatures, which are created on a surface during abrading.

A large difference in hardness between the abrasive and substrate allows the most efficient abrading to take place.

Materials, which are brittle, are more rapidly abraded than those which are malleable and ductile.

Brinell and Knoop hardness values are functions of materials resistance to indentation; whereas Moh's values are functions of materials resistance to abrasion.

Particle Size and Shape

Particle size: Particle size is an important factor in the rate of abrasion. The size of the abrasive particles plays an important role during abrasion. The larger the particle, the deeper the scratches in the surface and the faster the surface is worn away (Fig. 18.1A).

They are only used where large surface irregularities have to be removed since they leave a deeply scratched surface. A coarse abrasive must be followed by a finer one before the surface can be polished.

Size of abrasives is expressed in terms of μm. Based on the size the abrasive particles are classified into three types:

- Abrasives of fine particles: 0–10 μm.
- Abrasives of medium particles: 10–100 μm.
- Abrasives of coarse particles: 100–500 μm.

Particle shape: Particle shape also has an effect on rate of abrasion. Sharp, irregularly shaped particles will abrade a surface more rapidly than will more rounded particles having duller cutting angles. The former will produce deeper scratches than latter. The rate of abrasion of an abrasive decreases during use. This is partly due

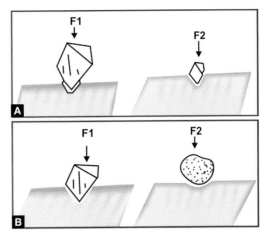

Figs 18.1A and B (A) Particles of same shape and are of different size (under same force (B) Particles of almost same size but of different shape under same force

to rounding of the particles and partly due to contamination of the abrasive with some of the substrate material (Fig. 18.1B).

Fracture of abrasive grains plays an important role in maintaining abrasive action. Because rounded part of abrasive undergoes fracturing producing new sharp cutting edge. The clogged fragments of abraded material must be removed by washing in water.

Pressure

The pressure of the abrasive against the surface being abraded is an important factor. Heavy pressure applied by the abrasive will cause deeper scratches and more rapid removal of the material. As the abrasive particles pass over the work piece, the back pressure of the work piece tends to dislodge or fracture the abrasive. The greater the pressure deeper is the scratch and greater is the tendency for the abrasive particle to be fractured or dislodged (Fig. 18.2).

Speed

A very important factor in the control of the rate of abrasion is the speed at which the particle travels across the work. The greater the speed the greater the frequency per unit time the particle contacts the surface.

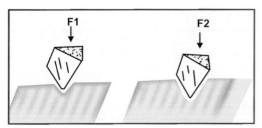

Fig. 18.2 Particles of same shape and size under different pressures (F1—less pressure and F2—greater pressure)

Increasing the speed is the logical method for increasing the rate of abrasion with a given abrasive without wearing away the abrasive tool. At higher speed, many abrasive particles pass across the work at a rapid rate; the pressure can be decreased without a decrease in the rate of abrasion.

The slower the speed of movement of the abrasive the deeper are the scratches which are produced, and the greater are the forces trying to fracture the abrasive or remove it from its bonding material.

Lubricants

For example, Silicone grease, water spray, glycerol, etc.

Lubricants are used during abrasion for two purposes:
- To reduce heat builds up.
- To wash away debris to prevent clogging of the abrasive instrument.

Too much lubrication can reduce the abrasion rate because it may prevent some of the abrasive from coming in contact with the substrate.

Properties of Abrasive and Substrate

If the abrasive material is brittle, its particles break and form a new cutting edge. Thus brittleness can be an advantage.

If the substrate is a brittle material, it can be abraded rapidly, whereas a malleable and ductile material will flow instead of being removed by the abrasive.

Desirable Characteristics of an Abrasive

- An abrasive should be irregular in shape.
- An abrasive should be harder than the work it abrades.
- An abrasive should possess a high impact strength or body strength.
- An abrasive should possess attrition resistance so that it does not wear.

Abrasive Materials

Abrasive materials are mainly classified as natural and synthetic abrasives.

Natural abrasives include Arkansas stone, chalk, corundum, diamond, emery, garnet, pumice, quartz, sand, tripoli, and zirconium silicate. Cuttle and Kieselguhr are derived from the remnants of living organisms.

Manufactured abrasives are synthesized materials that are generally preferred because of their more predictable physical properties. Silicon carbide, aluminum oxide, synthetic diamond, rouge and tin oxide are examples of manufactured abrasives.

Aluminum Oxide

It is a synthetic abrasive and is in pure form, which is manufactured as a white powder from bauxite (an impure alumina). It is much harder than natural alumina (corundum) because of its purity. Pure alumina is manufactured from bauxite. Synthetic alumina is made as a white powder.

Uses
- To make blended abrasives, coated abrasives and air propelled grit abrasives.
- Sintered aluminum oxide are used to make white stones, which is used for adjusting dental enamel and for finishing both metal alloys and ceramic materials.

Corundum

It is an impure form of ruby. This mineral form of aluminum oxide is usually white. Its physical properties are inferior to that of manufactured aluminum oxide.

Uses
- Used primarily for grinding metal alloys.
- Most commonly used in white stone.

Arkansas Stone

Arkansas stone mainly contains microcrystalline quartz and it is dense, hard, semitranslucent, and light gray. These are used to give various shapes for fine grinding of tooth enamel and metal alloys.

Chalk

It is composed of calcium carbonate and is used as a mild abrasive paste to polish tooth enamel (i.e. one of the polishing agents of commercial dentifrices), gold foil, amalgam and plastic materials.

Chromic Oxide

It is a hard abrasive and is mainly used for polishing a variety of metals especially for stainless steel.

Cuttle

It is a white calcareous powder and also called as "cuttle fish or cuttle bone." Cuttle powder is made from the internal shell of a Mediterranean marine mollusc of the genus "sepia". These are available as coated abrasives.

Uses
- Used for polishing of metal margins and dental amalgam restorations.

Diamond

It is called as "super abrasive" as it can abrade any other known substance and it is mainly composed of carbon. These abrasives are supplied as diamond abrasive rotary instruments, flexible metal backed abrasive strips, and diamond polishing pastes.

Uses
- Used on ceramic and resin-based composite materials.

Emery

This is a mixture of aluminum oxide (corundum) and iron. These are available in the form of coated abrasive disks.

Uses
- May be used for finishing metal alloys or plastic materials.

Garnet

Garnet is an extremely hard abrasive and is usually dark red in color. Garnet is a silicate mineral with the combination of any other minerals such as Al, Co, Mg, Fe, and Mn. It is usually coated on paper or cloth with glue or similar binder.

Uses
- Used in grinding metal alloys and plastic materials.

Kieselguhr

It is also called as diatomaceous earth and is composed of siliceous remains of minute aquatic plants known as diatoms. It is well used as a mild abrasive (hardness is about 800 KHN) and polishing agent. Diatomaceous earth is used as filler in many dental impression materials. The main disadvantage with this abrasive agent is a risk of respiratory silicosis when exposed to airborne particles.

Pumice

It is of volcanic origin, i.e. this material is obtained by crushing pumice stone, a porous volcanic rock.

Because of its moderate hardness pumice is used by dentist for cleaning away tartar deposits from the surface of the natural teeth. It abrades the tartar, but has little effect on the harder tooth enamel.

Inhaling pumice dust leads to chest complaints (silicosis). Pummy disease, which is mainly caused by pumice substitutes, is known to occur frequently in a person who performs great deal of polishing.

Uses
- Used in smoothening of denture bases.
- Removes the tartar deposits from the surface of the natural teeth.
- Polishes tooth enamel, gold foil and acrylic resins.

Quartz

It is very hard, colorless and transparent. Quartz particles are used for making coated abrasive disks. Quartz abrasives are mainly used to finish metal alloys and may be used to grind enamel.

Rouge

It is a fine red powder composed of iron oxide. It is usually used in cake form by blending with soft binders. It may be impregnated on paper or cloth, known as "crocus cloth". It is an excellent polishing agent for gold and noble metal alloys.

Sand

Sand is a mixture of small mineral particles predominately composed of silica. Its use in sand paper is a common example. They are applied under air pressure to remove refractory investment materials from base metal alloy castings.

Uses
- Used for grinding of metal alloys and plastic materials.
- Used as a powder in sand blasting equipment.

Silicon Carbide (Carborundum)

This is an extremely hard synthetic abrasive (2400 KHN). It is of two types—green and blue-black. Both are manufactured by fusing sand (silicon) and carbon at 2000°C. The green form is often preferred because substrates are more visible against the green color. Most of stone burs employed for cutting of tooth structure are made of silicon carbide.

Uses
- Used as an abrasive agent for metal alloys, ceramics and plastic materials.

Synthetic Diamond Abrasive

These are used in manufacture of diamond saws, wheels and burs. Diamond polishing pastes containing particles smaller than 5 μm in diameter are useful in polishing ceramic materials.

Uses
- Used primarily on tooth structure, ceramic materials, and resin-based composite materials.

Tin Oxide or Putty Powder

It is mixed with water, alcohol or glycerin to form mild abrasive paste.

Uses
- Used extensively as polishing agent for teeth and metallic restorations.

Tripoli

It is a kind of porous rock which is powdered and used as coated abrasives and polishing agent. These are available in different colors such as white, gray, pink, red and yellow. Gray and red are used frequently in dentistry. It was named so because it was first found in northern Africa near Tripoli.

Uses
- For polishing metal alloys, composite resins and acrylics.

Tungsten Carbide

Burs of tungsten carbide are made by embedding tungsten carbide particles in matrix of cobalt. These particles are harder and more efficient in cutting enamel. They are very rigid and more brittle.

Uses
- Used in manufacture of burs, chisels, etc.

Zirconium Silicate

It mainly occurs as Zircon or Zirconium silicate in nature.

Uses
- Used to make coated abrasive disks and strips.
- Used as a polishing agent.
- Used as a component of dental prophylactic paste.

Zinc Oxide

Zinc oxide in alcohol is used for polishing dental amalgam restorations.

POLISHING

Polishing is the production of a smooth mirror-like surfaces without much loss any external form, or polishing is the process of making a rough surface smooth to the touch and glossy which reflects most of the incident light, or polishing is a process which acts on an extremely thin region of the substrate surface and provides scratches so fine that they are not visible unless greatly magnified.

Metallographically speaking, polishing denotes the production of a smooth, mirror-like surface on a metal without the use of a film. A metallographic polish is accomplished by producing a virtually scratch-free surface.

If the abrasive particles are finer, smaller particles are removed from the surface finer scratches are produced. If the particle size of the abrasive is reduced sufficiently, the scratches become extremely fine and may disappear entirely. The surface then acquires a smooth shiny layer known as "a polish", such a layer is thought to be composed of minute crystals and is said to have a "microcrystalline structure".

The polishing agents actually remove material from the surface molecule by molecule and in the process fine scratches and irregularities are filled in by the powdered particulate being removed from the surface. This microcrystalline layer is referred to as "polish layer" or "Beilby layer". This is named so because such a microcrystalline surface layer after polishing was first noted by a scientist, "Beilby". It is probable that the rapid movement of a polishing agent across a surface heats the top layer of the material and causes it to flow and fill in the scratches producing "Beilby layer".

The coarse abrasives are used initially to remove gross surface irregularities produce deep scratches. When finer abrasives are used deep scratches are eliminated and replaced by finer scratches.

Difference between Abrasion and Polishing

The difference between an abrasive agent and a polishing agent is difficult to define. The terms are generally interchangeable. Differences between abrasion and polishing are discussed in Table 18.1.

Benefits of Polishing

- *Oral health:* A well-contoured and polished restoration promotes oral health by resisting the accumulation of food debris and pathogenic bacteria.
- *Oral function:* Oral function is enhanced with a well-polished restoration because food glides more freely over occlusal and the spaces on each side of the contact point surfaces during mastication.
- *Polished surface reduces the formation of dental calculus on smooth enamel surfaces.*
- Polished surfaces of metal restorations significantly reduce the tarnish and corrosion activity.
- A highly polished tooth will be more resistant to carcinogenic action than one that is not polished.
- A polished tooth surface is approximately 15% less soluble in acid than one with a rough surface.
- A polished restoration contact minimizes wear rates on opposing and adjacent teeth.
- Polishing increases enamel luster and smoothness.
- A rough surface leads to uncomfortability. Hence polished surface is desirable.

Polishing Agents

Whiting (Precipitated Chalk)

- Used for softer metals and plastics.
- Can also be used in dentifrices.
  Whiting is mixed with water during use.

Table 18.1 Differences between abrasion and polishing

Properties	Abrasion	Polishing
Particle size	A given agent having a large particle size acts as abrasive producing scratches.	The same agent with a smaller particle size acts as a polishing agent leaving a polish layer on the surface.
Amount of material removed	More amount of the material is removed greater than 5 μm and even up to 10 μm (i.e. 0.005 to 0.010 mm)	A very little amount of the material is removed from the surface during polishing. Not more than 5 μm (i.e. <5 μm) (i.e. 0.005 mm).
Speed	The optimum speed for abrasion is lower than that for polishing. The average speed is approximately 5000 feet per minute.	The optimum speed for polishing is higher than that for abrading. It varies with polishing agents. The average speed is approximately 7500 feet per minute. Linear speed as high as 10000 feet per minute also used.

Prepared Chalk

It is the purified natural material, used in dentifrices.

Rouge (Fe$_2$O$_3$)

Never to be used to polish stainless steel as it contaminates the surface with iron thus providing suitable conditions for corrosion.
• Give excellent shine on gold alloys.
• Dirty to use.

Chromium Oxide

• Green chromium oxide is dirty to use.
• Produces excellent polish on stainless steel.

Tin Oxide

• Tin oxide or putty powder is used for polishing glass or porcelain.
• It is not used in the mouth.

Some other polishing agents are pumice, tripoli, zinc oxide (for polishing amalgam restorations), cuttle and kieselguhr, etc.

Burnishing

Burnishing is somewhat related to polishing in that the surface is drawn or moved.

The surface of a metal can be smoothened by rubbing it with another small, highly polished, hard metal surface.

This action disturbs deeper layers of the metal than are affected by polishing and work hardens the metal surface. This technique is usually used to adapt the margins of a gold inlay.

Usually stainless steel or chromium-plated instruments are used either by hand or in the form of smooth, rotating engine burnishers.

The ability of an alloy to be burnished may depend on:
• High percentage elongation.
• Low proportional limit.
• A slow rate of work hardening.

Electropolishing or Electrolytic Polishing

This is the reverse procedure of electroplating. An electrolytic cell consists of two electrodes, and an electrolyte to carry current. The alloy to be polished is made the anode of an electrolytic cell. As the current is passed, some of the anode is dissolved leaving a bright surface. Very little material is removed in this process.

This is an excellent method for polishing the fitting surface of cobalt-chromium alloy denture, since little material is removed that the fit of the denture is virtually unaltered.

Table 18.2 Composition of dentifrices

Components	Weight percentage		Materials	Functions
	Pastes and gels	Powders		
Abrasive	20–55	90–98	$CaCO_3$, dibasic calcium phosphate, hydrated Al_2O_3, hydrated silica, Na bicarbonate, calcium pyrophosphate, insoluble Na metaphosphate, MgO	• Essential for adequate cleaning • Removes stain, plaque, etc. • Gives clean and polished surface
Detergent (surface active agents)	1–2	1–6	Sodium lauryl sulfate, sodium N-lauryl sacrosinate	• Decreases surface tension and improves the ability of dentifrice to wet the tooth surface • Aids in removing debris from tooth surface
Colorants	1–2	1–2	Food colorants	• To accentuate flavor • To promote consumer acceptance • Appearance
Flavoring agents	1–2	1–2	Oils of spearmint, peppermint, wintergreen or cinnamon	• To accentuate flavor
Humectants	20–35	0	Glycerine, sorbitol and propylene glycol	• Prevents paste or gel type from drying out, i.e. maintains moisture content • Improves the appearance and consistency of the product
Water	15–25	0	Deionized water or distilled water	It gives desired consistency.
Binder	1–3	0	Carrageenan, carboxy methyl cellulose, natural gums	• As a thickener • Prevents the separation of liquid and solid components • Maintains the consistency of the dentifrice
Fluorides	0–1	0	Na monofluorophosphate, NaF, Stannous fluoride	• Dental caries prevention
Tartar control agents	0–1	0	Di sodium pyrophosphate, tetra sodium pyrophosphate, tetra potassium pyrophosphate	Inhibits or reduces the rate at which new calculus deposits formation supragingivally
Desensitization agents	0–5	0	Potassium nitrate, strontium chloride	Promotes occlusion of dentinal tubules

Techniques for Polishing Restorative Materials

Dental Amalgam

A polished surface is desirable on dental amalgam to retard the collection of plaque and help to retard tarnish as well. Burnishing alone does not create as smooth surface as does polishing.

Polishing can be performed after 24 hrs with a rotary instrument with a fine abrasive mixed with water or alcohol in a slurry or paste, flour of pumice, or tin oxide may be used for this purpose.

Gold Alloys

Gold alloys can be finished by using coarse, medium and fine abrasives. Coarse scratches are removed with fine pumice (as an abrasive). The surface is then finished with a rubber wheel impregnated with a fine abrasive. Finally polishing is carried out by Tripoli and rouge on rag wheels.

Acrylic Resin Denture Bases

These are soft materials and can be finished easily with pumice followed by tripoli or tin oxide. Because of its softness, care should be taken not to alter the contour of the restoration.

Porcelain

Glazing gives a glossy, smooth surface on dental porcelain crown.

It can be polished by a series of coarse to fine abrasive rubber wheels, containing silicon carbide or aluminum oxide, followed by a fine-particle sized diamond paste applied on a felt wheel.

DENTIFRICES

No discussion of the action of abrasive or polishing agents in dentistry would be complete without mentioning the effect of dentifrices on tooth surfaces. Dentifrices are available in the form of pastes/gels/powders. The detailed composition of all the forms are discussed in Table 18.2.

Dentifrices are agents used along with a toothbrush to cleanse and polish natural teeth.

Dentifrices should have maximum cleansing efficiency with minimum tooth abrasion. Highly abrasive dentifrices should not be used specially when dentin or cementum is exposed. Dentifrices perform three important functions such as:

1. They assist the toothbrush to mechanically remove stains, debris, plaque and stained pellicle from the teeth.
2. They polish teeth to provide increased light reflectance and superior esthetic appearance. The high polish as an added benefit enables teeth to resist accumulation of microorganisms and stains better than rougher surface.
3. Finally, they act as vehicles for the delivery of therapeutic agents that provide known benefits.

   For example, Fluorides, tartar control agents, desensitizing agents, peroxides, and bicarbonates.

Dispension

Dentifrices supplied as powders, pastes and gels. Composition of dentifrices have been discussed in Table 18.2.

SUGGESTED READING

1. Ancowitz S, Torres T, Rostami H. Texturing and polishing: the final attempt at value control. Dent Clinics of America. 1998; 42(4):607-13.
2. Attin T, Müller T, Patyk A, Lennon AM. Influence of different bleaching systems on fracture toughness and hardness of enamel. Oper Dent. 2004;29(2):188-95.
3. Fine DH, Furgang D, Markowitz K, Sreenivasan PK, Klimpel K, De Vizio W. The antimicrobial effect of a triclosan/copolymer dentifrice on oral microorganisms in vivo. J Am Dent Assoc. 2006;137(10):1406-13.
4. Joiner A. The bleaching of teeth: A review of the literature. J Dent. 2006;34:412-9.
5. Mostafa Sadeghi, Shokrollah Assar. An *in vitro* antimicrobial activity of ten Iranian-made toothpastes. Dent Res J. 2009;6(2): 87-92.
6. Ozaki F, Pannuti CM, Imbronito AV, Pessotti W, Saraiva L, de Freitas NM, et al. Efficacy of a

herbal toothpaste on patients with established gingivitis a randomized controlled trial. Braz Oral Res. 2006;20(2):172-7.

7. Seghi RR, Denry I. Effects of external bleaching on indentation and abrasion characteristics of human enamel *in vitro*. J Dent Res. 1992; 71(6):1340-4.

8. White DJ, Kozak KM, Gibb R, Dunavent J, Klukowska M, Sagel PA. A 24-hour dental plaque prevention study with a stannous fluoride dentifrice containing hexametaphosphate. J Contemp Dent Pract. 2006;7(3):1-11.

9. Williams KR. Behind the scenes at the toothpaste aisle: the chemistry of dental materials. J Chem Edu. 2010;87(10):1007-8.

10. Zantner C, Beheim-Schwarzbach N, Neumann K, Kielbassa AM. Surface microhardness of enamel after different home bleaching procedures. Dent Mat. 2007;23(2):243-50.

Soldering and Welding

19

Metals joining operations are usually divided into three categories such as brazing, soldering, and welding.

SOLDERING

Process of building up a localized area with a filler metal or joining two or more metal components by heating them to a temperature and filling the gap between them to a molten with a liquidus temperature below 450°C (for brazing the liquidus temperature is more than 450°C).

WELDING

Process of fusing two or more metals parts through the application of heat, pressure or both, with or without a filler metal, to produce a localized union across the interface between the parts.

Soldering is often used in the construction of dental appliances.

Advantages

1. Fixed partial dentures are frequently casting parts that are soldered together after careful fitting to the master casting.
2. Wrought wire clasp arms can be soldered in place for partial dentures using investment-soldering technique.
3. Orthodontic wires and bands are often soldered together.
4. Soldering can be used to build up certain regions of crowns and inlays where the dimensions should be increased, such as for missing contact points.

5. Some casting defects can be corrected with soldering.

Clean oxide-free metal surfaces brought into intimate contact will bond together as a consequence of metallic bonding forces. However, this does not occur in most practically due to surface contamination and/or oxidation.

1. The basic technique of soldering is first to obtain metal surfaces that are free of contamination. This is accomplished by cleaning and by using fluxes, which also prevents oxidation during the soldering process.
2. A metal alloy with a lower melting point than the parts to be joined must be chosen.
3. The parts should be brought to the solder's melting temperature. If the molten metal wets the solid metal, it will spread between the flux and the metal part, providing intimate contact.

Upon solidification, the solder will still be in contact and metallic bonding will be established. Solder penetrates joints by capillary action.

Type of Solders

1. Gold solders
2. Silver solders.

Gold Solders

Composition of gold solders are given in Table 19.1.

Ni may be added instead of copper if a white alloy is desired. Copper is not used for "PFM" appliance because it colors the porcelain green, as does silver.

Table 19.1 Composition of gold solders

Ingredients	Weight %	Functions
Gold	65	Main ingredient.
Silver	16.3	• Improves the welding (spreading and penetration) of gold solders • Also whitens the alloy
Copper	13.4	• Lowers the fusion temperature • Improves strength • Makes solder amenable to age-hardening
Zinc	3.9	Lowers the fusion temperature
Tin	1.7	Lowers the fusion temperature

Table 19.2 Composition of silver solders

Ingredients	Weight %	Functions
Silver	10–80	Main ingredient
Copper	15–50	Improves the strength
Zinc	4–35	
Cadmium	Trace	Lowers the fusion temperature
Tin	Trace	Lowers the fusion temperature
Phosphorus	Trace	Lowers the fusion temperature

Silver Solders

Compositions of silver solders are given in Table 19.2.

FLUX

The Latin word "flux" means "flow".

"A flux is a material that is used to prevent oxidation, removes any preexisting oxide coat on the metal surface and allows free flow of solder".

Ideal Requirements

• Should be resistant to tarnish and corrosion.

• It should flow freely when it melts so that a layer of the solder should be formed over the parts united.
• It should be as strong as the parts joined.
• The fusion temperature of a solder should be less than that of the solidus temperature of the parent metals by at least 100°C.
• It should not cause pitting of the soldered joint.
• The solder should have a color that matches the color of the parts joined.

Classification

1. *According to their purpose*
   Fluxes may be divided into three types.
   Type-1: Surface protection—prevents oxidation.
   Type-II: Reducing agent—reduces any oxides present and exposes clean metal.
   Type-III: Solvent—dissolves any oxides present and carries them away.
2. *According to type of material*
   • Borax flux
   • Fluoride flux.

Borax Flux

Composition
   • Dehydrated borax ($Na_2B_4O_7$)
   • Boric acid (H_3BO_3)
   • Silica.

The fused borax flux produces oxide-free surfaces over which the solder will flow easily. The flux can be applied as a powder or a liquid (flux mixed with alcohol), or a paste. A paste gives the most control in application and is formed by mixing the powdered flux with petrolatum or a similar inert base.

Fluoride Flux

Composition
   • Potassium fluoride
   • Boric acid
   • Borax glass
   • Sodium carbonate or silica.

The ingredients are fused and grounded to fine powder, which is used either directly or as a liquid in alcohol or paste in petrolatum. These fluxes are used for soldering alloys containing chromium because fluorides dissolve the chromium oxide.

SOLDERING INVESTMENT MATERIALS

Soldering investments should not expand as for casting investments because soldering requires lower temperatures than casting.

Low fusing gold solders: Quartz based, rather than crystobalite based, gypsum investments are used.

Preceramic soldering: Phosphate bonded soldering investments are used.

TYPES OF SOLDERING TECHNIQUES

1. Investment soldering
2. Free-hand soldering.

Investment Soldering

Investment soldering is recommended for precise arrangement of parts for fixed partial dentures or partial dentures with wrought wire clasp arms.

Procedure

The parts are placed on the cast with the gap distance between them is at least 0.1 mm. Excessive gap distance can lead to distortion and pitting. The parts are securely fastened together with sticky wax before removal from master cast and subsequent placement in the soldering investment. Investment should cover metal parts where they are not to be soldered, but no investment in the soldering joint. Antiflux may be applied to confine the flow of solder. Flux can be applied to the joint area before or after preheating of the investment.

Soldering is accomplished with a reducing flame when the parts are at 750°C–870°C, giving them a yellowish red color. The solder flows smoothly into the joint area. The investment and appliance are allowed to cool for about 5 minutes before quenching. The flux cools to a glass that can be removed through pickling.

Precautions

1. The parts must be clean and secured properly on the master cast to prevent warping or porosity.
2. Sheets of paper should not be used as a gauge because they are often too thin, ranging from 0.005–0.1 mm.
3. The parts should be securely fastened together with sticky wax.
4. There should not be any investment material at the joint.
5. Over-heating may cause sulfur contamination.
6. Immediate quenching should be avoided because warpage could occur if the investment were quenched immediately.
7. Total bench cooling also should be avoided because that would make the solder too brittle through age-hardening.
8. Finishing instruments should not be used to remove the flux because the glass is harder than the metal, and surrounding metal will be removed along with the wax.

Free Hand Soldering

Soldering of orthodontic appliances is generally accomplished without the use of an investment. Orthodontic torches can be placed on the bench so that both hands are free to hold the parts in position. Solder is generally melted on one of the parts. Then they are held together and the joint is heated.

Precautions

• Thin wire parts must be held in contact to avoid narrowing of the joint caused by the surface tension of the solder. This decrease in diameter, concentrates stress is much more significant that for larger appliances.
• The wires should not be overheated because that deteriorates mechanical properties.
• Overheating of stainless steel wires should be avoided since they can lead carbide protection, which may soften the wire.

Defective Soldering

Microstructural changes result from prolonged heating or overheating. Overheating of wrought wires during soldering can lead to diffusion between solder and wire and recrystallization and grain growth. Microstructural changes, surface fitting and internal porosity all result in a weak joint.

When the solder does not flow properly resulting in an incomplete joint, it usually due to one or more of the following:

- The parts were too cool when the solder was applied.
- The parts were not at similar temperatures; the solder would flow over the heater part leaving an incomplete joint.
- Flux was insufficient to cover the joint.
- Contamination was present due to improper cleaning, poor placements of flux, sulfur released from overheated investment, oxidation from an improperly adjusted torch.
- The gap distance was too small (0.1 mm) for the solder to penetrate between the parts, which leads to the formation to voids.
- If the gap distance was too large, the solder may not bridge the gap or if it does, the diameter of the joint will be too small for an adequate strength.

Bonding will occur between two metallic surfaces placed in contact if they are free of surface films (including oxides and films of adsorbed gases) and surface roughness.

METHODS OF WELDING

The three methods of welding used in dentistry achieved metal-to-metal contact differently.

1. Spot welding or resistance welding
2. Pressure welding
3. Laser welding.

Spot welding

In spot welding the two clean metal surfaces to be welded are placed together under pressure. Metal-to-metal contact is obtained by passing a current through the joint to cause interfacial melting. If a pulse of sufficient voltage and duration is applied by means of copper electrodes, melting will begin at the interface between the parts and spread outward to form a weld.

Spot welding is used to join flat structures, such as orthodontic bands and brackets, and an electric pulse is applied. The magnitude of the pulse depends on the metals and their size and shape at the welding point, and on the size of the electrodes.

Pressure Welding

If two metal parts are placed together and a sufficiently large force is applied perpendicular to the surface, pressure welding occurs, e.g. pure gold and gold foil.

Laser Welding

In laser welding, the beam is focused at the joint to melt the opposing surfaces. The two liquid surfaces contact and form a weld on solidification.

Appendix

Units and conversion factors

Unit	SI equivalent
Angstrom (Å)	1×10^{-10} meter (m)
Angstrom (Å)	1×10^{-1} nanometer (nm)
Nanometer (nm)	1×10^{-9} meter (m)
Micrometer (mm)	1×10^{-6} meter (m)
Inch (in)	0.0254 meter (m)
Inch (in)	2.54 centimeter (cm)
Pound (lb)	0.4536 kilogram (kg)
Dyne	1×10^{-5} newton (N)
Pound force (lbf)	4.4482 newton (N)
Erg	1×10^{-7} joule (J)
Calorie (Cal)	4.1868 joule (J)
Btu	1055.06 joule (J)
Dyne/cm^2	1×10^{-1} newton/meter^2 (N/m^2)
Atmosphere	1.013×10^5 N/m^2 (Pascal, Pa)
Pound per square inch (psi)	6.895×10^3 N/m^2 (Pascal, Pa)
Pound per square inch (psi)	6.895×10^3 N/m^2 (Pascal, Pa)
Kg/cm^2	9.804×10^4 MN/m^2 (Pa)
1 pennyweight (dwt) (Troy) = 1.555 g	
20 dwt = 1 ounce (Troy) = 1.097 ounce (Avoirdupois)	
Photomicrograph distance: µm/cm = $\dfrac{10{,}000}{\text{magnification}}$	
Temperature	(°C × 1.8) + 32 = °F
	$\dfrac{(°F - 32)}{1.8} = °C$

Prefixes for SI units

Multiply by this factor	Symbol	Prefix
10^{12}	T	Tera
10^{9}	G	Giga
10^{6}	M	Mega
10^{3}	k	Kilo
10^{2}	h	Hector
10	da	Deca
10^{-1}	d	deci
10^{-2}	c	Centi
10^{-3}	m	Milli
10^{-6}	m	Micro
10^{-9}	n	nano
10^{-12}	P	Pico
10^{-15}	f	Femto
10^{-18}	a	Atto

Index

Page numbers followed by *f* refer to figure and *t* refer to table, respectively.